Oxford Medical Publications

Health measurement scales

Oxford University Press makes no representation, express or implied, that the drug dosages in this book are correct. Readers must therefore always check the product information and clinical procedures with the most up to date published product information and data sheets provided by the manufacturers and the most recent codes of conduct and safety regulations. The authors and the publishers do not accept responsibility or legal liability for any errors in the text or for the misuse or misapplication of material in this work.

Health Measurement Scales
A Practical Guide to Their Development and Use

THIRD EDITION

David L. Streiner
Kunin-Lunenfeld Applied Research Unit,
Baycrest Centre for Geriatric Care,
Toronto, Ontario, Canada

and

Geoffrey R. Norman
Department of Clinical Epidemiology and Biostatistics,
McMaster University,
Hamilton, Ontario, Canada

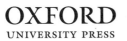

OXFORD
UNIVERSITY PRESS

OXFORD

UNIVERSITY PRESS

Great Clarendon Street, Oxford OX2 6DP

Oxford University Press is a department of the University of Oxford.
It furthers the University's objective of excellence in research, scholarship,
and education by publishing worldwide in

Oxford New York

Auckland Bangkok Buenos Aires Cape Town Chennai
Dar es Salaam Delhi Hong Kong Istanbul Karachi Kolkata
Kuala Lumpur Madrid Melbourne Mexico City Mumbai Nairobi
São Paulo Shanghai Taipei Tokyo Toronto

Oxford is a registered trade mark of Oxford University Press
in the UK and in certain other countries

Published in the United States
by Oxford University Press Inc., New York

© Oxford University Press, 2003

A catalogue record for this title is available from the British Library

ISBN 0 19 852847 7 (Pbk)

10 9 8 7 6 5 4 3 2

Typeset by Newgen Imaging Systems (P) Ltd., Chennai, India
Printed in Great Britain
on acid-free paper by
Biddles Ltd, King's Lynn, Norfolk

Preface to the third edition

Over the past 30 years or so, there have been two major advances in the field of measurement: generalizability theory and item response theory (IRT). The former was first developed in 1972, and IRT can be traced back to Lord and Novick's seminal work in 1968. Both of these topics were included in earlier editions of this book. Why, then, did we write a new edition eight years after the previous one? In the preface to the second edition, we spoke of the 'dynamism of the field'. While there have not been any breakthroughs over the past decade that rival those of generalizability theory or IRT in terms of their influence on the field, the dynamism continues, with both positive and negative consequences.

On the positive side, cognitive psychology has become even more important in explaining how people address the difficult task of interpreting questions and framing answers. In particular, the concepts of *optimizing* and *satisficing* are now used to account for some of the biases in responding to questions, such as yea-saying and acquiescence. Research into the cognitive processes people use while filling out questionnaires have elucidated why people have such difficulty in accurately recalling past events; and work in the area of *response shift* have tried to explain seemingly unusual patterns in measuring change in health status over time. The greater availability of sophisticated statistical techniques such as *structural equation modeling* has resulted in a better conceptualization of an area rife with misunderstanding: when internal consistency is important in the construction of a scale, and when it is not. A related technique, *confirmatory factor analysis*, has led to better ways of testing the equivalence of test responses across different groups, such as men and women, or between original and translated versions of a scale. All of these have been added to or expanded in this version.

Unfortunately, the growth in the psychometric literature has also resulted in much that is confusing, misleading, or simply wrong. For example, in 1987, the noted clinical epidemiologist, Alvan R. Feinstein, wrote a book whose title introduced a new term into the measurement field, *Clinimetrics*. Clinimetric scales were purportedly different from psychometric ones, in that the correlations among the items are low with the former but high with the latter; and the items in clinimetric scales are selected on the basis of 'clinical justification' and 'clinical applicability', whereas items in psychometric scales are chosen solely on statistical considerations. As we point out in various places in this book, this portrayal of psychometrics *may* have been true before the 1950s, but seriously misrepresents how scales have been developed over the past half century.

Another development that we feel is unfortunate was the attempt to classify scales as 'evaluative', 'discriminative', or 'predictive'. While there is no doubt that scales can be used for different purposes, a mythology arose around these terms that held that different techniques of item selection, reliability testing, and validity assessment were necessary for each 'type' of test, and that scales are to be developed and used for only one of these aims. As we explain in Chapter 10: Validity, we believe that this classification ignores the reality that nearly all scales developed for one purpose are put to other uses; and that it mistakenly assumes that it is tests that are validated, rather than the uses to which the tests are put.

A misunderstanding of the concept of validity also underlies a third area of confusion. Until about 10 years ago, articles about scale development said that they were assessing the 'reliability and validity' of a test. With greater frequency now, we read that they are assessing the 'reliability, validity, and responsiveness' (or 'sensitivity to change'), as if these latter two terms were unique properties, somehow different from validity. We discuss in the Validity chapter that responsiveness and sensitivity to change are simply two aspects of validity testing.

We continue to be extremely gratified by students' and professionals' reactions to this book (at our last count, it has been cited well over 400 times), and by the willingness of people to tell us how it has helped them (and their seemingly greater readiness to point out typographical errors). We welcome both, and encourage readers to contact us at:

dstreiner@klaru-baycrest.on.ca or norman@mcmaster.ca

Finally, we hope the readers learn as much about scale development by reading this book as we have learned by writing it.

November 2002   D. L. S.
G. R. N.

Preface to the second edition

This second edition of *Health measurement scales: a practical guide to their development and use* was initiated in recognition of some significant developments in the field of measurement since the first printing in 1989. This in itself is remarkable: psychological measurement is as mature as any of the social sciences, and much of the pioneering work in the field dates to the beginning of the century. That the span of only five years could witness significant changes speaks for the dynamism of the field.

In particular, when we wrote the first edition, generalizability theory, although developed by Cronbach in 1972, was largely a technical curiosity in health measurement. Since then, prompted in part by research efforts surrounding the widespread implementation of the Objective Structured Clinical Examination in North America, generalizablity theory has become an accepted and conventional approach to the investigation of test reliability. As a consequence, whereas the first edition deliberately treated the topic in a cursory manner, in order to merely familiarize the reader with the general concept, the chapter in the present edition (Chapter 9) is much more extensive. Accompanying these changes, we have completely revised Chapter 8: Reliability, in order to cover new topics and to present these difficult concepts in a more coherent manner.

Measuring change has been a continuing source of debate amongst researchers in measurement for many decades. However, the past decade or so has witnessed a new and elegant approach to the problem, based on individual growth curves, which was initially identified by Rogosa (1981) and has since been refined by a number of investigators. These new techniques are described in Chapter 11.

Ethics in research is not a new topic, but the past decade has witnessed growing concern about the issue, and a number of governmental and non-governmental agencies have issued specific guidelines. Because researchers in measurement must be aware of these issues, a new chapter, Chapter 13, is devoted to a discussion of ethical problems which may be encountered in developing measurement tools.

In addition to these major changes, there have been many minor ones; too many, in fact, for us to list more than a sampling. New sections have been added on Goal Attainment Scaling (GAS) and multidimensional scaling. As is the case with generalizability theory, these are not new techniques, but ones which have seen something of a resurgence in the past few years. On the other hand, the difficulties encountered when two scores (such as the frequency and importance of symptoms) are multiplied together to form a multiplicative composite have only recently been examined in depth, and these are discussed in Chapter 7. We have also expanded the appendix pointing out where to find existing scales to include a wider range of topics and recent additions, and have tried to bring empirical findings on scale development and use up to date.

We have been very gratified by the positive comments we have received about the first edition of this book, and hope that the current edition makes it ever more useful to those who want to develop their own scales, or just to learn more about how others have (or should have) gone about this task.

December 1994   D. L. S.
G. R. N.

Contents

Chapter 1

Introduction

The act of measurement is an essential component of scientific research, whether in the natural, social, or health sciences. Until recently, however, discussion regarding issues of measurement was noticeably absent in the deliberations of clinical researchers. Certainly, measurement played as essential a role in research in the health sciences as in other scientific disciplines. However, measurement in the laboratory disciplines presented no inherent difficulty. Like other natural sciences, measurement was a fundamental part of the discipline, and was approached through the development of appropriate instrumentation. Subjective judgement played a minor role in the measurement process; any issue of reproducibility or validity was therefore amenable to a technological solution. It should be mentioned, however, that expensive equipment does not, of itself, eliminate measurement error.

Conversely, clinical researchers were acutely aware of the fallibility of human judgement as evidenced by the errors involved in such processes as radiological diagnosis (Garland 1959; Yerushalmy 1955). Fortunately the research problems approached by many clinical researchers—cardiologists, epidemiologists, and the like—frequently did not depend on subjective assessment. Trials of therapeutic regimens focused on the prolongation of life and the prevention or management of such life-threatening conditions as heart disease, stroke, or cancer. In these circumstances, measurement is reasonably straightforward. 'Objective' criteria, based on laboratory or tissue diagnosis where possible, can be used to decide whether a patient has the disease, and warrants inclusion in the study. The investigator then waits an appropriate period of time and counts those who did or did not survive—and the criteria for death are reasonably well established, even though the exact cause of death may be a little more difficult.

In the past few decades, the situation in clinical research has become more complex. The effects of new drugs or surgical procedures on *quantity* of life is likely to be marginal indeed. Conversely, there is increased awareness of the impact of health and health care on the *quality* of human life. Therapeutic efforts in many disciplines of medicine—psychiatry, respirology, rheumatology, oncology—other health professions—nursing, physiotherapy, occupational therapy—are directed equally if not primarily to the improvement of quality, not quantity of life. If the efforts of these disciplines are to be placed on a sound scientific basis, methods must be devised to measure what was previously thought to be unmeasurable, and assess in a reproducible and valid fashion those subjective states which cannot be converted into the position of a needle on a dial.

The need for reliable and valid measures was clearly demonstrated by Marshall *et al.* (2000). After examining 300 randomized controlled trials in schizophrenia, they found that the studies were nearly 40 per cent more likely to report that treatment was effective when they used unpublished scales rather than validated ones; and in non-drug studies, one-third of the claims of treatment superiority would not have been made if the studies had used published scales.

The challenge is not as formidable as it may seem. Psychologists and educators have been grappling with the issue for many years, dating back to the European attempts at the turn of the century to assess individual differences in intelligence (Galton, cited in Allen and Yen 1979; Stern 1979). Since that time, and particularly since the 1930s, much has been accomplished, so that a sound methodology for the development and application of tools to assess subjective states now exists. Unfortunately, much of this literature is virtually unknown to most clinical researchers. Health science libraries do not routinely catalog *Psychometrica* or *The British Journal of Statistical Psychology*. Nor should they—the language would be incomprehensible to most readers, and the problems of seemingly little relevance.

Similarly, the textbooks on the subject are directed at educational or psychological audiences. The former is concerned with measures of achievement applicable to classroom situations, and the latter is focused primarily on personality or aptitude measures, again with no apparent direct relevance. In general, textbooks in these disciplines are directed to the development of achievement, intelligence, or personality tests.

By contrast, researchers in health sciences are frequently faced with the desire to measure something that has not been approached previously—arthritic pain, return to function of post-MI patients, speech difficulties of aphasic stroke patients, or clinical competence of junior medical students. The difficulties and questions raised in developing such instruments range from the straightforward (e.g. How many boxes do I put on the response?) to the complex (e.g. How do I establish whether the thing is measuring what I hope it is?). Nevertheless, to a large degree, the answers are known, although frequently difficult to access.

The intent of this book is to introduce researchers in health sciences to these concepts of measurement. It is not an introductory textbook, in that we do not confine ourselves to a discussion of introductory principles and methods; rather, we attempt to make the book as current and comprehensive as possible. The book does not delve as heavily into mathematics as many books in the field; such side trips may provide some intellectual rewards for those so inclined, but frequently at the expense of losing the majority of readers. Similarly, we emphasize applications, rather than theory, so that some theoretical subjects (like Thurstone's Law of Comparative Judgement), which are of historical interest but little practical importance, are omitted. Nevertheless, we spend considerable time in explanation of the concepts underlying current approaches to measurement. One other departure from current books is that our focus is on those attributes of interest to researchers in health sciences—subjective states, attitudes, response to illness, etc., rather than the topics such as personality or achievement familiar to readers in education and psychology. As a result, our examples are drawn from the literature in health sciences.

Finally, some understanding of certain selected topics in statistics is necessary to learn many essential concepts of measurement. In particular, the *correlation coefficient* is used in many empirical studies of measurement instruments. Discussion of reliability is based on the methods of *repeated measures analysis of variance*. Item analysis and certain approaches to test validity use the methods of *factor analysis*. It is not by any means necessary to have detailed knowledge of these methods to understand the concepts of measurement discussed in this book. Still, it would be useful to have some conceptual understanding of these techniques. If the reader requires some review of statistical topics, we have suggested a few appropriate resources in Appendix A.

The book is organized in a sort of chronological sequence; that is, we are attempting to cover topics in the order they might be confronted by someone faced with the problem of developing a new instrument. Chapter 2 provides an overview of the criteria that should be used to assess any measurement instrument; by reviewing this section, the reader should be able to peruse the literature to see if any available instrument is suitable. In the remaining chapters, we assume an unsuccessful search, and provide detailed information regarding the steps involved in developing a new scale. Finally, the appendix provides additional resources for locating further information about issues in measurement, including an annotated bibliography of references for existing scales (Appendix B).

References

Galton, F. (1979). Cited in M. J. Allen and W. M. Yen, *Introduction to measurement theory*. Brooks Cole, Monterey.

Garland, L. H. (1959). Studies on the accuracy of diagnostic procedures. *American Journal of Roentgenology*, **82**, 25–38.

Marshall, M., Lockwood, A., Bradley, C., Adams, C., Joy, C., and Fenton, M. (2000). Unpublished rating scales: A major source of bias in randomised controlled trials of treatments for schizophrenia. *British Journal of Psychiatry*, **176**, 249–52.

Stern, W. (1979). Cited in M. J. Allen and W. M. Yen, *Introduction to measurement theory*. Brooks Cole, Monterey.

Yerushalmy, J. (1955). Reliability of chest radiography in diagnosis of pulmonary lesions. *American Journal of Surgery*, **89**, 231–40.

Chapter 2

Basic concepts

One feature of the health sciences literature devoted to measuring subjective states is the daunting array of available scales. Whether one wishes to measure depression, pain, or patient satisfaction, it seems that every article published in the field has used a different approach to the measurement problem. This proliferation impedes research, since there are significant problems in generalizing from one set of findings to another.

Paradoxically, if you proceed a little further in the search for existing instruments to assess a particular concept, you may conclude that none of the existing scales is quite right, so it is appropriate to embark on the development of one more scale to add to the confusion in the literature. Most researchers tend to magnify the deficiencies of existing measures and underestimate the effort required to develop an adequate new measure. Of course, scales do not exist for all applications; if this were so, there would be little justification for writing this book. Nevertheless, perhaps the most common error committed by clinical researchers is to dismiss existing scales too lightly, and embark on the development of a new instrument with an unjustifiably optimistic and naive expectation that they can do better. As will become evident, the development of scales to assess subjective attributes is not easy and requires considerable investment of both mental and fiscal resources. Therefore, a useful first step is to be aware of any existing scales that might suit the purpose. The next step is to understand and apply criteria for judging the usefulness of a particular scale. In subsequent chapters, these will be described in much greater detail for use in developing a scale; however, the next few pages will serve as an introduction to the topic and a guideline for a critical literature review.

The discussion that follows is necessarily brief. A much more comprehensive set of standards, which is widely used for the assessment of standardized tests used in psychology and education, is the manual called *Standards for educational and psychological tests*, published by the American Psychological Association (1985).

Searching the literature

An initial search of the literature to locate scales for measurement of particular variables might begin with the standard bibliographic sources, particularly Medline. However, depending on the application, one might wish to consider bibliographic reference systems in other disciplines, particularly *PsycINFO* for psychological scales and ERIC for instruments designed for educational purposes.

In addition to these standard sources, there are a number of compendia of measuring scales. These are described in Appendix B. We might particularly highlight the volume entitled *Measuring health: a guide to rating scales and questionnaires* (McDowell and Newell 1996), which is a critical review of scales designed to measure a number of characteristics of interest to researchers in the health sciences, such as pain, illness behavior, and social support.

Critical review

Having located one or more scales of potential interest, it remains to choose whether to use one of these existing scales or to proceed to development of a new instrument. In part this decision can be guided by a judgement of the appropriateness of the items on the scale, but this should always be supplemented by a critical review of the evidence in support of the instrument. The particular dimensions of this review are described below:

Face and content validity

The terms *face validity* and *content validity* are technical descriptions of the judgement that a scale looks reasonable. Face validity simply indicates whether, on the face of it, the instrument appears to be assessing the desired qualities. The criterion represents a subjective judgement based on a review of the measure itself by one or more experts, and rarely are any empirical approaches used. Content validity is a closely related concept, consisting of a judgement whether the instrument samples all the relevant or important content or domains. These two forms of validity consist of a judgement by experts whether the scale appears appropriate for the intended purpose. Guilford (1954) calls this approach to validation 'validity by assumption', meaning the instrument measures such-and-such because an expert says it does. However, an explicit statement regarding face and content validity, based on some form of review by an expert panel or alternative methods described later, should be a minimum prerequisite for acceptance of a measure.

Having said this, there are situations where face and content validity may not be desirable, and may be consciously avoided. For example, in assessing behavior such as child abuse or excessive alcohol consumption, questions like 'Have you ever hit your child with a blunt object?' or 'Do you frequently drink to excess?' may have face validity, but are unlikely to elicit an honest response. Questions designed to assess sensitive areas are likely to be less obviously related to the underlying attitude or behavior, and may appear to have poor face validity. It is rare for scales not to satisfy minimal standards of face and content validity, unless there has been a deliberate attempt from the outset to avoid straightforward questions.

Nevertheless, all too frequently, researchers dismiss existing measures on the basis of their own judgements of face validity—they did not like some of the questions, or the scale was too long, or the responses were not in a preferred format. As we have indicated, this judgement should comprise only one of several used in arriving at an overall judgement of usefulness, and should be balanced against the time and cost of developing a replacement.

Reliability

The concept of *reliability* is, on the surface, deceptively simple. Before one can obtain evidence that an instrument is measuring what is intended, it is first necessary to gather evidence that the scale is measuring *something* in reproducible fashion. That is, a first step in providing evidence of the value of an instrument is to demonstrate that measurements of individuals on different occasions, or by different observers, or by similar or parallel tests, produce the same or similar results.

That is the basic idea behind the concept—an index of the extent to which measurements of individuals obtained under different circumstances yield similar results. However, the concept is refined a bit further in measurement theory. If we were considering the reliability of, for example, a set of bathroom scales, it might be sufficient to indicate that the scales are accurate to ±1 kg. From this information, we can easily judge whether the scales will be adequate to distinguish among adult males (probably yes) or to assess weight gain of premature infants (probably no), since we have prior knowledge of the average weight and variation in weight of adults and premature infants.

Such information is rarely available in the development of subjective scales. Each scale produces a different measurement from every other. Therefore, to indicate that a particular scale is accurate to ±3.4 units provides no indication of its value in measuring individuals unless we have some idea about the likely range of scores on the scale. To circumvent this problem, reliability is usually quoted as a ratio of the variability between individuals to the total variability in the scores; in other words, the reliability is a measure of the proportion of the variability in scores which was due to true differences between individuals. Thus, the reliability is expressed as a number between 0 and 1, with 0 indicating no reliability, and 1 indicating perfect reliability.

An important issue in examining the reliability of an instrument is the manner in which the data were obtained that provided the basis for the calculation of a reliability coefficient. First of all, since the reliability involves the ratio of variability between subjects to total variability, one way to ensure that a test will look good is to conduct the study on an extremely heterogeneous sample, for example to measure knowledge of clinical medicine using samples of first year, third year, and fifth year students. Examine the sampling procedures carefully, and assure yourself that the sample used in the reliability study is approximately the same as the sample you wish to study.

Second, there are any number of ways in which reliability measures can be obtained, and the magnitude of the reliability coefficient will be a direct reflection of the particular approach used. Some broad definitions are described below:

1. *Internal consistency.* Measures of internal consistency are based on a single administration of the measure. If the measure has a relatively large number of items addressing the same underlying dimension, e.g. Are you able to dress yourself?', 'Are you able to shop for groceries?', 'Can you do the sewing?' as measures of physical function,

then it is reasonable to expect that scores on each item would be correlated with scores on all other items. This is the idea behind measures of internal consistency—essentially, they represent the average of the correlations among all the items in the measure. There are a number of ways to calculate these correlations, called *Cronbach's alpha*, *Kuder-Richardson*, or *split halves*, but all yield similar results. Since the method involves only a single administration of the test, such coefficients are easy to obtain. However, they do not take into account any variation from day to day or from observer to observer, and thus lead to an optimistic interpretation of the true reliability of the test.

2. *Stability*. There are various ways of examining the reproduceability of a measure administered on different occasions. For example, one might ask about the degree of agreement between different observers (inter-observer reliability); the agreement between observations made by the same rater on two different occasions (intra-observer reliability); observations on the patient on two occasions separated by some interval of time (test–retest reliability), and so forth. As a minimum, any decision regarding the value of a measure should be based on some information regarding stability of the instrument. Internal consistency, in its many guises, is not a sufficient basis upon which to make a reasoned judgement.

3. *Standards of acceptable reliability*. One difficulty with the reliability coefficient is that it is simply a number between 0 and 1, and does not lend itself to common-sense interpretations. Various authors have made different recommendations regarding the minimum accepted level of reliability. Certainly, internal consistency should exceed 0.8, and it might be reasonable to demand stability measures greater than 0.5. Depending on the use of the test, and the cost of misinterpretation, higher values might be required.

Finally, although there is a natural concern that many instruments in the literature are too long to be practical, the reason for the length should be borne in mind. If we assume that every response has some associated error of measurement, then by averaging or summing responses over a series of questions, we can reduce this error. For example, if the original test has a reliability of 0.5, doubling the test will increase the reliability to 0.67, and quadrupling it will result in a reliability of 0.8. As a result, we must recognize that there is a very good reason for long tests; brevity is not necessarily a desirable attribute of a test, and is achieved at some cost.

Empirical forms of validity

Reliability simply assesses that a test is measuring something in a reproducible fashion; it says nothing about *what* is being measured. To determine that the test is measuring what was intended requires some evidence of 'validity'. To demonstrate validity requires more than peer judgements; empirical evidence must be produced to show that the tool is measuring what is intended. How is this achieved?

Although there are many approaches to assessing validity, and myriad terms used to describe these approaches, eventually the situation reduces to two circumstances:

1. *Other scales of the same or similar attributes are available*. In the situation where measures already exist, then an obvious approach is to administer the experimental

instrument and one of the existing instruments to a sample of people and see whether there is a strong correlation between the two. As an example, there are many scales to measure depression. In developing a new scale, it is straightforward to administer the new and old instruments to the same sample. This approach is described by several terms in the literature including *convergent validity, criterion validity,* and *concurrent validity.* The distinction among the terms will be made clear in Chapter 10.

Although this method is straightforward it has two severe limitations. First, if other measures of the same property already exist, then it is difficult to justify developing yet another unless it is cheaper or simpler. Of course, many researchers believe that the new instrument that they are developing is better than the old, which provides an interesting bit of circular logic. If the new method is better than the old, why compare it to the old method? And if the relationship between the new method and the old is less than perfect, which one is at fault?

In fact, the nature of the measurement challenges we are discussing in this book usually precludes the existence of any conventional 'gold standard'. Although there are often measures which have, through history or longevity, acquired criterion status, a close review usually suggests that they have less than ideal reliability and validity. Any measurement we are likely to make will have some associated error; as a result we should expect that correlations among measures of the same attribute should fall in the midrange of 0.4–0.8. Any lower correlation suggests that either the reliability of one or the other measure is likely unacceptably low, or that they are measuring different phenomena.

2. *No other measure exists.* This situation is the more likely, since it is usually the justification for developing a scale in the first instance. At first glance, though, we seem to be confronting an impossible situation. After all, if no measure exists, how can one possibly acquire data to show that the new measure is indeed measuring what is intended?

The solution lies in a broad set of approaches labeled *construct validity.* We begin by linking the attribute we are measuring to some other attribute by a hypothesis or construct. Usually this hypothesis will explore the difference between two or more populations who would be expected to have differing amounts of the property assessed by our instrument. We then test this hypothetical construct by applying our instrument to the appropriate samples. If the expected relationship is found, then the hypothesis and the measure are sound; conversely, if no relationship is found, the fault may lie with either the measure or the hypothesis.

Let us clarify this with an example. Suppose that the year is 1920, and a biochemical test of blood sugar has just been devised. Enough is known to hypothesize that diabetics have higher blood sugar values than normal subjects; but no other test of blood sugar exists. Here are some likely hypotheses which could be tested empirically:

individuals diagnosed as diabetic on clinical criteria will have higher blood sugar on the new test than comparable controls;

dogs whose pancreases are removed will show increasing levels of blood sugar in the days from surgery until death;

individuals who have sweet-tasting urine will have higher blood sugar than those who do not;

diabetics injected with insulin extract will show a decrease in blood sugar levels following the injection.

These hypotheses certainly do not exhaust the number of possibilities, but each can be put to an experimental test. Further, it is evident that we should not demand a perfect relationship between blood sugar and the other variable, or even that each and all relationships are significant. But the weight of the evidence should be in favour of a positive relationship.

Similar constructs can be developed for almost any instrument, and in the absence of a concurrent test, some evidence of construct validity should be available. However, the approach is non-specific, and is unlikely to result in very strong relationships. Therefore, the burden of evidence in testing construct validity arises not from a single powerful experiment, but from a series of converging experiments.

The two traditions of assessment

Not surprisingly, medicine on the one hand, and psychology and education on the other, have developed different ways of evaluating people; ways that have influenced how and why assessment tools are constructed in the first place, and the manner in which they are interpreted. This has led each camp to ignore the potential contribution of the other: the physicians contending that the psychometricians do not appreciate how the results must be used to abet clinical decision-making, and the psychologists and educators accusing the physicians of ignoring many of the basic principles of test construction, such as reliability and validity. It has only been within the last decade that some rapprochement has been reached; a mutual recognition that we feel is resulting in clinical instruments that are both psychometrically sound as well as clinically useful. In this section, we will explore two of these different starting points—categorical vs. dimensional conceptualization and the reduction of measurement error—and see how they are being merged.

Categorical vs. dimensional conceptualization

Medicine traditionally has thought in terms of diagnoses and treatments. In the most simplistic terms, a patient either has a disorder or does not, and is either prescribed some form of treatment or is not. Thus, diastolic blood pressure (DBF), which is measured on a continuum of millimetres of mercury, is often broken down into just two categories: normotensive (under 90 mm in North America), in which case nothing needs to be done; and hypertensive (90 mm and above), which calls for some form of intervention.

Test constructors who come from the realm of psychology and education, though, look to the writings of S. Smith Stevens (1951) as received wisdom. He introduced the concept of 'levels of measurement', which categorizes variables as *nominal, ordinal, interval,* or *ratio*—a concept we will return to in greater depth in Chapter 4.

The basic idea is that the more finely we can measure something, the better; rating an attribute on a scale in which each point is equally spaced from its neighbors is vastly superior to dividing the attribute into rougher categories with fewer divisions. Thus, psychometricians tend to think of attributes as continua, with people falling along the dimension in terms of how much of the attribute they have.

The implications of these two different ways of thinking have been summarized by Devins (1993), and are presented in modified form in Table 2.1. In the categorical mode, the diagnosis of, for example, major depression in the *Diagnostic and statistical manual* (DMS-IV; American Psychiatric Association 1994) requires that the person exhibit at least five of nine symptoms (one of which, depressed mood or loss of interest/pleasure, must be among the five) and that none of four exclusion criteria be present. In turn, each of the symptoms, such as weight change or sleep disturbance, has its own minimum criterion for being judged to be demonstrated (the threshold value). A continuous measure of depression, such as the Center for Epidemiological Studies – Depression scale (CES-D; Radloff 1977), uses a completely different approach. There are 20 items, each scored 1 through 4, and a total score over 16 is indicative of depression. No specific item must be endorsed, and there are numerous ways that a score of 16 can be achieved—a person can have four items rated 4, or 16 items rated 1, or any combination in between. Thus, for diagnostic purposes, having many mild symptoms is equivalent to having a few severe ones.

Second, DSM-IV differentiates among various types of depressions according to their severity and course. A bipolar depression is qualitatively and quantitatively different from a dysthymic disorder; different sets of criteria must be met to reflect that the former is not only more severe than the latter, but that it is cyclical in its time course, whereas dysthymia is not. On the other hand, the CES-D quantifies the depressive symptomatology, but does not differentiate among the various types.

Table 2.1 Categorical and dimensional conceptualization

Categorical model	Dimensional model
1. Diagnosis requires that multiple criteria, each with its threshold value, be satisfied.	Occurrence of some features at high intensities can compensate for non-occurrence of others.
2. Phenomenon differs qualitatively and quantitatively at different severities.	Phenomenon differs only quantitatively, at different severities.
3. Differences between cases and non-cases are implicit in the definition.	Differences between cases and non-cases are less clearly delineated.
4. Severity is lowest in instances that minimally satisfy diagnostic criteria.	Severity is lowest among non-disturbed individuals.
5. One diagnosis often precludes others.	A person can have varying amounts of different disorders.

Consequently, it would reflect that one person's symptoms may be more extensive than another's, irrespective of category.

One implication of this difference is that there is a clear distinction between cases and non-cases with the categorical approach, but not with the dimensional. In the former, one either meets the criteria and is a case, or else the criteria are not satisfied, and one is not a case. With the latter, 'caseness' is a matter of degree, and there is no clear dividing line. The use of a cut point on the CES-D is simply a strategy so that it can be used as a diagnostic tool. The value of 16 was chosen only because, based on empirical findings, using this score maximized agreement between the CES-D and clinical diagnosis; the number is not based on any theoretical argument. Furthermore, there would be less difference seen between two people, one of whom has a score of 15 and the other 17, than between two other people with scores of 30 and 40, although one is a 'case' and the other not in the first instance, and both would be 'cases' in the second.

Another implication is that, since people who do not meet the criteria are said to be free of the disorder with the categorical approach, differences in severity are seen only among those who are diagnosed (point 4 in Table 2.1). Quantification of severity is implicit, with the assumption that those who meet more of the criteria have a more severe depression than people who satisfy only the minimum number. With the dimensional approach, even 'normal' people may have measurable levels of depressive symptomatology; a non-depressed person whose sleep is restless would score higher on the CES-D than a non-depressed person without sleep difficulties.

Last, using the categorical approach, it is difficult (at least within psychiatry) for a person to have more than one disorder. A diagnosis of major depression, for example, cannot be made if the patient has a psychotic condition, or shows evidence of delusions or hallucinations. The dimensional approach does permit this; some traits may be present, albeit in a mild form, even when others coexist.

The limitations of adhering strictly to one or the other of these ways of thinking are becoming more evident. The categorical mode of thinking is starting to change, in part due to the expansion of the armamentarium of treatment options. Returning to the example of hypertension, now patients can be started on salt-restricted diets, followed by diuretics at higher levels of the DBP, and finally placed on vasodilators. Consequently, it makes more sense to measure blood pressure on a continuum, and to titrate the type and amount of treatment to smaller differences, than to simply dichotomize the reading. On the other hand, there are different treatment implications, depending on whether one has a bipolar or a non-cyclical form of depression. Simply measuring the severity of symptomatology does not allow for this. One resolution, which will be discussed in Chapter 4, called multidimensional scaling, is an attempt to bridge these two traditions. It permits a variety of attributes to be measured dimensionally, in such a way that the results can be used to both categorize and determine the extent to which these categories are present.

The reduction of measurement error

Whenever definitive laboratory tests do not exist, physicians rely primarily on the clinical interview to provide differential diagnoses. The clinician is the person who both elicits the information and interprets its significance as a sign or symptom (Dohrenwend and Dohrenwend 1982). Measurement error is reduced through training, interviewing skills, and especially clinical experience. Thus, older physicians are often regarded as 'gold standards', since they presumably have more experience and therefore would make fewer errors. (In a different context, though, Caputo (1980, p. 370) wrote, 'They haven't got seventeen years' experience, just one year's experience repeated seventeen times'.)

In contrast, the psychometric tradition relies on self-reports of patients to usually close-ended questions. It is assumed that the response to any one question is subject to error: the person may misinterpret the item, respond in a biased manner, or make a mistake in transcribing his or her reply to the answer sheet. The effect of these errors is minimized in a variety of ways. First, each item is screened to determine if it meets certain criteria. Second, the focus is on the consistency of the answers across many items, and for the most part, disregarding the responses to the individual questions. Last, the scale as a whole is checked to see if it meets another set of criteria.

The 'medical' approach is often criticized as placing unwarranted faith in the clinical skills of the interviewer. Indeed, as was mentioned briefly in Chapter 1, the reliability (and hence the validity) of the clinical interview leaves much to be desired. Conversely, psychometrically sound tests may provide reliable and valid data, but do not yield the rich clinical information and the ways in which patients differ from one another which come from talking to them in a conversational manner. These two 'solitudes' are starting to merge, especially in psychiatry, as is seen in some of the more recent structured interviews, such as the Diagnostic Interview Schedule (DIS; Robins *et al.* 1981). The DIS is derived from the clinical examination used to diagnose psychiatric patients, but is constructed in such a way that it can be administered by trained lay people, not just psychiatrists. It also relies on the necessity of answering a number of questions before an attribute is judged to be present. Thus, elements of both traditions guided its construction, although purists from both camps will be dissatisfied with the compromises.

Summary

The criteria we have described are intended as a guideline for reviewing the literature, and as an introduction to the remainder of this book. We must emphasize that the research enterprise involved in development of a new method of measurement requires time and patience. Effort expended to locate an existing measure is justified, because of the savings if one can be located and the additional insights provided in the development of a new instrument if none prove satisfactory.

References

American Psychiatric Association (1994). *Diagnostic and statistical manual of mental disorders* (4th edn, revised). American Psychiatric Association, Washington DC.
American Psychological Association (1985). *Standards for educational and psychological testing.* American Psychological Association, Washington.

Caputo, P. (1980). *Horn of Africa.* Holt, Rinehart and Winston, New York.

Devins, G. (1993). *Psychiatric rating scales.* Paper presented at the Clarke Institute of Psychiatry, Toronto, Ontario.

Dohrenwend, B. P. and Dohrenwend, B. S. (1982). Perspectives on the past and future of psychiatric epidemiology. *American Journal of Public Health,* 72, 1271–9.

Guilford, J. P. (1954). *Psychometric methods.* McGraw-Hill, New York.

McDowell, I. and Newell, C. (1996). *Measuring health* (2nd edn). Oxford University Press, Oxford.

Radloff, L. S. (1977). The CES-D scale: A self-report depression scale for research in the general population. *Applied Psychological Measurement,* 1, 385–401.

Robins, L. N., Helzer, J. E., Crougham, R., and Ratcliff, K. S. (1981). National Institute of Mental Health Diagnostic Interview Schedule: Its history, characteristics, and validity. *Archives of General Psychiatry,* 38, 381–9.

Stevens, S. S. (1951). Mathematics, measurement, and psychophysics. In *Handbook of experimental psychology* (ed. S. S. Stevens) pp. 1–49. Wiley, New York.

Chapter 3

Devising the items

The first step in writing a scale or questionnaire is, naturally, devising the items themselves. This is far from a trivial task, since no amount of statistical manipulation after the fact can compensate for poorly chosen questions; those that are badly worded, ambiguous, irrelevant, or—even worse—not present. In this chapter we explore various sources of items, and the strengths and weaknesses of each of them.

The first step is to look at what others have done in the past. Instruments rarely spring full grown from the brows of their developers. Rather, they are usually based on what other people have deemed to be relevant, important, or discriminating. Wechsler (1958), for example, quite openly discussed the patrimony of the subtests that were later incorporated into his various IQ tests. Of the 11 subtests which comprise the adult version, at least nine were derived from other widely used indices. Moreover, the specific items that make up the individual subtests are themselves based on older tests. Both the items and the subtests were modified and new ones added to meet his requirements, but in many cases the changes were relatively minor. Similarly, the *Manifest Anxiety Scale* (Taylor 1953) is based in large measure on one scale from the *Minnesota Multiphasic Personality Inventory* (MMPI; Hathaway and McKinley 1951).

The long, and sometimes tortuous, path by which items from one test end up in others is beautifully described by Goldberg (1971). He wrote that (p. 335):

> Items devised around the turn of the century may have worked their way via Woodworth's Personal Data Sheet, to Thurstone and Thurstone's Personality Schedule, hence to Bernreuter's Personality Inventory, and later to the Minnesota Multiphasic Personality Inventory, where they were borrowed for the California Personality Inventory and then injected into the Omnibus Personality Inventory—only to serve as a source of items for the new Academic Behavior Inventory.

Angleitner *et al.* (1986) expanded this to, 'and, we may add, only to be translated and included in some new German personality inventories' (p. 66).

There are a number of reasons that items are repeated from previous inventories. First, it saves work and the necessity of constructing new ones. Second, the items have usually gone through repeated processes of testing, so that they have proven themselves to be useful and psychometrically sound. Third, there are only a limited number of ways to ask about a specific problem. If we were trying to tap depressed mood, for instance, it is difficult to ask about sleep loss in a way that has not been used previously.

Hoary as this tradition may be, there are (at least) two problems in adopting it uncritically. First, it may result in items which use outdated terminology. For example, the original version of the MMPI (in use until 1987) contained such quaint terms such as 'deportment', 'cutting up', and 'drop the handkerchief'. Endorsement of these items most likely told more about the person's age than about any aspect of his or her personality. Perhaps more importantly, the motivation for developing a new tool is the investigator's belief that the previous scales are inadequate for one reason or another, or do not completely cover the domain under study. At this point, new items can come from five different sources: the patients or subjects themselves, clinical observation, theory, research, and expert opinion; although naturally the lines between these categories are not firm.

The source of items

A point often overlooked in scale development is the fact that patients and potential research subjects are an excellent source of items. Whereas clinicians may be the best observers of the outward manifestations of a trait or disorder, only those who have it can report on the more subjective elements. Over the years, a variety of techniques have been developed, which can elicit these viewpoints in a rigorous and systematic manner; these procedures are used primarily by 'qualitative' researchers, and are only now finding their way into more 'quantitative' types of studies. Here, we can touch only briefly on two of the more relevant techniques; greater detail is provided in texts such as Taylor and Bogden (1984) and Willms and Johnson (1993).

Focus groups

Willms and Johnson (1993) describe a focus group as (p. 61):

> ...a discussion in which a small group of informants (six to twelve people), guided by a facilitator, talk freely and spontaneously about themes considered important to the investigation. The participants are selected from a target group whose opinions and ideas are of interest to the researcher. Sessions are usually tape recorded and an observer (recorder) also takes notes on the discussion.

In the area of scale development, the participants would be patients who have the disorder, or subjects representative of those whose opinions would be elicited by the instrument. At first, their task would not be to generate the specific items, but rather to suggest general themes that the research team can use to phrase the items themselves. Usually, no more than two or three groups would be needed. Once the items have been written, focus groups can again be used to discuss whether these items are relevant, clear, unambiguous, written in terms that are understood by potential respondents, and if all the main themes have been covered. These groups are much more focused than during the theme generation stage, since there is a strong externally generated agenda; discussing the items themselves.

Key informant interviews

As the name implies, these are in-depth interviews with a small number of people, chosen because of their unique knowledge. These can be patients who have, or have had, the disorder, for example, and who can articulate what they felt; or clinicians who have extensive experience with the patients and can explain it from their perspective. The interviews can range from informal or unstructured ones, which are almost indistinguishable from spontaneous conversations, to highly structured ones, where the interviewer has a preplanned set of carefully worded questions. Generally, the less that is known about the area under study, the less structured the interview. There is no set number of people who should be interviewed. The criterion often used in this type of research is 'sampling to redundancy'; that is, interviewing people until no new themes emerge.

Clinical observation is perhaps one of the most fruitful sources of items. Indeed, it can be argued that observation, whether of patients or students, precedes theory, research, or expert opinion. Scales are simply a way of gathering these clinical observations in a systematic fashion, so that all observers are ensured of looking for the same thing, or all subjects of responding to the same items. As an example, Kruis *et al.* (1984) devised a scale to try to differentiate between irritable bowel syndrome (IBS) and organic bowel disease. The first part of their questionnaire consists of a number of items asked by the clinician of the patient—presence of abdominal pain and flatulence, alteration in bowel habits, duration of symptoms, type and intensity of pain, abnormality of the stools, and so forth. The choice of these items was predicated on the clinical experience of the authors, and their impressions of how IBS patients' symptomatology and presentation differ from other patients'. Similarly, the *Menstrual Distress Questionnaire* (Moos 1984) consists of 47 symptoms, such as muscle stiffness, skin blemishes, fatigue, and feeling sad or blue, which have been reported clinically to be associated with premenstrual syndrome (PMS).

This is not to say that these groups of researchers are necessarily correct, in that the items they selected *are* different between patients with organic or functional bowel disease, or between women who do and do not have PMS. In fact, perhaps the major drawback of relying solely on clinical observation to guide the selection of items is the real possibility that the clinicians may be wrong. The original rationale for electroconvulsive shock therapy, for instance, was based on a quite erroneous 'observation' that the incidence of epilepsy is far lower in the schizophrenic population than with normals. Any scale that tried to capitalize on this association would be doomed to failure. A related problem is that the clinician, because of a limited sample of patients, or narrow perspective imposed by a particular model of the disorder, may not be aware of other factors which may prove to be better descriptors or discriminators.

Clinical observation rarely exists in isolation. Individual laboratory results or physical findings convey far more information if they are components of a more global theory of an illness or behavior. The term *theory*, in this context, is used very broadly, encompassing not only formal, refutable models of how things relate to one another, but also to vaguely formed hunches of how or why people behave, if only within a relatively narrow domain. A postulate that patients who believe in the efficacy of therapy will be more compliant with their physician's orders, for example, may not rival the theory of relativity in its scope or predictive power, but can be a fruitful source of items in this limited area. A theory or model can thus serve a heuristic purpose, suggesting items or subscales.

At first glance, it may appear as if theory is what we rely on until data are available; once studies have been done, it would be unnecessary to resort to theory and the scale developer can use facts to generate items or guide construction of the scale. Indeed, this was the prevailing attitude among test designers until relatively recently. However, there has been an increasing appreciation of the role that theory can play in scale and questionnaire development. This is seen most clearly when we are trying to assess attitudes, beliefs, or traits. For example, if we wanted to devise a scale that could predict those post-MI patients who would comply with an exercise regimen, our task would be made easier (and perhaps more accurate) if we had some model or theory of compliance. The Health Belief Model (Decker *et al.* 1979), for instance, postulates that compliance is a function of numerous factors, including the patient's perception of the severity of the disorder and his susceptibility to it, and his belief in the effectiveness of the proposed therapy, as well as external cues to comply and barriers which may impede compliance. If this model has any validity, then it would make sense for the scale to include items from each of these areas, some of which may not have occurred to the investigator without the model.

The obverse side is that a model which is wrong can lead us astray, prompting us to devise questions which ultimately have no predictive or explanatory power. While the inadequacy of the theory may emerge later in testing the validity of the scale, much time and effort can be wasted in the interim. For example, Patient Management Problems (PMPs) were based on the supposition that physician competence is directly related to the thoroughness and comprehensiveness of the history and physical examination. The problems, therefore, covered every conceivable question that could be asked of a patient and most laboratory tests that could be ordered. The scoring system similarly reflected this theory; points were gained by being obsessively compulsive, and lost if the right diagnosis were arrived at by the 'wrong' route, one which used short cuts. While psychometrically sound, the PMPs did not correlate with any other measure of clinical competence, primarily for the reason that the model was wrong—expert physicians do not function in the way envisioned by the test developers (Feightner 1985).

Just as naked observations need the clothing of a theory, so a theory must ultimately be tested empirically. *Research findings* can be a fruitful source of items and subscales. For the purposes of scale construction, research can be of two types: a literature review of studies that have been done in the area, or new research carried out specifically for the purpose of developing the scale. In both cases, the scale or questionnaire would be comprised of items which have been shown empirically to be characteristic of a group of people, or which differentiate them from other people.

As an example of a scale based on previous research, the second part of the Kruis *et al.* (1984) scale for IBS is essentially a checklist of laboratory values and clinical history, e.g. erythrocyte sedimentation rate, leucocytes, and weight loss. These were chosen on the basis of previous research which indicated that IBS and organic patients differed on these variables. This part of the scale, then, is a summary of empirical findings based on research done by others.

In a different domain, Ullman and Giovannoni (1964) developed a scale to measure the 'process–reactive' continuum in schizophrenia. A number of items on the questionnaire relate to marriage and parenthood, because there is considerable evidence that process schizophrenics, especially males, marry at a far lower rate than do reactive schizophrenics. Another item relates to alcohol consumption, since among schizophrenics at least, those who use alcohol tend to have shorter hospital stays than those who do not drink.

When entering into a new area, though, there may not be any research which can serve as the basis for items. Under these circumstances, it may be necessary for the scale developer to conduct some preliminary research, which can then be the source of items. For example, Brumbach and Howell (1972) needed an index to evaluate the clinical effectiveness of physicians working in federal hospitals and clinics. Existing scales were inadequate or inappropriate for their purposes, and did not provide the kind of information they needed in a format that was acceptable to the raters. The checklist portion of the scale they ultimately developed was derived by gathering 2500 descriptions of critical incidents from 500 people; classifying these into functional areas; and then using various item analytic techniques (to be discussed in Chapter 6) to arrive at the final set of 37 items. While this study is unusual in its size, it illustrates two points. First, it is sometimes necessary to perform research prior to constructing the scale itself, in order to determine key aspects of the domain under investigation. Second, the initial item pool is often much larger than the final set of items. Again, the size of the reduction is quite unusual in this study (only 1. 5 per cent of the original items were ultimately retained), but the fact that reduction occurs is not.

The use of *expert opinion* in a given field was illustrated in a similar study by Cowles and Kubany (1959) to evaluate the performance of medical students. Experienced faculty members were interviewed to determine what they felt were the most important characteristics students should have in preparing for general practice, ultimately resulting in eight items. This appears quite similar to the first step taken by Brumbach and Howell, which was labeled 'research'; indeed, the line between the two is a very fine one and the distinction somewhat arbitrary. The important point is that, in both cases, information had to be gathered prior to the construction of the scale.

There are no hard and fast rules governing the use of expert judgements: how many experts to use, how they are found and chosen, or even more important, how differences among them are reconciled. The methods by which the opinions are gathered can run the gamut from having a colleague scribble some comments on a rough draft of the questionnaire to holding a conference of recognized leaders in the field, with explicit rules governing voting. Most approaches usually fall between these two extremes; somewhere in the neighbourhood of three to ten people known to the scale developer as experts are consulted, usually individually. Since the objective is to generate as many potential items as possible for the scale, those suggested by even one person should be considered, at least in the first draft of the instrument.

The advantage of this approach is that if the experts are chosen carefully, they probably represent the most recent thinking in an area. Without much effort, the scale developer has access to the accumulated knowledge and experience of others who have worked in the field. The disadvantages may arise if the panel is skewed in some way, and does not reflect a range of opinions. Then, the final selection of items may represent one particular viewpoint, and there may be glaring gaps in the final product.

It should be borne in mind that these are not mutually exclusive methods of generating items. A scale may consist of items derived from some or all of these sources. Indeed, it would be unusual to find any questionnaire derived from only one of them.

Content validity

Once the items have been generated from these various sources, the scale developer is ideally left with far more items than will ultimately end up on the scale. In Chapter 5 we will discuss various statistical techniques to select the best items from this pool. For the moment, though, we address the converse of this, ensuring that the scale has enough items and adequately covers the domain under investigation. The technical term for this is *content validity*, although some theorists have argued that 'content relevance' and 'content coverage' would be more accurate descriptors (Messick 1980). These concepts arose from achievement testing, where students are assessed to determine if they have learned the material in a specific content area; final examinations are the prime example. With this in mind, each item on the test should relate to one of the course objectives (content relevance). Items that are not related to the content of the course introduce error in the measurement, in that they discriminate among the students on some dimension other than the one purportedly tapped by the test; a dimension that can be totally irrelevant to the test. Conversely, each part of the syllabus should be represented by one or more questions (content coverage). If not, then students may differ in some important respects, but this would not be reflected in the final score. Table 3.1 shows how these two components of content validity can be checked in a course of, for example, cardiology. Each row reflects a different item on the test, and each column a different content area. Every item is examined in turn, and a mark placed in the appropriate column(s). Although a single number does not emerge at the end, as with other types of validity estimates, the visual display yields much information.

First, each item should fall into at least one content area represented by the columns. If it does not, then either that item is not relevant to the course objectives, or the list of objectives is not comprehensive. Second, each objective should be represented by at least one question; otherwise, it is not being evaluated by the test. Last, the number of questions in each area should reflect its actual importance in the syllabus (this is referred to as the *representativeness* of the content area). The reason for checking this is that it is quite simple to write items in some areas, and far more difficult in others. In cardiology, for example, it is much easier to write multiple-choice items to find out if the students know the normal values of obscure enzymes than to devise questions tapping their ability to deal with the rehabilitation of cardiac

Table 3.1 Checking content validity for a course in cardiology

Question	Content area				
	Anatomy	Physiology	Function	...	Pathology
1		x			
2	x				
3			x		
4	x				
5					x
.					
.					
.					
20		x			

patients. Thus, there may be a disproportionately large number of the former items on the test and too few of the latter in relation to what the students should know. The final score, then, would not be an accurate reflection of what the instructor hoped the students would learn.

Depending on how finely one defines the course objectives, it may not be possible to assess each one, as this would make the test too long. Under these conditions, it would be necessary to *randomly sample* the domain of course objectives; that is, select them in such a way that each has an equal opportunity of being chosen. This indeed is closer to what is often done in measuring traits or behaviours, since tapping the full range of them may make the instrument unwieldy.

Although this matrix method was first developed for achievement tests, it can be applied equally well to scales measuring attitudes, behaviours, symptoms, and the like. In these cases, the columns are comprised of aspects of the trait or disorder that the investigator wants the scale to cover, rather than course objectives. Assume, for example, that the test constructor wanted to develop a new measure to determine whether living in a home insulated with urea formaldehyde foam (UFFI) leads to physical problems. The columns in this case would be those areas she felt would be affected by UFFI (and perhaps a few that should *not* be affected, if she wanted to check on a general tendency to endorse symptoms). So, based on previous research, theory, expert opinion, and other sources, these may include upper respiratory symptoms, gastrointestinal complaints, skin rash, sleep disturbances, memory problems, eye irritation, and so forth. This would then serve as a check that all domains were covered by at least one question, and that there were no irrelevant items. As can be seen, content validity applies to the scale as a whole, not to the separate items individually. Bear in mind, though, that content validity is a 'state' of the instrument, not a 'trait' (Messick 1993). That is, how relevant and representative the content is depends on the use to which the scale is put. One that has good content validity as a screening test for depression may have poor content coverage if it is used to measure response to treatment. Further, content validity may decrease over time, as we learn more about the construct under study or as the nature of the underlying theory evolves (Haynes *et al.* 1995). For example, it was once believed that cardiovascular problems were associated with the 'Type-A personality', which was defined by a constellation of attitudes (e.g. time pressure, anger), behaviours (e.g. finishing the sentences of others), and physical characteristics. More recent research, though, has shown that only the destructive expression of anger is the key ingredient (Seligman 1993). Consequently, any scale that tries to tap psychological correlates of heart disease, based on the old model of Type-A personality, would suffer from content irrelevance in light of more recent research.

Let us use a concrete example to illustrate how these various steps are put into practice. As part of a study to examine the effects of stress (McFarlane *et al.* 1980), a scale was needed to measure the amount of social support that the respondents felt they had. Although there were a number of such instruments already in existence, none met the specific needs of this project, or matched closely enough our theoretical model of social support. Thus, the first step, although not clearly articulated as such at the time, was to elucidate our *theory* of social support; what areas we wanted to tap, and which we felt were irrelevant or unnecessary for our purposes. This was augmented by *research* done in the field by other groups, indicating aspects of social support which served as buffers, protecting the person against stress. The next step was to locate *previous instruments*, and cull from them those questions or approaches which met our needs. Finally, we showed a preliminary draft of our scale to a number of highly experienced family therapists, whose *expert opinion* was formed on the basis of their years of *clinical observation*. This last step actually served two related purposes: they performed a *content validity* study, seeing if any important areas were missed by us, and also suggested additional items to fill these gaps. The final draft (McFarlane *et al.* 1981) was then subjected to a variety of reliability and validity checks, as outlined in subsequent chapters.

Some people, primarily in the area of nursing research, have advocated a more rigorous approach to evaluating content validity (e.g. Lynn 1986; Waltz and Bausell 1981). Each expert is given an explicit description of each of the domains, and rates the content relevance on a four-point scale, where 1 indicates totally irrelevant content and 4 reflects extremely relevant content. Then, a *content validity index* (CVI) is derived for each item, which is the proportion of judges who rate the item 3 or 4. Lynn (1986) recommends a minimum of five raters, in which case the CVI should be 1.00 for each item. If there are more raters (to a maximum of 10), she recommends that there be no more than one rater who scores an item less than 3 for the CVI to be statistically significant. A very comprehensive guide to determining content validity is given by Haynes *et al.* (1995).

How many items should be written? At this first stage in scale development, our interest is in creating the item pool. Our aim is to be as inclusive as possible, even to the point of being overinclusive; poor items can be detected and weeded out later, but as we said in the opening paragraph of this chapter, nothing can be done after the fact to compensate for items we neglected to include. In a classic article on test construction, Loevinger (1957) wrote that (p. 659, italics in the original):

> The items of the pool should be chosen so as to sample all possible contents which might comprise the putative trait according to all known alternative theories of the trait.

Generic versus specific scales and the 'fidelity versus bandwidth' issue

Let us say you want to find or develop a test to measure the quality of life (QOL) of a group of rheumatoid arthritis (RA) patients. Should you look for (or develop) a QOL instrument that is tailored to the characteristics of these RA patients, or should it be a scale which taps QOL for patients with a variety of disorders, of which RA is only one? Indeed, should we go even further, and tailor the scale to the unique requirements of the individual patients? There are some scales (e.g. Guyatt *et al.* 1993) which are constructed by asking the patient to list five activities which he or she feels have been most affected by the disorder. Thus, the items on one patient's scale may be quite different from those on anyone else's instrument.

The argument in favour of disease-specific and patient-specific questionnaires is two-fold. The first consideration is that if an instrument has to cover a wide range of disorders, many of the questions may be inappropriate or irrelevant for any one specific problem. A generic scale, for example, may include items tapping incontinence, shortness of breath, and problems in attention and concentration. These are areas which may present difficulties for patients with Crohn's disease, asthma, or depression, but rarely for arthritics. Consequently, these non-useful items contribute nothing but noise when the questionnaire is used for one specific disorder. This argument is simply carried to its logical extreme with patient-specific instruments; here, all of the items are, by definition, relevant for the patient, and there should be no items which are not applicable, or should not change with effective therapy.

The second reason for using disease- or patient-specific scales follows directly from the first problem. In order to keep the length of a generic questionnaire manageable, there cannot be very many items in each of the areas tapped. Thus, there will be fewer relevant questions to detect real changes within patients, or differences among them.

On the opposite side of the argument, the cost of the greater degree of specificity is a reduction in generalizability (Aaronson 1988, 1989). That is, generic scales allow comparisons across different disorders, severities of disease, interventions, and perhaps even demographic and cultural groups (Patrick and Deyo 1989), as well as being able to measure the burden of illness of populations suffering from chronic medical and psychiatric conditions as compared with normals (McHorney *et al.* 1994). This is much harder, or even impossible, to do when each study uses a different scale. Especially in light of the recent increase in the use of meta-analysis to synthesize the results of different studies (e.g. Glass *et al.* 1981), this can be a major consideration. Furthermore, since any one generic scale tends to be used more frequently than a given specific instrument, there are usually more data available regarding its reliability and validity.

Dowie (2002a, 2002b) raises a different argument in favour of generic scales. He states that researchers are most often interested in the 'main' effect of an intervention (i.e. did it improve the patients' condition), relegating adverse or side-effects to secondary outcomes. However, patients simply experience 'effects,' which include the direct positive changes produced by the treatment; possibly other, indirect, gains (e.g. a greater feeling of independence following hip replacement); as well as any negative ones. Thus, from a clinical and decision-making perspective, disease-specific scales may miss aspects of the intervention that are important to the patient.

These problems are even more acute with patient-specific scales. Since no two people have exactly the same scale, it is difficult to establish psychometric properties such as reliability and validity, or to make any comparisons across people, much less across different disorders. Another problem is a bit more subtle. Since all patients choose their most troublesome symptoms, this means that they will all start off with very similar scores, even if they differ among themselves quite considerably in other areas. That is, even if Patient A has problems in six areas, and Patient B in 11, they will be identical on the scale if each can choose only the five most bothersome. Furthermore, since they both will start off at the test's ceiling, they have nowhere to go but down, making any intervention look effective.

Another way of conceptualizing the difference between specific and generic scales is related to what Cronbach (1990) labeled the 'bandwidth versus fidelity' dilemma. The term comes from communication theory (Shannon and Weaver 1949), and refers to the problem faced in designing radios. If we build a receiver that covers all of the AM and FM stations, plus the short-wave bands, and also allows us to monitor police and fire calls, then we have achieved a wide bandwidth. The trade-off, though, is that no one station is heard very well. The opposite extreme is to design a receiver that will pick up only one station. The fidelity of the reception will be superb, since all of the components are designed for that one specific part of the spectrum, but the radio will be useless for any other station we may want to hear. Thus, we achieve bandwidth at the cost of fidelity, and vice versa.

The issue is the proper balance between a narrow scale with low bandwidth and (presumably) good fidelity versus a generic scale with greater bandwidth but (again presumably) poorer fidelity. The literature comparing these two types of scales is somewhat limited. However, the general conclusion is that the advantages of disease-specific scales may be more apparent than real; well-designed, reliable, and valid generic questionnaires appear to yield results that are comparable to disease-specific ones across a number of illnesses and instruments (e.g. Bombardier *et al.* 1986; Liang *et al.* 1985; Parkerson *et al.* 1993).

The safest option, then, would likely be to use a generic instrument such as the SF-36 (Ware *et al.* 1993) or the Sickness Impact Profile (Gilson *et al.* 1975) in all studies of QOL, and to supplement it with a disease-specific one if it does not impose too much of a burden on the subjects.

Translation

Although it is not directly related to the problem of devising items, translation into another language is a problem that may have to be addressed. In most large studies, especially those located in major metropolitan centers, it is quite probable that

English will not be the first language of a significant proportion of respondents. This raises one of two possible alternatives, both of which have associated problems. First, such respondents can be eliminated from the study. However, this raises the possibility that the sample will then not be a representative one, and the results may have limited generalizability. The second alternative is to translate the scales and questionnaires into the languages most commonly used within the catchment area encompassed by the study.

The goal of translation is to achieve equivalence between the original version and the translated version of the scale. The first problem is what is meant by 'equivalence'. Herdman *et al.* (1997) list 19 different types of equivalencies that have been proposed by various authors, but most agree that there are five or six key ones (although they often differ regarding which five or six), and that they form a hierarchy (Herdman *et al.* 1998; Sechrest *et al.* 1972).

First it is necessary to establish *conceptual equivalence*; that is, do people in the two cultures see the concept in the same way? At one extreme, both the source and the target cultures agree completely on what the elements are that constitute the construct, indicating that the translators can proceed to the next step. At the other extreme, the concept may not exist in the target culture. Hunt (1986), for example, reported that poor Egyptian women had difficulty responding to an item about enjoying themselves, because it did not have 'much existential relevance in a context where the concept of enjoyment is not present. Living in, or on, the edge of poverty, most of the day is taken up with work, finding food, doing chores, and just subsisting' (p. 156). Most often, what is found falls between these extremes; the concept exists in the target culture, but there may be differences with regard to the constituent elements or the weight given to each element. As an example, one of our students (Aracena *et al.* 1994) wanted to translate a child abuse scale into Spanish. As a first step, she conducted some focus groups to determine if the meaning of abuse was similar in Chile as in the US, where the scale was developed. She found that behaviours that would be considered abusive (both physically and sexually) in North America were seen as part of the continuum of normal child-rearing practices in Chile. This meant that some of the items from the original scale should not be included in the translated version, because they would not fall within the Chilean concept of abuse.

If conceptual equivalence exists, even partially, it is possible to move to looking for *item equivalence*. This determines whether the specific items are relevant and acceptable in the target population. It does not make sense, for instance, to ask about a person's ability to climb a flight of stairs if the questionnaire will be used in a setting consisting solely of single-story dwellings. Also, it may be taboo in some cultures to inquire about certain topics, such as sexual problems, negative feelings directed toward family members, or income. These questions may have to be reworded or replaced before translation can begin.

Semantic equivalence refers to the meaning attached to each item. For example, we generally associate the colour blue with sadness, and black with depression. In China, though, white is the colour of mourning, a shade we use to connote purity.

Consequently, a literal translation of the phrase, 'I feel blue,' or 'The future looks black to me' would not convey the same semantic meaning in many other cultures. Similarly, Anglo-Saxons often associate mild physical discomfort with stomach problems, whereas the French would be more prone to attribute it to their liver, and Germans to their circulation. This problem exists even within the same language as spoken in different countries. The word 'comadre' has the dictionary definition of a child's godmother; in Mexican and Texan Spanish, though, it means a close personal advisor and friend; but in Nicaragua, it can also refer to 'the other woman'. Obviously, a scale measuring who is available for social support will yield different responses (and reactions) when used in these different countries.

Operational equivalence goes beyond the items themselves, and looks at whether the same format of the scale, the instructions, and the mode of administration can be used in the target population. For example, it is impolite in many North American Indian groups to ask a direct question; and in some Asian and African cultures for younger people to question their elders. Needless to say, self-administered scales would be totally inappropriate in places with low literacy levels. Even the format of the items may present difficulties. We found that elderly people in Canada had difficulty grasping the concept of putting an X on a 10-cm line (a Visual Analogue Scale, discussed in the next chapter) corresponding to their degree of discomfort. They were able to use this type of scale reliably only when we turned it on its side and made it resemble a thermometer that could be filled in with a red marker (Mohide *et al.* 1990).

Finally, *measurement equivalence* investigates whether the psychometric properties of the test—its various forms of reliability and validity—are the same in both versions. Of course, this can be done only after the test has been translated.

Once it has been determined that the scale can be translated (i.e. if conceptual equivalence exists, and items that may present problems for item and semantic equivalence can be changed), it is time to begin the translation process itself. Guillemin *et al.* (1993) recommend at least two independent translations, and state that it is even better if each translation is done by a team. The people should translate into their native tongue, and be aware of the intent of each item and of the scale as a whole. This allows them to go beyond a strictly semantic translation, and to use more idiomatic language that would be better understood by the respondents.

The next step is called 'back-translation'. Each item is now translated back into the source language, again by independent teams who have not seen the originals and are not aware of the purpose of the scale. This time, the members should be familiar with idiomatic use of the source language. Finally, a committee should look at the original and the back-translated items, and resolve any discrepancies.

As mentioned under *measurement equivalence*, it is now necessary to establish the psychometric properties of the translated scale. This can be as simple as determining its reliability and doing some validity studies. A more thorough testing would also see if the norms and cut-points used in the original scale are appropriate for the translated one. At the most sophisticated level, statistical testing using confirmatory factor analysis (CFA) can be used to determine if the individual items perform in the same way in both versions. A very brief description of CFA is given in Appendix C; people who are interested in a basic introduction can read Norman and Streiner (2000), or Byrne (2001) for a more detailed explanation.

The question that therefore arises is whether translating a scale is worth the effort. It requires the translation itself, back-translation, and then re-establishing the reliability and validity within the new context; in essence, exactly the same steps that are required for developing a new scale. The only difference is that the devising of new items has been replaced by the translating of old ones. Many scales have been translated, but problems still remain. For example, in two studies we have been involved in (O'Brien *et al.* 1994; Streiner *et al.* 1994), we used 'validated' versions of tests translated into French. The results, though, showed a lower incidence of migraine headaches in one study, and a higher self-reported quality of life in the other. The unresolved issue is whether these differences are due to cultural and other factors, or reflect subtle variations in the instruments used to measure them. Although questions may not have arisen had the prevalence rates been similar, there would still have been the issue of whether there actually are differences, but our translated instrument may have missed them.

The conclusion is that translating an instrument *can* be done, but it is as time-consuming as developing a new tool. Further, both similarities and differences in results must be interpreted with extreme caution.

References

Aaronson, N. K. (1988). Quantitative issues in health-related quality of life assessment. *Health Policy*, 10, 217–30.

Aaronson, N. K. (1989). Quality of life assessment in clinical trials: Methodological issues. *Controlled Clinical Trials*, 10, 195S–208S.

Angleitner, A., John, O. P., and Löhr, F-J. (1986). It's *what* you ask and *how* you ask it: An item metric analysis of personality questionnaires. In *Personality assessment via questionnaires* (ed. A. Angleitner and J. S. Wiggins) pp. 61–107. Springer-Vela, New York.

Aracena, M., Balladares, E., and Román, F. (1994). *Factores de riesgo para maltrato infantil, a nivel del sistema familiar: Una mirador cualitativa.* Documento de Trabajo N.1. Universidad de la Frontera, Temuco, Chile.

Becker, M. H., Maiman, L. A., Kirscht, J. P., Haefner, D. P., Drachman, R. H., and Taylor, D. W. (1979). Patient perception and compliance: Recent studies of the health belief model. In *Compliance in health care* (ed. R. B. Haynes and D. L. Sackett) pp. 78–109. Johns Hopkins University Press, Baltimore.

Bombardier, C., Ware, J., Russell, I. J., Larson, M., Chalmers, A., and Read, J. L. (1986). Auranofin therapy and quality of life in patients with rheumatoid arthritis: Results of a multicenter trial. *American Journal of Medicine*, 81, 565–78.

Brumback, G. B., and Howell, M. A. (1972). Rating the clinical effectiveness of employed physicians. *Journal of Applied Psychology*, 56, 241–4.

Byrne, B. M. (2001). *Structural equation modeling with AMOS: Basic concepts, applications, and programming.* Lawrence Erlbaum, Mahwah NJ.

Cowles, J. T. and Kubany, A. J. (1959). Improving the measurement of clinical performance of medical students. *Journal of Clinical Psychology*, 15, 139–42.

Cronbach, L. J. (1990). *Essentials of psychological testing* (5th edn.). Harper and Row, New York.

Dowie, J. (2002a). Decision validity should determine whether a generic or condition-specific HRQOL measure is used in health care decisions. *Health Economics*, 11, 1–8.

Dowie, J. (2002b). 'Decision validity...': a rejoinder. *Health Economics*, 11, 21–2.

Feightner, J. W. (1985). Patient management problems. In *Assessing clinical competence* (ed. V. R. Neufeld and G. R. Norman) pp. 183–200. Springer–Verlag, New York.

Gilson, B. S., Gilson, J. S., Bergner, M., Bobbit, R. A., Kressel, S., Pollard, W. E., and Vesselago, M. (1975). The Sickness Impact Profile: Development of an outcome measure of health care. *American Journal of Public Health*, 65, 1304–10.

Glass, G. V., McGraw, B., and Smith, M. L. (1981). *Meta-analysis in social research*. Sage, Beverly Hills, CA.

Goldberg, L. R. (1971). A historical survey of personality scales and inventories. In *Advances in psychological assessment*, Vol. 2 (ed. P. McReynolds) pp. 293–336. Science and Behavior, Palo Alto, CA.

Guillemin, F., Bombardier, C., and Beaton, D. (1993). Cross-cultural adaptation of health-related quality of life measures: Literature review and proposed guidelines. *Journal of Clinical Epidemiology*, 46, 1417–32.

Guyatt, G. H., Eagle, D. J., Sackett, B., Willan, A., Griffith, L., McIlroy, W., *et al.* (1993). Measuring quality of life in the frail elderly. *Journal of Clinical Epidemiology*, 46, 1433–44.

Hathaway, S. R. and McKinley, J. C. (1951). *Manual for the Minnesota Multiphasic Personality Inventory* (rev.) Psychological Corporation, New York.

Haynes, S. N., Richard, D. C. S., and Kubany, E. S. (1995). Content validity in psychological assessment: A functional approach to concepts and methods. *Psychological Assessment*, 7, 238–47.

Herdman, M., Fox-Rushby, J., and Badia, X. (1997). 'Equivalence' and the translation and adaptation of health-related quality of life questionnaires. *Quality of Life Research*, 6, 237–47.

Herdman, M., Fox-Rushby, J., and Badia, X. (1998). A model of equivalence in the cultural adaptation of HRQoL instruments: The universalist approach. *Quality of Life Research*, 7, 323–35.

Hunt, S. M. (1986). Cross-cultural issues in the use of socio-medical indicators. *Health Policy*, 6, 149–58.

Kruis, W., Thieme, C., Weinzierl, M., Schuessler, P., Holl, J., and Paulus, W. (1984). A diagnostic score for the irritable bowel syndrome: Its value in the exclusion of organic disease. *Gastroenterology*, 87, 1–7.

Liang, M. H., Larson, M. G., Cullen, K. E., and Schwartz, J. A. (1985). Comparative measurement efficiency and sensitivity of five health status instruments for arthritis research. *Arthritis and Rheumatism*, 28, 542–7.

Loevinger, J. (1957). Objective tests as instruments of psychological theory. *Psychological Reports*, 3, 635–94.

Lynn, M. R. (1986). Determination and quantification of content validity. *Nursing Research*, 35, 382–5.

McFarlane, A. H., Norman, G. R., Streiner, D. L., Roy, R. G., and Scott, D. J. (1980). A longitudinal study of the influence of the psychosocial environment on health status: A preliminary report. *Journal of Health and Social Behavior*, 21, 124–33.

McFarlane, A. H., Neale, K. A., Norman, G. R., Roy, R. G., and Streiner, D. L. (1981). Methodological issues in developing a scale to measure social support. *Schizophrenia Bulletin*, 7, 90–100.

McHorney, C. A., Ware, J. E., Lu, J. F. R., and Sherbourne, C. D. (1994). The MOS 36-item short form health survey (SF-36): III. Tests of data quality, scaling assumptions, and reliability across diverse patient groups. *Medical Care*, 32, 40–66.

Messick, S. (1980). Test validity and the ethics of assessment. *American Psychologist*, 35, 1012–27.

Messick, S. (1993). Validity. In *Educational measurement* (2nd edn) (ed. R. L. Linn) pp. 13–104. Oryx Press, Phoenix.

Moos, R. H. (1984). *Menstrual distress questionnaire*. Stanford University Medical Center, Palo Alto, CA.

Mohide, E. A., Pringle, D. M., Streiner, D. L., Gilbert, J. R., Muir, G., and Tew, M. (1990). A randomized trial of family caregiver support in the home management of dementia. *Journal of the American Geriatric Society*, 38, 446–54.

Norman, G. R. and Streiner, D. L. (2000). *Biostatistics: The bare essentials* (2nd edn). B. C. Decker, Toronto.

O'Brien, B., Goeree, R., and Streiner, D. L. (1994). Prevalence of migraine headache in Canada: A population-based survey. *International Journal of Epidemiology*, 23, 1020–6.

Parkerson, G. R., Connis, R. T., Broadhead, W. E., Patrick, D. L. Taylor, T. R., and Tse, C. J. (1993). Disease-specific versus generic measurement of health-related quality of life in insulin-dependent diabetic patients. *Medical Care*, 31, 629–39.

Patrick, D. L. and Deyo, R. A. (1989). Generic and disease-specific measures in assessing health status and quality of life. *Medical Care*, 27 (Supplement), S217–32.

Sechrest, L., Fay, T. L., and Hafeez Zaidi, S. M. (1972). Problems of translation in cross-cultural research. *Journal of Cross-Cultural Psychology*, 3, 41–56.

Shannon, C. and Weaver, W. (1949). *The mathematical theory of communication*. University of Illinois Press, Urbana, IL.

Seligman, A. W. (1993). Cardiovascular consequences of expressing, experiencing, and repressing anger. *Journal of Behavioral Medicine*, 16, 539–69.

Streiner, D. L., O'Brien, B., and Dean, D. (1994). *Quality of life in major depression: A comparison of instruments*. Paper presented at the 19th Annual Meeting of the Collegium Internationale Neuro-Psychopharmacologicum, Washington DC.

Taylor, J. A. (1953). A personality scale of manifest anxiety. *Journal of Abnormal and Social Psychology*, 48, 285–90.

Taylor, S. J. and Bogden, R. (1984). *Introduction to qualitative research methods*. Wiley, New York.

Ullman, L. P. and Giovannoni, J. M. (1964). The development of a self-report measure of the process-reactive continuum. *Journal of Nervous and Mental Disease*, 138, 38–42.

Waltz, C. W. and Bausell, R. B. (1981). *Nursing research: Design, statistics and computer analysis*. F. A. Davis, Philadelphia.

Ware, J. E. Jr., Snow, K. K., Kosinski, M., and Gandek, B. (1993). *SF-36 health survey manual and interpretation guide*. The Health Institute, New England Medical Center, Boston.

Wechsler, D. (1958). *The measurement and appraisal of adult intelligence* (4th edn). Williams and Wilkins, Baltimore.

Willms, D. G. and Johnson, N. A. (1993). *Essentials in qualitative research: A notebook for the field*. Unpublished manuscript.

Chapter 4

Scaling responses

Introduction

Having devised a set of questions using the methods outlined in the previous chapter, we must choose a method by which responses will be obtained. The choice of method is dictated, at least in part, by the nature of the question asked. For example, a question like 'Have you ever gone to church?' leads fairly directly to a response method consisting of two boxes, one labeled 'Yes' and the other 'No'. By contrast, the question 'How religious are you?' does not dictate a simple two-category response, and a question like 'Do you believe that religious instruction leads to racial prejudice?' may require the use of more subtle and sophisticated techniques to obtain valid responses.

There has been a bewildering amount of research in this area, in disciplines ranging from psychology to economics. Often the results are conflicting, and the correct conclusions are frequently counter-intuitive. In this chapter, we describe a wide variety of scaling methods, indicate their appropriate use, and make recommendations regarding a choice of methods.

Some basic concepts

In considering approaches to the development of response scales, it is helpful to first consider the kinds of possible responses which may arise. A basic division is between those responses that are categorical, such as race, religion or marital status, and those that are continuous variables like hemoglobin, blood pressure, or the amount of pain recorded on a 100-mm line. A second related feature of response scales is commonly referred to as the *level of measurement*. If the response consists of named categories, such as particular symptoms, a job classification, or religious denomination, the variable is called a *nominal* variable. Ordered categories, such as staging in breast cancer, educational level (less than high school, high school diploma, some college or university, university degree, postgraduate degree) are called *ordinal* variables. By contrast, variables in which the interval between responses and constant is known are called *interval* variables. Temperature, measured in degrees Celsius or Fahrenheit, is an interval variable. Generally speaking, rating scales, where the response is on a five-point or seven-point scale, are not considered interval-level measurement, since we can never be sure that the distance between 'strongly disagree' and 'disagree' is the same as between 'agree' and 'strongly agree'. However, some methods have been devised to achieve interval-level measurement with subjective scales, as will be discussed. Finally, variables where there is a meaningful zero point, so that the ratio of two responses has some meaning, are called *ratio* variables. Temperature measured in Kelvin is a ratio variable, temperature degrees in Fahrenheit or Celsius is not.

What is the significance of these distinctions? The important difference lies between nominal and ordinal data on one hand, and interval and ratio variables on the other. In the latter case, measures such as means, standard deviations, and differences among means can be interpreted and the broad class of techniques called 'parametric statistics' can therefore be used for analysis. By contrast, since it makes no sense to speak of the average religion or average sex of a sample of people, nominal and ordinal data must be considered as frequencies in individual categories, and 'non-parametric' statistics must be used for analysis. The distinction between these two types of analysis is described in any introductory statistics book, such as those listed in Appendix A.

Categorical judgements

One form of question frequently used in health sciences requires only a categorical judgement by the respondent, either as a 'yes/no' response, or as a simple check. The responses would then result in a *nominal* scale of measurement. Some examples are shown in Fig. 4.1. Care must be taken to ensure that questions are written clearly and unambiguously, as discussed in Chapter 5. However, there is little difficulty in deciding on the appropriate response method.

Perhaps the most common error when using categorical questions is that they are frequently employed in circumstances where the response is not, in fact, categorical. Attitudes and behaviors often lie on a continuum. When we ask a question like 'Do

---

Have you ever had a chest X-ray?   yes __ no __

Which of the following symptoms are you currently experiencing?

    Headaches __
    Dizziness   __
    Cough   __
    Colds   __
    Other   (please write in) _____

Are you able to climb the stairs?   yes __ no __

I think that people are watching me.   true __ false __

Fig. 4.1 Examples of questions requiring categorical judgements.

you have trouble climbing stairs?', we ignore the fact that there are varying degrees of trouble. Even the best athlete might have difficulty negotiating the stairs of a skyscraper at one run without some degree of discomfort. What we wish to find out presumably, is *how much* trouble the respondent has in negotiating an ordinary flight of stairs.

Ignoring the continuous nature of many responses leads to three difficulties. The first is fairly obvious: since different people may have different ideas about what constitutes a positive response to a question, there will likely be error introduced into the responses, as well as uncertainty and confusion on the part of respondents.

The second problem is perhaps more subtle. Even if all respondents have a similar conception of the category boundaries, there will still be error introduced into the measurement because of the limited choice of response levels. For example, the statement in Fig. 4.2 might be responded to in one of two ways, as indicated in (a) and (b): the first method effectively reduces all positive opinions, ranging from strong to mild, to a single number, and similarly for all negative feelings. The effect is a potential loss of information and a corresponding reduction in reliability.

The third problem, which is a consequence of the second, is that dichotomizing a continuous variable leads to a loss of *efficiency* of the instrument, and a reduction in its correlation with other measures. A more efficient instrument requires fewer subjects in order to show an effect than a less efficient one. Suissa (1991) calculated that a dichotomous outcome is, at best, 67 per cent as efficient as a continuous one; depending on how the measure was dichotomized, this can drop to under 10 per cent. Under the best of circumstances, then, if you needed 67 subjects to show an effect when the outcome is measured along a continuum, you would need 100 subjects to demonstrate the same effect when the outcome is dichotomized. When circumstances are not as ideal, the inflation in required sample size can be 10 or more. Similarly, Hunter and Schmidt (1990) showed that if the dichotomy resulted in a 50–50 split, with half of the subjects in one group and half in the other, the correlation of that instrument with another is reduced by 20 per cent. Any other split results in a greater attenuation; if the result is that 10 per cent of the subjects are in one group and 90 per cent in the other, then the reduction is 41 per cent.

Doctors carry a heavy responsibility

(a) agree __   disagree __

(b) strongly agree	agree	mildly agree	mildly disagree	disagree	strongly disagree
__	__	__	__	__	__

Fig. 4.2 Example of a continuous judgement.

We have demonstrated this result with real data on several occasions. In a recent study of the certification examinations in internal medicine in Canada, the reliability of the original scores, inter-rater and test–retest, was 0.76 and 0.47, respectively. These scores were then converted to a pass–fail decision and the reliability recalculated. The comparable statistics for these decisions were 0.69 and 0.36, a loss of about 0.09 in reliability.

An even more dramatic demonstration of the phenomenon derives from a standardized clinical skills test called the Objective Structured Clinical Examination or OSCE (Harden and Gleeson 1979). In this examination, students are required to pass through a series of brief encounters with simulated patients, and perform circumscribed maneuvers, such as auscultating a patient or taking a brief history of chest pain. The examiner is furnished with a standard checklist of required actions, and scores such as 'Done' versus 'Not done', or alternatively, 'Done well', 'Done poorly', or 'Not done' are assigned by observers. These scores are then summed to create a total score for the station. One appeal of the method is its apparent objectivity; however, several studies (van der Vleuten *et al.* 1991) comparing the summary score from the checklist to a single global rating on a five- or seven-point scale, have shown that the global rating has consistently equal or better reliability than the checklist score, despite the fact that the latter may be based on 10 to 30 items, whereas the former is derived from a single score. The illusion of objectivity may not be reflected in reliability.

There are two common, but invalid, objections to the use of multiple response levels. The first is that the researcher is only interested in whether respondents agree or disagree, so it is not worth the extra effort. This argument confuses measurement with decision-making; the decision can always be made after the fact by establishing a cutoff point on the response continuum, but information lost from the original responses cannot be recaptured.

A second argument is that the additional categories are only adding noise or error to the data; people cannot make finer judgements than 'agree–disagree'. Although there may be particular circumstances where this is true, in general the evidence indicates that people are capable of much finer discriminations; this will be reviewed in a later section of the chapter where we discuss the appropriate number of response steps (p. 37).

Continuous judgements

Accepting that many of the variables of interest to health care researchers are continuous rather than categorical, methods must be devised to quantify these judgements.

The approaches that we will review fall into three broad categories:

Direct Estimation techniques, in which subjects are required to indicate their response by a mark on a line or check in a box;

Comparative methods, in which subjects choose among a series of alternatives that have been previously calibrated by a separate criterion group; and

Econometric methods, in which the subjects describe their preference by anchoring it to extreme states (perfect health–death).

Direct estimation methods

Direct estimation methods are designed to elicit from the subject a direct quantitative estimate of the magnitude of an attribute. The approach is usually straightforward, as in the example used above, where we asked for a response on a six-point scale ranging from 'strongly agree' to 'strongly disagree'. This is one of many variations, although all share many common features. We begin by describing the main contenders, then we will explore their advantages and disadvantages.

Visual analog scales

The visual analog scale (VAS) is the essence of simplicity—a line of fixed length, usually 100 mm, with anchors like 'No pain' and 'Pain as bad as it could be' at the extreme ends, and no words describing intermediate positions. An example is shown in Fig. 4.3. Respondents are required to place a mark, usually an 'X' or a vertical line, on the line corresponding to their perceived state. The VAS technique was introduced over 80 years ago (Hayes and Patterson 1921), at which time it was called the 'graphic rating method,' but became popular in clinical psychology only in the 1960s. The method has been used extensively in medicine to assess a variety of constructs; pain (Huskisson 1974), mood (Aitken 1969), and functional capacity (Scott and Huskisson 1978), among many others.

The VAS has also been used for the measurement of change (Scott and Huskisson 1979). In this approach, researchers are interested in perceptions of the degree to which patients feel they have improved as a result of treatment. The strategy used is to show patients, at the end of a course of treatment, where they had marked the line prior to commencing treatment, and then asking them to indicate, by a second line, their present state. There are a number of conceptual and methodological issues in the measurement of change, by VAS or other means, which will be addressed in Chapter 11.

Proponents are enthusiastic in their writings regarding the advantages of the method over its usual rival, a scale in which intermediate positions are labeled (e.g. 'mild', 'moderate', 'severe'); however, the authors frequently then demonstrate a substantial correlation between the two methods (Downie *et al.* 1978) suggesting that the advantages are more perceived than real. One also suspects that the method provides an illusion of precision, since a number given to two decimal places (e.g. a length measured in millimetres) has an apparent accuracy of 1 per cent. Of course,

How severe has your arthritic pain been today?

pain as
bad as it _____ no
could be   pain

Fig. 4.3 The visual analogue scale (VAS).

although one can measure a response to this degree of precision, there is no guarantee that the response accurately represents the underlying attribute to the same degree of resolution. In fact, Jensen *et al.* (1994) found that when pain patients were given a 101-point numerical scale, almost all of the people grouped the numbers in multiples of 5 or 10; in essence treating it as if it were an 11- or 21-point scale. Moreover, little information was lost using these 'coarser' gradations.

The simplicity of the VAS has contributed to its popularity, although there is some evidence that patients may not find it as simple and appealing as researchers; in one study described above (Huskisson 1974), 7 per cent of patients were unable to complete a VAS, as against 3 per cent for a graphic rating scale. Similarly, Bosi Ferraz *et al.* (1990) found that in Brazil, illiterate subjects had more difficulty with a VAS than with numerical or adjectival scales; their test-retest reliabilities, although statistically significant, were below an acceptable level. Some researchers in geriatrics have concluded that there may be an age effect in the perceived difficulty in using the VAS, leading to a modification of the technique. Instead of a horizontal line, they have used a vertical 'thermometer', which is apparently easier for older people to complete.

Even among people who are comfortable with the method, the VAS has a number of serious drawbacks. Scale constructors tend to give little thought to the wording of the end-points, yet patients' ratings of pain are highly dependent on the exact wording of the descriptors (Seymour *et al.* 1985). While the lower limit is often easy to describe (none of the attribute being measured), the upper end is more problematic. What is the maximum amount of dizziness; is it a function of time (e.g. 'dizzy all of the time'), or of intensity (we have no idea how to word that), or both? For that matter, how does a person know what is 'The most intense pain imaginable' if he or she has never experienced it? This also means that everyone will have a different end-point, dependent on his or her imagination.

Perhaps the most serious problem with the VAS is not inherent in the scale at all. In many applications of the VAS in health sciences, the attribute of interest, such as pain, is assessed with a single scale, as in the example shown earlier. However, the reliability of a scale is directly related to the number of items in the scale, so that the one-item VAS test is likely to demonstrate low reliability in comparison to longer scales. The solution, of course, is to lengthen the scale by including multiple VASs, to assess related aspects of the attribute of interest.

In conclusion, although the VAS approach has the merit of simplicity, there appears to be sufficient evidence that other methods may yield more precise measurement, and possibly increased levels of satisfaction among respondents.

Adjectival scales

Adjectival scales, as the name implies, use descriptors along a continuum, rather than simply labeling the end-points, as with the VAS. Two examples of this are shown in Fig. 4.4. The top scale uses discrete boxes, forcing the respondent to select among the four alternatives (the actual number of boxes is arbitrary), while the

How much of a role should the courts have in deciding whether to end life-support measures?

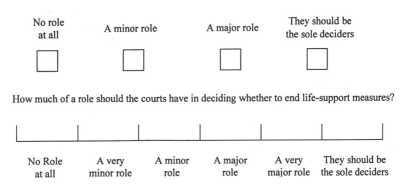

How much of a role should the courts have in deciding whether to end life-support measures?

| No Role at all | A very minor role | A minor role | A major role | A very major role | They should be the sole deciders |

Fig. 4.4 Examples of adjectival scales.

10	Certain, practically certain	(99 in 100 chance)
9	Almost sure	(9 in 10 chance)
8	Very probably	(8 in 10 chance)
7	Probable	(7 in 10 chance)
6	Good possibility	(6 in 10 chance)
5	Fairly good possibility	(5 in 10 chance)
4	Fair possibility	(4 in 10 chance)
3	Some possibility	(3 in 10 chance)
2	Slight possibility	(2 in 10 chance)
1	Very slight possibility	(1 in 10 chance)
0	No chance, almost no chance	(1 in 100 chance)

Fig. 4.5 Example of a Juster scale.

bottom scale looks more like a continuous line, allowing the person to place the mark even on a dividing line. This gives more an illusion of greater flexibility than the reality, as the person who scores the scale usually uses some rule to assign the answer into one of the existing categories (e.g. always use the category on the left, or the one closer to the middle). Adjectival scales are used very often in rating scales, such as those used for student evaluations (e.g. unsatisfactory/satisfactory/ excellent/superior) or self-reported health (excellent/very good/good/fair/poor).

A variant of this, used primarily for estimating the probability of an event, is called the *Juster scale* (Hoek and Gendall 1993). As seen in Fig. 4.5, it combines adjectival descriptors of probabilities with numerical ones, and appears to have good psycho-metric properties.

It is evident that the rating scale, with continuous responses, bears close resemblance to the VAS, with the exception that additional descriptions are introduced at interme-diate positions. Although proponents of the VAS eschew the use of descriptors, an opposite position is taken by psychometricians regarding rating scales. Guilford (1954) states 'Nothing should be left undone to give the rater a clear, unequivocal conception of the continuum along which he is to evaluate objects…' (p. 292).

Likert scales

Likert scales (Likert 1952) are similar to adjectival scales, with one exception. Adjectival scales are unipolar, in that the descriptors range from none or little of the attribute at one end to a lot or the maximal amount at the other. In contrast, Likert scales are bipolar, as in Fig. 4.6. The descriptors most often tap agreement (Strongly agree to Strongly disagree), but it is possible to construct a Likert scale measuring almost any attribute, such as acceptance (Most agreeable–Least agreeable), similar-ity (Most like me–Least like me), or probability (Most likely–Least likely).

There are two important points in designing Likert scales. The first is that the adjectives should be appropriate for the stem. Test constructors often want to keep the labels under the boxes the same from one item to another in order to reduce the burden on the respondents. However, this may lead to situations where descriptors for agreement appear on items that are better described with adjectives for similar-ity, for example (e.g. 'I am very easy going'). It is far better to have the stem and adjectives make sense than to have consistency. A second point is what to label the middle position. It should reflect a middle amount of the attribute, and not an inability to answer the question. For instance, 'Cannot say' may reflect:

(1) a middle amount;

(2) that the item does not apply;

(3) that the person does not understand the item; or

(4) that the person is unable to make up his or her mind.

Better terms would be Neither agree nor disagree, or Neutral.

A variant of the Likert scale, used primarily with children, is called a *Harter scale* (Harter 1982). A typical item is shown in Fig. 4.7. The child first decides whether he or she is more like the kid on the right or on the left, and then whether the description is

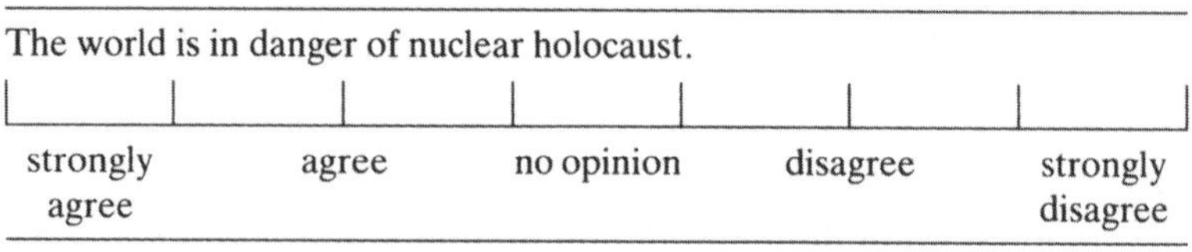

The world is in danger of nuclear holocaust.

| strongly agree | agree | no opinion | disagree | strongly disagree |

Fig. 4.6 Examples of a Likert scale.

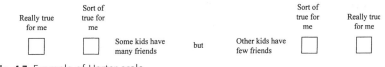

Fig. 4.7 Example of Harter scale.

True or Really true for him or her; there is no neutral position. Harter claims that this format reduces bias in responding, because contrasting two types of children reduces the possibility that one of the alternatives is seen as less normal or desirable than the other. We have successfully used this format with children as young as eight years of age. By the same token, their parents, who filled out the scale as they thought their kids would, did not feel that the format was too 'infantile' for them (Ronen *et al.* 2003).

There are a number of issues that have to be considered in constructing Likert scales, such as the number of boxes or scale divisions, whether there should be a neutral category and, if so, where it should be placed, and whether all of the divisions need be labeled. These are discussed in the following sections.

General issues in the construction of continuous scales

Regardless of the specific approach adopted, there are a number of questions that must be addressed in designing a rating scale to maximize precision and minimize bias.

1. *How many steps should there be?* The choice of the number of steps or boxes on a scale is not primarily an aesthetic issue. We indicated earlier in the discussion of categorical ratings that the use of two categories to express an underlying continuum will result in a loss of information. The argument can be extended to the present circumstances; if the number of levels is less than the rater's ability to discriminate, the result will be a loss of information.

Although the ability to discriminate would appear to be highly contingent on the particular situation, there is evidence that this is not the case. A number of studies have shown that for reliability coefficients in the range normally encountered, from 0.4 to 0.9, the reliability drops as fewer categories are used. Nishisato and Torii (1970) studied this empirically by generating distributions of two variables with known correlations, ranging from 0.1 to 0.9 in steps of 0.2. They then rounded off the numbers as if they were creating a scale of a particular number of steps. For example, if the original numbers fell in the range from 1.000 to 10.000, a two-point scale was created by calling any number less than 5.000 a 0, and any number greater than or equal to 5.000 a 1. A 10-point scale was created by rounding off up to the decimal point, resulting in discrete values ranging from 1 to 10. The final step in this simulation was to recalculate the correlation using the rounded numbers. Since the rounding process resulted in the loss of precision, this should have the effect of reducing the correlation between the sets of numbers. The original correlation corresponds to the test–retest reliability of the original data, and the recalculated

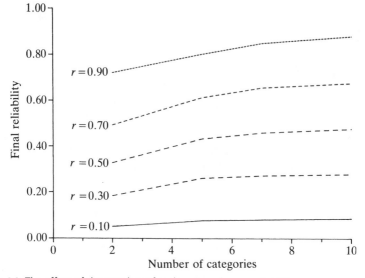

Fig. 4.8 The effect of the number of scale categories on reliability.

correlation, using the rounded-off numbers is equivalent to the reliability which would result from a scale with 2, 5 or 10 boxes, with everything else held constant.

As can be seen from Fig. 4.8, the loss in reliability for 7 and 10 categories is quite small. However, the use of five categories reduces the reliability by about 12 per cent, and the use of only two categories results in an average reduction of the reliability coefficient of 35 per cent. These results were confirmed by other studies, and suggest that the minimum number of categories used by raters should be in the region of five to seven. Of course, a common problem of ratings is that raters seldom use the extreme positions on the scale, and this should be taken into account when designing the scale, as discussed in Chapter 6.

Two other consideration are the preference of the respondents, and how easy they find it to complete scales with different numbers of options. Jones (1968) found that, even though they were the easiest to use, people did not like dichotomous items. They found them less 'accurate', 'reliable', and 'interesting' and more 'ambiguous' than items with more options. At the other end, Preston and Colman (2000) said that respondents found scales with 10 or 11 options less easy to use, and they required more time to fill out, than scales with fewer steps. Thus, respondent preferences are congruent with the statistical results; five to nine steps is ideal in most circumstances.

2. *Is there a maximum number of categories?* From a purely statistical perspective, the answer is 'No', since the actual reliability approaches the theoretical maximum asymptotically. However, there is good evidence that, in a wide variety of tasks,

people are unable to discriminate much beyond seven levels. In a now classic article entitled 'The magic number seven plus or minus two: Some limits on our capacity for processing information', Miller (1956) showed that the limit of short-term memory is of the order of seven 'chunks' (hence seven digit telephone numbers). Interestingly, the first two-thirds of the article is devoted to discussion of discrimination judgements. In an impressive number of situations, such as judging the pitch or loudness of a sound, the saltiness of a solution, the position of a point on a line, or the size of a square, the upper limit of the number of categories that could be discriminated was remarkably near seven (plus or minus two).

There is certainly no reason to presume that people will do any better in judgements of sadness, pain, or interpersonal skill. Thus it is reasonable to presume that the upper practical limit of useful levels on a scale, taking into account human foibles, can be set at seven. Certainly these findings clearly suggest that the 'one in a hundred' precision of the VAS is illusory; people are probably mentally dividing it into about seven segments.

There are two caveats to this recommendation. First, recognizing the common 'end-aversion bias' described in Chapter 6, where people tend to avoid the two extremes of a scale, there may be some advantage to designing nine levels on the scale. Conversely, when a large number of individual items are designed to be summed to a create a scale score, it is likely that reducing the number of levels to five or three will not result in significant loss of information.

3. *Should there be an even or odd number of categories?* Where the response scale is unipolar, that is to say, scale values range from zero to a maximum, then the question is of little consequence, and can be decided on stylistic grounds. However for bipolar scales (like Strongly agree–Strongly disagree) the provision of an odd number of categories allows raters the choice of expressing no opinion. Conversely, an even number of boxes forces the raters to commit themselves to one side or the other. There is no absolute rule; depending on the needs of the particular research it may or may not be desirable to allow a neutral position.

4. *Should all the points on the scale be labeled, or only the ends?* Most of the research indicates that there is relatively little difference between scales with adjectives under each box and end-anchored scales (e.g. Dixon *et al.* 1984; Newstead and Arnold 1989). In fact, subjects seem to be more influenced by the adjectives on the ends of the scales than those in the intermediate positions (e.g. Frisbie and Brandenburg 1979; Wildt and Mazis 1978). Respondents, though, are more satisfied when many or all of the points on the scale are labeled (Dickinson and Zellinger 1980). There is some tendency for end-anchored scales to pull responses to the ends, producing greater variability. Similarly, if only every other box is defined (usually because the scale constructor cannot think of enough adjectives), the labeled boxes tend to be endorsed more often than the unlabeled ones. The conclusion seems to be that it is better to label all of the points if you are able to think of descriptors.

5. *Should the neutral point always be in the middle?* As with many of the recommendations, the answer is a very definite, 'It all depends'. In situations where positive and negative responses to the item are equally likely, it makes sense to have the

neutral option (e.g. neither agree nor disagree) in the middle; and respondents tend to place themselves near the centre of rating scales, where they assume the 'typical' or 'normal' person falls (Schwarz *et al* 1985). However, ratings of students or residents, of satisfaction with care, and of many other targets, show a very strong skew toward the positive end. For example, Erviti *et al.* (1979) found a mean score of 3.3 on a four-point scale rating medical students; and Linn (1979) reported a mean of 4.11 with a five-point scale. This is understandable to a large degree. We do not have to make judgements about how unsatisfactory the bad students actually are; just that the do not pass muster. Ideally they are (we hope) weeded out early, leaving us to make distinctions among the remaining ones, who are at least satisfactory. The result is, in essence, that the bottom half of the scale is not used at all, truncating a seven-point scale into a two- or three-point one. Earlier, we recommended an unbalanced scale in such circumstances, with one box for the negative end, and five or six for the positive side, to allow the raters to make finer distinctions (Streiner 1985). There is some evidence that, combined with more points on the scale, this leads to greater discrimination, a lower mean score, and higher correlations with a gold standard (Klockars and Yamagishi 1988), although the effect is relatively modest (Klockars and Hancock 1993). We discuss this further, and give some examples of unbalanced scales, in Chapter 6.

6. *Do the adjectives always convey the same meaning?* Many adjectival scales use words or phrases like 'Almost always', 'Often', 'Seldom', or 'Rarely' in order to elicit judgements about the frequency of occurrence of an event or the intensity of a feeling. The question that arises from this is: to what extent do people agree on the meanings associated with these adjectives? Most research regarding agreement has focused on people's estimations of probabilities which they assign to words like 'Highly probable' or 'Unlikely', and the data are not encouraging. The estimated probability of a 'Highly probable' event ranged from 0.60 to 0.99. Other phrases yielded even more variability: 'Usually' went from 0.15 to 0.99, 'Rather unlikely' from 0.01 to 0.75, and 'Cannot be excluded' from 0.07 to 0.98 (Bryant and Norman 1980; Lichtenstein and Newman 1967). Part of the problem is the vagueness of the terms themselves. Another difficulty is that the meanings assigned to adjectives differ with the context. For example, the term 'Often' connotes a higher absolute frequency for common events as opposed to rare ones; and 'Not too often' carries different meanings depending on whether the activity described is an exciting or a boring one (Schaeffer 1991). As Parducci (1968) showed, the meaning of 'often' is different depending on whether one is describing the frequency of contraceptive failure or missing classes. Further, the interpretation of quantifiers such as 'quite a bit' or 'hardly ever' is strongly influenced by the respondent's own frequency of engaging in such behaviours. When asked how much television they watch, those who have the set on most of the day have a different interpretation of 'Often' from those who watch only one hour a day (Wright *et al.* 1994), much like the definition of an alcoholic as 'Someone who drinks more than I do'. The conclusion is that it is difficult to make comparisons among people when vague quantifiers of frequency are used. Under such circumstances, it would be better to use actual numbers, except when the

objective is to measure the person's *perception* of frequency. Bear in mind, though, that the format of the frequency scale itself may influence the responses, because it serves as a frame of reference (Schwarz 1999). People tend to think that values in the middle of the range reflect 'average' or 'typical' frequencies. When the answers consisted of low-frequency options in the middle, only 16. 2 per cent of respondents reported watching TV more than $2\frac{1}{2}$ hours a day; when higher-frequency options were in the middle, 37.5 per cent of the respondents reported doing so (Schwarz *et al.* 1985).

7. *Do numbers placed under the boxes influence the responses?* Some adjectival scales also put numbers under the words, to help the respondent find an appropriate place along the line. Does it matter whether the numbers range from 1 to 7 or from -3 to $+3$? What little evidence exists suggests that the answer is 'Yes'. Schwarz *et al.* (1991) gave subjects a scale consisting of a series of 11-point Likert scales. In all cases, one extreme was labeled 'Not at all successful' and the other end 'Extremely successful'. However, for some subjects, the numbers under the adjectives went from -5 to $+5$, while for others they went from 0 to 10. Although the questionnaire was completed anonymously, minimizing the chances that the respondents would attempt to present themselves well to the examiner (see *social desirability* bias in Chapter 6), the numbers made a large difference. When only positive integers were used, 34 per cent of the subjects used the lower (relatively unsuccessful) half of the scale (0 to 5), and had a mean value of 5.96. However, when the -5 to $+5$ numbering scheme was used, only 13 per cent used the lower half, and the mean value was pushed up to 7.38. Thus, it appeared as if the subjects were using the numbers to help them interpret the meaning of the adjectives, and that the negative scale values conveyed a different meaning from the positive ones.

8. *Should the order of successive question responses change?* Some scales reverse the order of responses at random, so that successive questions may have response categories which go from low to high or high to low, in order to avoid 'yea-saying' bias (discussed in Chapter 6). The dilemma is that a careless subject may not notice the change, resulting in almost totally uninterpretable responses. Of course, with reversed order, the researcher will *know* that the responses are uninterpretable due to carelessness, whereas if order is not reversed the subject looks consistent whether or not he paid attention to individual questions.

9. *Do questions influence the response to other questions?* The answer is definitely 'Yes'. Not only do earlier questions affect people's responses to later ones (e.g. Schuman and Presser 1981) but, when the person is able to go back and forth in the questionnaire, later ones can influence previous ones (Schwarz and Hippler 1995). There are at least three reasons for this. First, people try to appear consistent. If they believe that the answer to one question may contradict their response to a previous one, they may alter the earlier response to remove the inconsistency; and similarly, may respond to a new question in light of how they answered previously. Second, as Schwarz (1999) points out, respondents try to intuit what the intention of the questionnaire is, in order to respond appropriately. If later items change their interpretation, they may again go back and modify their responses in light of this different

understanding. Finally, according to cognitive theory, people do not retrieve all of their relevant knowledge about a topic at one time, but only what is *temporarily accessible* (Higgins 1996). Subsequent questions may alter what is remembered, and thus influence their responses.

10. *Can it be assumed that the data are interval?* As we indicated earlier, one issue regarding the use of rating scales is that they are, strictly speaking, on an ordinal level of measurement. Although responses are routinely assigned numerical values, so that 'Strongly agree' becomes a 7 and 'Strongly disagree' becomes a 1, we really have no guarantee that the true distance between successive categories is the same; i.e. that the distance between 'Strongly agree' and 'Agree' is really the same as the distance between 'Strongly disagree' and 'Disagree'. The matter is of more than theoretical interest, since the statistical methods that are used to analyze the data, such as analysis of variance, rest on this assumption of equality of distance. Considerable debate has surrounded the dangers inherent in the assumption of interval properties. The arguments range from the extreme position that the numbers themselves are interval (e.g. $1, 2, \ldots, 7$) and can be manipulated as interval-level data regardless of their relationship to the underlying property being assessed (Gaito 1982) to the opposite view that the numbers must be demonstrated to have a linear relationship with the underlying property before interval-level measurement can be assumed (Townsend and Ashby 1984). The debate shows no sign of resolution. Nevertheless, from a pragmatic viewpoint, it appears that under most circumstances, unless the distribution of scores is severely skewed, one can analyze data from rating scales as if they were interval without introducing severe bias.

Specter (1976) attempted to use a variation of Thurstone scaling in order to assign interval scale values to a variety of adjectives. He came up with three lists of categories: evaluation (consisting of words such as 'Terrible', 'Unsatisfactory', and 'Excellent'); agreement (e.g. 'Slightly', moderately', 'Very much'); and frequency ('Rarely' through 'Most of the time'). Each list contains 13 words or phrases, allowing the scale constructor to select five or seven with equal intervals. While these lists may help in rank ordering the adjectives, Specter unfortunately did not provide any indices of the agreement among the judges.

In Chapter 12, we will discuss statistical methods that allow us to determine the degree to which rating scales approach interval level status.

Critique of direct estimation methods

Direct estimation methods, in various forms, are pervasive in research involving subjective judgements. They are relatively easy to design, require little pre-testing in contrast to the comparative methods described next, and are easily understood by subjects. Nevertheless, the ease of design and administration is both an asset and a liability: because the intent of questions framed on a rating scale is often obvious to both researcher and respondent, bias in response can result. The issue of bias is covered in more detail in Chapter 6; but we mention some problems briefly here. One bias of rating scales is the *halo effect*; since items are frequently ordered in a single column on a page it is possible to rapidly rate all items on the basis of a global impression, paying little attention to the individual categories. People also rarely commit themselves to the extreme categories on the scale, effectively reducing the precision of measurement. Finally, it is common in ratings of other people, staff or students, to have a strong negative skew, so that the average individual is rated well above average, again sacrificing precision.

In choosing among specific methods, the scaling methods we have described differ for historical rather than substantive reasons, and it is easy to find examples which have features of more than one approach. The important point is to follow the general guidelines: specific descriptors, seven or more steps, and so forth, rather than becoming preoccupied with choosing among alternatives.

Comparative methods

Although rating scales have a number of advantages—simplicity, ease and speed of completion—there are occasions where their simplicity would be a deterrent to acquiring useful data. For example, in a study of predictors of child abuse (Shearman *et al.* 1983), one scale questioned parents on the ways they handled irritating child behaviours. A number of infant behaviours were presented, and parents were to specify how they dealt with each problem. Casting this scale into a rating format (which was not done) might result in items like those in Fig. 4.9.

The ordered nature of the response scale would make it unlikely that parents would place any marks to the left of the neutral position. Instead, we would like the respondent to simply indicate her likely action, or select it from a list. If we could then assign a value to each behaviour, we could generate a score for the respondent based on the sum of the assigned values.

The approach that was used was one of a class of *comparative* methods, called the *paired-comparison* technique, whereby respondents were simply asked to indicate which behaviour—'punish', 'cuddle', 'hit', 'ignore', 'put in room'—they were likely to do in a particular circumstance. These individual responses were assigned a numerical value in advance on the basis of a survey of a group of experts (in this case day care workers), who had been asked to compare each parental response to a situation to all other possible responses, and select the most appropriate response for each of these pairwise comparisons.

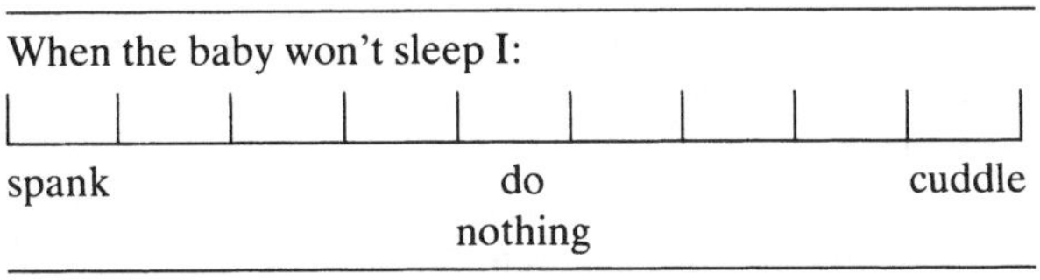

Fig. 4.9 Possible scaling of a question about child abuse.

The comparative methods also address a general problem with all rating scales, the ordinal nature of the scale. Comparative methods circumvent the difficulty by directly scaling the value of each description before obtaining responses, to ensure that the response values are on an interval scale.

There are three comparative methods commonly used in the literature: *Thurstone's method* of equal-appearing intervals, *Guttman scaling*, and the *paired-comparison* technique. Each is discussed below.

Thurstone's method of equal-appearing intervals

The method begins with the selection of 100–200 statements relevant to the topic about which attitudes are to be assessed. Following the usual approaches to item generation, these statements are edited to be short and to the point. Each statement is then typed on a separate card, and a number of judges are asked to sort them into a single pile from the lowest or least desirable to highest. Extreme anchor statements, at the opposite ends of the scale, may be provided. Following the completion of this task by a large number of judges, the median rank of each statement is computed, which then becomes the scale value for each statement.

As an example, if we were assessing attitude to doctors, we might assemble a large number of statements like 'I will always do anything my doctor prescribes', 'I think doctors are overpaid', and 'Most doctors are aware of their patients' feelings'. Suppose we gave these statements to nine judges (actually, many more would be necessary for stable estimates) and the statement 'I think nurses provide as good care as doctors' was ranked respectively by the nine judges 17, 18, 23, 25, 26, 27, 28, 31, and 35, of 100 statements. The median rank of this statement is the rank of the fifth person, in this case 26, so this would be the value assigned to the statement.

The next step in the procedure is to select a limited number of statements, about 25 in number, in such a manner that the intervals between successive items are about equal and they span the entire range of values. These items then comprise the actual scale.

Finally, in applying the scale to an individual, the respondent is asked to indicate which statements apply to him/her. The respondents' score is then calculated as the average score of items selected.

Paired comparison technique

The paired-comparison method is directed at similar goals, and uses a similar approach to the Thurstone method. In both methods, the initial step is to calibrate a limited set of items so that they can be placed on an interval scale. Subjects' responses to these items are then used in developing a score by simply summing or averaging the calibration weights of those items endorsed by a subject.

Where the two methods differ is in their approach to calibration. Thurstone scaling begins with a large number of items, and asks people to judge each item against all others by explicitly ranking the items. By contrast, the paired-comparison method, as the name implies, asks judges to explicitly compare each item one at a time to each of the remaining items, and simply judge which of the two has more of the property under study. Considering the example which began this chapter, our child care workers would be asked to indicate the more desirable parental behaviour in pairwise fashion as follows:

punish–spank

punish–cuddle

punish–ignore

spank–cuddle

spank–ignore

cuddle–ignore.

In actual practice, a larger sample of parental behaviours would be used, order from right to left would be randomized, and the order of presentation of the cards would be randomized.

If such a list of choices were given to a series of ten judges, the data would be then displayed as in Table 4.1, indicating the proportion of times each alternative was chosen over each other option.

Reading down the first column, the table shows, for example that 'punish' was chosen over 'spank' by 40 per cent of the subjects. Note that the diagonal entries are assumed equal to 0.50, i.e. 'punish' is selected over 'punish' 50 per cent of the time; also, the top right values are the 'mirror image' of those in the bottom left.

The next step is to use the property of the normal curve to convert this table to z-values. This bit of sleight-of-hand is best illustrated by reference to Fig. 4.10, which shows the 40 per cent point on a normal curve; that is, the point on the curve where 40 per cent of the distribution falls to the left. If the mean of the curve is set to zero, and the standard deviation to 1, this occurs at a value of −0.26. As a result, the probability value of 0.40 is replaced by a z-value of −0.26. In practice, these values are determined by consulting a table of the normal curve in any statistical text. The resulting values are shown in Table 4.2.

The z-scores for each column are then summed and averaged, yielding the z-score equivalent to the average probability of each item being selected over all other items. The resulting z-score for 'punish' now becomes −0.52, and for 'cuddle' it is +0.66. The range of negative and positive numbers is a bit awkward, so a constant (usually 3)

Table 4.1 Probability of selecting behaviour in column over behaviour in row

Behaviour	1 Punish	2 Spank	3 Ignore	4 Cuddle
1. Punish	0.50	0.60	0.70	0.90
2. Spank	0.40	0.50	0.70	0.80
3. Ignore	0.30	0.30	0.50	0.70
4. Cuddle	0.10	0.20	0.30	0.50

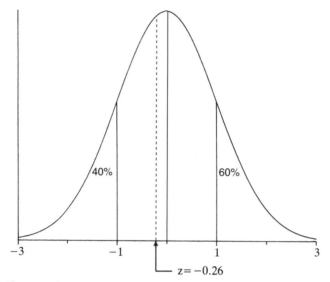

Fig. 4.10 The normal curve.

Table 4.2 z-values of the probabilities

Behaviour	1	2	3	4
1. Punish	0.00	0.26	0.53	1.28
2. Spank	−0.26	0.00	0.53	0.85
3. Ignore	−0.53	−0.53	0.00	0.53
4. Cuddle	−1.28	−0.85	−0.53	0.00
Total z	−2.07	−1.12	+0.53	+2.66
Average z	−0.52	−0.28	+0.13	+0.66

is often added to all the values to avoid negative weights. These weights can be assumed to have interval properties.

All this manipulation is directed to the assignment of weights to each option. To use these weights for scoring a subject is straightforward; the score is simply the weight assigned to the option selected by the subject. If the questionnaire is designed in such a way that a subject may endorse multiple-response options, for example by responding to various infant behaviours like crying, not going to sleep, refusing to eat, the weights for all responses can be added or averaged since they are interval level measurements.

The Guttman method

The Guttman method begins, as does the Thurstone method, with a large sample of items. However, this is reduced by judgement of the investigator to a relatively small sample of 10–20 items, which are thought to span the range of the attitude or behaviour assessed. As we shall see, in Guttman scaling, it is crucial that the items address only a single underlying attribute, since an individual score arises from the accumulated performance on all items.

These items are then administered directly to a sample of subjects, who are asked to endorse those items applicable to them. Unlike the alternative methods discussed in this section, there is no separate calibration step. The items are then tentatively ranked according to increasing amount of the attribute assessed, and responses are displayed in a subject-by-item matrix, with 1's indicating those items endorsed by a subject and O's indicating the remaining items.

As an example, suppose we were assessing function of the lower limbs in a sample of people with osteo-arthritis. A display of the responses of five subjects to the following four items might resemble Table 4.3.

In this example, subject A gets a score of 4, subject B a score of 3, C and D attain scores of 2, and subject E a score of 1. This is an idealized example, since no 'reversals' occur, in which a subject endorsed a more difficult item (e.g. walk more than a mile) but not an easier one (e.g. climb the stairs). In reality, such reversals do occur, detracting from the strict ordering of the items implied by the method. There are a number of indices which reflect how much an actual scale deviates from perfect cumulativeness, of which the two most important are the *coefficient of reproducibility* and the *coefficient of scalability*.

The first, reproducibility, indicates the degree to which a person's scale score is a predictor of his or her response pattern. To calculate it, we must know the total number of subjects (N), the number for whom there was some error in the ordering (n_e), and the number of items (I). The coefficient is then:

$$Reproducibility = 1 - \frac{n_e}{I \times N}$$

Table 4.3 Guttman scaling

I am able to:	Subject				
	A	B	C	D	E
Walk across the room	1	1	1	1	1
Climb the stairs	1	1	1	1	0
Walk one block outdoors	1	1	0	0	0
Walk more than one mile	1	0	0	0	0

If we gave our four-item scale to 150 people, and found that the order was correct for 109 cases and incorrect for 41, then the coefficient in this case would be:

$$1 - \frac{41}{150 \times 4} = 0.932$$

Reproducibility can vary between 0 and 1, and should be higher than 0.9 for the scale to be valid.

The coefficient of scalability reflects whether the scale is truly unidimensional and cumulative. Its calculation is complex and best left to computer programs. It, too, varies between 0 and 1, and should be at least 0.6.

Guttman scaling is best suited to behaviours which are developmentally determined (e.g. crawling, standing, walking, running), where mastery of one behaviour virtually guarantees mastery of lower order behaviours. Thus it is useful in assessing development in children, decline due to progressively deteriorating disease, functional ability, and the like. It is *not* appropriate in assessing the kind of loss in function due to focal lesions that arises in stroke patients, where impairment of some function may be unrelated to impairment of other functions. Unlike the other methods discussed in this section, Guttman scales are unlikely to have interval scale properties.

Guttman scaling is also the basis of *item response theory* (discussed in Chapter 12), which has emerged as a very powerful scaling method, and begins with a similar assumption of ordering of item difficulty and candidate ability. However, in contrast to Guttman scaling, item response scaling explicitly assigns values to both items and subjects on an interval scale, and also deals successfully with the random processes which might result in departures from strict ordering demanded by the Guttman scale.

Critique of comparative methods

It is clear that any of the three comparative methods we have described requires considerably more time for development than any of the direct scaling methods. Nevertheless, this investment may be worthwhile under two circumstances:

(1) if it is desirable to disguise the ordinal property of the responses, as in the child abuse example, then the additional resources may be well spent;

(2) the Thurstone and paired-comparison methods guarantee interval-level measurement, which may be important in some applications, particularly when there are relatively few items in the scale.

With regard to choice among the methods, as we have indicated, the Guttman method has several disadvantages in comparison to other methods. It is difficult to select items with Guttman properties, and the scale has only ordinal properties. The choice between Thurstone and paired-comparison is more difficult. However, the Thurstone method is more practical when there are a large number of items desired in the scale, since the number of comparisons needed in the paired-comparison technique is roughly proportional to the square of the number of items.

Goal attainment scaling

Goal attainment scaling (GAS) is an attempt to construct scales that are tailored to specific individuals, yet can yield results which are measured on a common, ratio scale across all people. It got its start in the area of program evaluation (Kiresuk and Sherman 1968), but has been widely applied in clinical settings (e.g. Santa-Barbara *et al.* 1974; Stolee *et al.* 1992), where the criteria for 'success' may vary from one patient to another.

The heart of GAS is the 'goal attainment follow-up guide', which is a matrix having a series of goals across the top, and five levels down the left side. For each individual, three to five goals are identified; the number of goals need not be the same for all people. The five levels are comparable to a Likert scale, ranging from the 'most favourable outcome thought likely' (given a score of +2) to the 'least favourable outcome thought likely' (a score of −2), with the mid-point labeled 'expected level of success' (a score of 0). Within each box of the matrix are written the criteria for determining whether or not that level of outcome for the specific goal has been attained for the person. Since good research technique demands that outcome evaluation be done by a rater who is blind with respect to which group a subject is in, the criteria must be written in terms of concrete, observable outcomes. For example, if one of the goals for a subject in a geriatric reactivation program is 'meal preparation', then an expected level of success (a score of 0) may be 'Has cooked her own supper every night for the past week'. The most favourable outcome (+2) may be 'Has cooked all her meals for the past week', and the criterion for a score of +1 may be 'Has cooked all suppers and some of the other meals during the past week'. Conversely, the least favourable outcome (−2) could be that the person has not cooked at all, and a score of −1 is given if some cooking was done, but not every night.

There are three points to note:

1. If the intervention works as intended, the experimental subjects should score 0 for all goals; a higher mean score for all people probably indicates that the goals were set too low, not that the program was wildly successful.

2. The criteria may vary from one person to the next; what is an 'expected level of success' for one individual may be somewhat favourable for a second, and least favourable for a third.

3. Not all subjects need have the same goals.

After the goals have been selected, they can each be given a weight (which traditionally ranges between 1 and 9), reflecting the importance of that goal relative to the others. To compensate for the fact that people may have a different number of goals, and to make the final score have a mean of 50 with an SD of 10, the GAS score is calculated using the equation:

$$GAS = 50 + \frac{10 \, \Sigma \, w_i x_i}{\sqrt{(1 - r) \, \Sigma w_i^2 + r \, (\Sigma w_i)^2}}$$

where x, is the score for scale i, w_i is the weight for scale i, and r is the average correlation among the scales.

The major advantage of GAS is its ability to tailor the scale to the specific goals of the individuals. However, this can also be one of its major limitations. Each subject has his or her own scale, with different numbers of goals, and varying criteria for each one. At the end of the study, it is possible to state that the intervention worked or did not work, but much more difficult to say where it did well and where it did poorly; poor scores on some scales may reflect more a bad choice of goals or criteria rather than a failure of the program. Moreover, comparisons across studies, and especially of different varieties of the intervention (e.g. various types of anti-inflammatory agents), become nearly impossible, since all successful trials will, by definition, have a mean of 50 and an SD of 10; less 'powerful' interventions will simply set more lenient criteria for success.

A second limitation of the technique is that it is extremely labour-intensive. The clinicians or researchers must be taught how to formulate goals, and write criteria in objective, observable terms. Then, the raters have to be trained and tested to ensure that they reach adequate levels of reliability in scoring the goals. Thus, it seems as if GAS is potentially useful when:

(1) the objective is to evaluate an intervention as a whole, without regard to *why* it may work, or in comparing it to any other program;

(2) the goals for each person are different; and

(3) there are adequate resources for training goal setters and raters.

Econometric methods

The final class of scaling methods we will consider has its roots in a different discipline, economics, and has become increasingly popular in the medical literature in applications ranging from clinical trials to decision analysis. The problem for which these methods were devised involves assigning a numerical value to various health states. This arises in economics and health in the course of conducting cost/benefit studies, where it becomes necessary to scale benefits along a numerical scale so that cost/benefit ratios can be determined.

Note that economists are generally not interested in a specific individual's choice, but rather tend to obtain ratings of health states by averaging judgements from a large number of individuals in order to create a utility score for the state. Thus the focus of measurement is the described health state, not the characteristic of the individual respondent. This creates interesting problems for the assessment of reliability, which are explicitly dealt with in Chapter 9.

For example, consider a clinical trial comparing medical management of angina to coronary bypass surgery. Surgery offers a potential benefit in quality of life, but the trade-off is the finite possibility that the patient may not survive the operation or immediate post-operative period. How, then, does one make a rational choice between the two alternatives?

The first approach to the problem was developed in the 1950s, and is called the *Von Neumann–Morgenstern standard gamble* (1953). The subject is asked to consider the following scenario:

> You have been suffering from 'angina' for several years. As a result of your illness, you experience severe chest pain after even minor physical exertion such as climbing stairs, or walking one block in cold weather. You have been forced to quit your job, and spend most days at home watching TV. Imagine that you are offered a possibility of an operation that will result in complete recovery from your illness. However, the operation carries some risk. Specifically, there is a probability 'p' that you will die during the course of the operation. How large must 'p' be before you will decline the operation and choose to remain in your present state?

Clearly, the closer the present state is to perfect health, the smaller the risk of death one would be willing to entertain. Having obtained an estimate of 'p' from subjects, the value of the present state can be directly converted to a 0–1 scale by simply subtracting 'p' from 1, so that a tolerable risk of 1 per cent results in a value (called a 'utility') of 0.99 for the present state, and a risk of 50 per cent results in a utility of 0.50.

One difficulty with the 'standard gamble' is that few people, aside from statisticians and professional gamblers, are accustomed to dealing in probabilities. In order to deal with this problem, a number of devices are used to simplify the task. Subjects may be offered specific probabilities; e.g. 10 per cent chance of perioperative death, and 90 per cent chance of complete recovery, until they reach a point of indifference between the two alternatives. Visual aids, such as 'probability wheels', have also been used.

This difficulty in handling probabilities led to the development of an alternative method, called the *time trade-off technique* (Torrance *et al.* 1972), which avoids the use of probabilities. One begins by estimating the likely remaining years of life for a healthy subject, using actuarial tables; i.e. if the patient is 30 years old we could estimate that he has about 40 years remaining. The previous question would then be rephrased as follows:

> Imagine living the remainder of your natural lifespan (40 years) in your present state. Contrast this with the alternative that you can return to perfect health for fewer years. How many years would you sacrifice if you could have perfect health?

In practice, the respondent is presented with the alternatives of 40 years in her present state versus 0 years of complete health. The upper limit is decreased, and the lower limit increased, until a point of indifference is reached. The more years a subject is willing to sacrifice in exchange for a return to perfect health, presumably the worse he perceives his present health. The response (call it Y) can be converted to a scaled utility by the simple formula:

$$U = (40 - Y)/40.$$

A thorough example of the application of this method in a clinical trial of support for relatives of demented elderly is given in Mohide *et al.* (1988).

Critique of econometric methods

We have presented the two methods as a means to measure individual health states. Although they are limited to the measurement of health states, they have been used both with real patients and with normal, healthy individuals imagining themselves to be ill.

The methods are quite difficult to administer and require a trained interviewer, so it remains to see whether they possess advantages over simpler techniques. One straightforward alternative would be a direct estimation of health state, using an adjectival or visual analog scale. Torrance (1976) has shown that the time trade-off and standard gamble methods yield similar results, which differed from the direct estimation method, suggesting that these methods may indeed be a more accurate reflection of the underlying state.

However, the methods are based on the notion that people make rational choices under conditions of uncertainty. There is an accumulation of evidence, reviewed in Chapter 6, which suggests that responses on rating scales can be influenced by a variety of extraneous factors. The methods reviewed in this section are no more immune to seemingly irrational behaviour, as reviewed by Llewellyn-Thomas and Sutherland (1986). As one example, framing a question in terms of 40 per cent survival instead of 60 per cent mortality will result in a shift of values. The problem addressed by the econometric methods assumed that context-free values could be elicited. It seems abundantly clear that such 'value-free' values are illusory, and a deeper understanding of the psychological variables which influence decisions and choices is necessary. Moreover, it appears that real patients assign higher (more positive) utilities to states of ill health than do normals imagining themselves in that state, casting doubt on the analog studies.

Ever since Von Neumann and Morgenstern's (1953) theoretical work, one of the main selling points of econometric methods is that they yield results that are at an interval or ratio level of measurement. This was an unproven (and, for many years, unprovable) assertion. However, with the introduction of item response theory (discussed in Chapter 12), techniques have been developed to evaluate whether scales actually do have interval or ratio level properties. The limited research is not encouraging. Cook *et al.* (2001) found that 'None of the utility scales functioned as interval-level scales in our sample' (p. 1275).

Last, the lower anchor is usually assumed to be death. There has been little work to examine conditions which some people (e.g. Richard Dreyfuss in the movie *Whose Life Is It Anyway*) see as worse than death.

On psychometric grounds, the Standard Gamble (SG) may not bear close scrutiny, either. While early studies appeared to show that the test–retest reliability of the SG was superior to a rating scale (RS) (Torrance 1987), it turns out that this may have been a consequence of an incorrect approach to computing reliability, as we will discuss in Chapter 9. More recent studies have shown that the test–retest reliability of the SG is worse than the RS (0.45 versus 0.67; Moore *et al.* 1999). Juniper *et al.* (2001) showed substantially lower concurrent validity than the RS against a disease-specific quality of life measure (-0.08 to $+0.12$ versus $+0.21$ to $+0.46$), as did Rutten-van Molken *et al.* (1995; 0.13 to 0.19 versus 0.47 to 0.59). Of course, it could be claimed that the SG remains the gold standard, since it alone is consistent with rational choice theory. Perhaps, but one suspects that while the researchers may appreciate these theoretical distinctions, they are lost on participants. Indeed, one problem with the SG and TTO is that respondents find them difficult to complete. In one study, it took three years of schooling to complete the RS against six years for the SG.

To rate or to rank

The goal of many of the techniques discussed so far, such as adjectival and Likert scales, VASs, and the various econometric methods, is to assign a numerical value to an item; i.e. the respondents rate themselves as to the degree to which they have an attribute or endorse a statement. Even the comparative techniques (Thurstone's method, Guttman scaling, and paired-comparison), which begin by ranking items, have as their ultimate aim the construction of a scale that has specific numbers (i.e. ratings) assigned to each item or step. However, in some areas, particularly the assessment of values, another approach is possible; that of *ranking* a series of alternatives. For example, one of the measures in our study of the effect of social support on morbidity (McFarlane *et al.* 1980) tapped how highly people valued good health in relation to nine other qualities. We gave the respondents 10 index cards, on each of which was printed one quality, such as Wealth, Happiness, and Health, and their task was to arrange the cards from the most highly valued to the least. The outcome measure was the rank assigned to Health.

One major advantage of ranking, as opposed to rating, is that it forces people to differentiate among the responses. If the respondents are poorly motivated, or are low in 'cognitive sophistication', they can minimize their effort in responding (a phenomenon called *satisficing*, which we discuss in more detail in Chapter 6) by rating all qualities equally high or low (Krosnick and Alwin 1988). Forcing the respondents to rank the attributes in order of desirability or value lessens the possibility of nondifferentiation, because the person must make choices among the alternatives. It does not totally eliminate the problem of poor motivation, as the subject can simply order them randomly, but this can be detected by having the person do the task twice.

However, there is a price to pay for this. First, it is cognitively more difficult to rank order a list of items than to rate each one. In face-to-face interviews, subjects can be given cards, with one attribute on each, and they can rearrange them until they are satisfied. This cannot be done, though, if the questionnaire is mailed, and especially if it administered over the telephone. A more important problem is statistical in nature. If all of the values are used (as opposed to the situation in the example, where only the value of Health was recorded), then the scale becomes *ipsative*. An ipsative scale has the property that the sum of the individual items is always the same, and therefore is also the same for every person. For example, if the respondent has to rank five attributes, then the sum of the ranks will be 15 (i.e. $1 + 2 + 3 + 4 + 5$; more generally, with k items, the sum will be $k(k + 1)/2$, and the mean will be

$(k + 1)/2)$. This means that there must be a negative correlation among the items (Jackson and Alwin 1980), and the sum of the correlations between individual items and some other variable will always be zero (Clemans 1966). Related to this is another problem, that the rankings are not independent. If we know the ranks assigned to four of the five attributes, then we would be able to perfectly predict the last one. This lack of independence violates assumptions of most statistical tests.

Alwin and Krosnick (1985) conclude that the correlation between ratings and rankings is extremely high, but the relationships among the individual items are quite different. Because of the statistical problems mentioned above as well as others (e.g. traditional forms of techniques such as factor analysis, the intra-class correlation, and generalizability theory—all discussed in later chapters—cannot be used with ranked data), ratings are usually preferred.

Multidimensional scaling

In the previous sections of this chapter, we discussed various techniques for creating scales, which differentiate attributes along one dimension; such as a Guttman scale, which taps mobility. However, there are situations in which we are interested in examining the similarities of different 'objects', which may vary along a number of separate dimensions. These objects can be diagnoses, occupations, social interactions, stressful life events, pain experiences, countries, faces, or almost anything else we can imagine (Weinberg 1991). The dimensions themselves are revealed by the analysis; that is, they are 'hidden' or 'latent', in that they are not directly observable from the data but inferred from the patterns that emerge in the way the objects group together. (For a more complete description of latent variables, see the chapter on Factor Analysis in Norman and Streiner (2000).) The family of techniques for performing this type of analysis is called *multidimensional scaling* (MDS). Very briefly, MDS begins with some index of how 'close' each object is to every other object, and then tries to determine how many dimensions underlie these evaluations of closeness.

To illustrate the technique, imagine that we want to determine what dimensions may underlie the similarities or differences among nine symptoms experienced by patients with various types of depression. The first step is to construct a *similarity matrix* (also called a *proximity matrix*). This can be done in a number of different ways. First, patients or clinicians can be given all possible pairs of symptoms, as with the paired comparison technique. But now, rather than choosing one or the other, they would indicate how similar the two symptoms are on, say, a 10-point scale, with 1 meaning not at all similar to 10 meaning most similar. Another way of constructing the matrix is to determine the frequency with which the symptoms co-occur in a sample of patients. A third method may be to ask patients to rate the perceived severity of each of the nine symptoms on some form of scale, and then correlate each symptom with all of the others. The mathematics of MDS do not care how the similarity matrix is formed—rating or judgements, frequency of co-occurrence, correlations, or any one of a number of other techniques. The difference shows up only in terms of how we interpret the results.

For the purposes of this example, let us assume that we used the frequency of co-occurrence, and obtained the results shown in Table 4.4. A score of 1 means that the symptoms always occur together, and 0 indicates that they never occur together. As would be expected, the maximum coefficient occurs along the main diagonal; sadness is more related to itself than to any other symptom. Conversely, coefficients of 0 reflect mutually exclusive symptoms, such as insomnia and hypersomnia.

MDS uses this matrix to determine the number of dimensions that underlie the similarities among the symptoms. There are a number of different computer programs which do this. They vary according to various assumptions which are made: whether the objects are differentiated holistically or in terms of separate attributes; and whether the proximities among the objects are measured on an ordinal or an interval scale. A description of the programs is given in an article by Weinberg (1991) and a monograph by Kruskal and Wish (1978). Irrespective of which program is used, the results are usually displayed in a graph, with each axis representing one dimension. The researcher then tries to determine what the dimensions represent, in terms of the underlying properties of the objects. For example, assume that the similarity matrix yielded just two interpretable dimensions. We can then plot the location of each symptom along these two dimensions, as in Fig. 4.11.

The closer the symptoms are on the graph, the more similar they are to one another. It would appear as if the first dimension is differentiating symptoms which are

Table 4.4 Similarity matrix of nine symptoms of depression

	A	B	C	D	E	F	G	H	I
A	1.00								
B	0.865	1.00							
C	0.495	0.691	1.00						
D	0.600	0.823	0.612	1.00					
E	0.125	0.135	0.402	0.127	1.00				
F	0.201	0.129	0.103	0.111	0.000	1.00			
G	0.125	0.581	0.513	0.578	0.713	0.399	1.00		
H	0.312	0.492	0.192	0.487	0.303	0.785	0.000	1.00	
I	0.105	0.223	0.332	0.201	0.592	0.762	0.414	0.185	1.00

A = Feeling of sadness
B = Pessimism
C = Decreased libido
D = Suicidal ideation
E = Weight gain
F = Weight loss
G = Hypersomnia
H = Early morning wakening
I = Psychomotor retardation

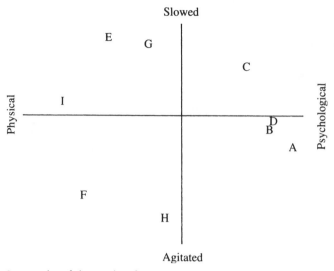

Fig. 4.11 Scatter plot of the results of MDS.

primarily psychological from those which are more physiological in nature, while the second dimension reflects a continuum of psychomotor retardation versus agitation.

Most researchers stop at this point, and are content to have determined the number and characteristics of the underlying dimensions. The scale developer, however, can use MDS as a first step, to reveal the 'psychological dimensions' people use in evaluating different stimuli, which are then used to construct scales that measure the various dimensions separately.

MDS and exploratory factor analysis (EFA) are very similar in terms of what they hope to accomplish: reduce a large number of variables into a smaller number of latent, explanatory factors. In fact, EFA is a special case of one form of MDS, called smallest space analysis (Guttman 1982). The question, then, is when to use each. If the responses are dichotomous (e.g. True/False, Yes/No), then the choice is obvious; traditional forms of EFA should never be used with dichotomous items, and MDS is definitely an option (e.g. Brazill and Grofman 2002). When the data are continuous and appropriate for EFA, then it appears that MDS results in fewer factors than EFA. Some argue that this makes the solution easier to interpret, but carries the risk that some important factors may be overlooked.

References

Aitken, R. C. B. (1969). A growing edge of measurement of feelings. *Proceedings of the Royal Society of Medicine*, **62**, 989–92.

Alwin, D. F. and Krosnick, J. A. (1985). The measurement of values in surveys: A comparison of ratings and rankings. *Public Opinion Quarterly*, **49**, 535–52.

Bosi Ferraz, M., Quaresma, M. R., Aquino, L. R. L., Atra, E., Tugwell, P., and Goldsmith, C. H. (1990). Reliability of pain scales in the assessment of literate and illiterate patients with rheumatoid arthritis. *Journal of Rheumatology*, **17**, 1022–4.

Brazill, T. J. and Grofman, B. (2002). Factor analysis versus multi-dimensional scaling: Binary choice roll-call voting and the US Supreme Court. *Social Networks*, **24**, 201–29.

Bryant, G. D. and Norman, G. R. (1980). Expressions of probability: Words and numbers. *New England Journal of Medicine*, **302**, 411.

Clemans, W. V. (1966). An analytical and empirical examination of some properties of ipsative measures. *Psychometric Monographs*, **14**.

Cook, K. F., Ashton, C. M., Byrne, M. M., Brody, B., Geraci, J., Giesler, R. B., Hanita, M., Souchek, J., and Wray, N. P. (2001). A psychometric analysis of the measurement level of the rating scale, time trade-off, and standard gamble. *Social Science & Medicine*, **53**, 1275–85.

Dickinson, T. L. and Zellinger, P. M. (1980). A comparison of the behaviorally anchored rating mixed standard scale formats. *Journal of Applied Psychology*, **65**, 147–54.

Dixon, P. N., Bobo, M., and Stevick, R. A. (1984). Response differences and preferences for all-category-defined and end-defined Likert formats. *Educational and Psychological Measurement*, **44**, 61–6.

Downie, W. W., Leatham, P. A., Rhind, V. M., Wright, V., Branco, J. A., and Anderson, J. A. (1978). Studies with pain rating scales. *Annals of Rheumatic Diseases*, **37**, 378–81.

Erviti, V., Fabrey, L. J., and Bunce, J. V. (1979). The development of rating scales to assess the clinical performance of medical students. *Proceedings, 18th Annual Conference on Research in Medical Education*, Washington.

Frisbie, D. A. and Brandenburg, D. C. (1979). Equivalence of questionnaire items with varying response formats. *Journal of Educational Measurement*, **16**, 43–8.

Gaito, J. (1982). Measurement scales and statistics: Resurgence of an old misconception. *Psychological Bulletin*, **87**, 564–7.

Guilford, J. P. (1954). *Psychometric methods*. McGraw-Hill, New York.

Harden, R. M. and Gleeson, F. A. (1979). Assessment of clinical experience using an objective structured clinical examination (OSCE). *Medical Education*, **13**, 41–54.

Guttman, L. (1982). Facet theory, smallest space analysis, and factor analysis. *Perceptual and Motor Skills*, **54**, 491–3.

Harter, S. (1982). The Perceived Competence Scale for Children. *Child Development*, **53**, 87–97.

Hayes, M. H. S. and Patterson, D. G. (1921). Experimental development of the graphic rating method. *Psychological Bulletin*, **18**, 98–9.

Higgins, E. T. (1996). Knowledge activation: Accessibility, applicability, and salience. In *Social psychology: Handbook of basic principles* (ed. E. T. Higgins and A. Kruglanski), pp. 133–68. Guilford Press, New York.

Hoek, J. A. and Gendall, P. J. (1993). A new method of predicting voting behavior. *Journal of the Market Research Society*, **35**, 361–73.

Hunter, J. E. and Schmidt, F. L. (1990). Dichotomization of continuous variables: The implications for meta-analysis. *Journal of Applied Psychology*, **75**, 334–49.

Huskisson, E. C. (1974). Measurement of pain. *Lancet*, **ii**, 1127–31.

Jackson, D. J. and Alwin, D. F. (1980). The factor analysis of ipsative measures. *Sociological Methods and Research*, **9**, 218–38.

Jensen, M. P., Turner, J. A., and Romano, J. M. (1994). What is the maximum number of levels needed in pain intensity measurement? *Pain*, **58**, 387–92.

Jones, R. R. (1968). Differences in response consistency and subjects' preferences for three personality response formats. In *Proceedings of the 76th annual convention of the American Psychological Association* (pp. 247–8). Washington.

Juniper, E. F., Norman, G. R., Cox, F. M., and Roberts, J. N. (2001). Comparison of the standard gamble, rating scale, AQLQ and SF-36 for measuring quality of life in asthma. *European Respiratory Journal*, 18, 38–44.

Kiresuk, T. J. and Sherman, R. E. (1968). Goal attainment scaling: A general method for evaluating comprehensive community health programs. *Community Mental Health Journal*, 4, 443–53.

Klockars, A. J. and Hancock, G. R. (1993). Manipulations of evaluative rating scales to increase validity. *Psychological Reports*, 73, 1059–66.

Klockars, A. J. and Yamagishi, M. (1988). The influence of labels and positions in rating scales. *Journal of Educational Measurement*, 25, 85–96.

Krosnick, J. A. and Alwin, D. F. (1988). A test of the form-resistant correlation hypothesis: Ratings, rankings, and the measurement of values. *Public Opinion Quarterly*, 52, 526–38.

Kruskal, J. B. and Wish, M. (1978). *Multidimensional scaling*. Sage, Beverly Hills, CA.

Lichtenstein, S. and Newman, J. R. (1967). Empirical scaling of common verbal phrases associated with numerical probabilities. *Psychonomic Science*, 9, 563–4.

Likert, R. A. (1952). A technique for the development of attitude scales. *Educational and Psychological Measurement*, 12, 313–15.

Linn, L. (1979). Interns' attitudes and values as antecedents of clinical performance. *Journal of Medical Education*, 54, 238–40.

Llewellyn-Thomas, H. and Sutherland, H. (1986). Procedures for value assessment. In *Recent advances in nursing: Research methodology* (ed. M. Cahoon). Churchill-Livingstone, London.

McFarlane, A. H., Norman, G. R., Streiner, D. L., Roy, R. G., and Scott, D. J. (1980). A longitudinal study of the influence of the psychosocial environment on health status: A preliminary report. *Journal of Health and Social Behavior*, 21, 124–33.

Miller, G. A. (1956). The magic number seven plus or minus two: Some limits on our capacity for processing information. *Psychological Bulletin*, 63, 81–97.

Mohide, E. A., Torrance, G. W., Streiner, D. L., Pringle, D. M., and Gilbert, J. R. (1988). Measuring the well-being of family caregivers using the time trade-off technique. *Journal of Clinical Epidemiology*, 41, 475–82.

Moore, A. D., Clarke, A. E., Danoff, D. S., Joseph, L., Belisle, P., Neville, C. and Fortin, P. R. (1999). Can health utility measures be used in lupus research? A comparative validation and reliability study of 4 indices. *Journal of Rheumatology*, 26, 1285–90.

Newstead, S. E. and Arnold, J. (1989). The effect of response format on ratings of teachers. *Educational and Psychological Measurement*, 49, 33–43.

Nishisato, N. and Torii, Y. (1970). Effects of categorizing continuous normal distributions on the product-moment correlation. *Japanese Psychological Research*, 13, 45–9.

Norman, G. R. and Streiner, D. L. (2000). *Biostatistics: The bare essentials* (2nd edn). B. C. Decker, Toronto.

Osgood, C., Suci, G., and Tannenbaum, P. (1957). *The measurement of feeling*. University of Illinois Press, Urbana.

Parducci, A. (1968). Often is often. *American Psychologist*, 25, 828.

Preston, C. C. and Colman, A. M. (2000). Optimal number of response categories in rating scales: Reliability, validity, discriminating power, and respondent preferences. *Acta Psychologica*, 104, 1–15.

Ronen, G. M., Streiner, D. L., Rosenbaum, P., and the Canadian Pediatric Epilepsy Network (in press). Health-related quality of life in childhood epilepsy: The development of self-report and proxy-response measures. *Epilepsia*, **44**, 598–612.

Rutten–van Molken, M. P. M. H., Custers, F., van Doorslaer, E. K. A., Jansen, C. C. M., Heurman, L., Maesen, F. P. *et al.* (1995). Comparison of performance of four instruments in evaluating the effects of salmeterol on asthma quality of life. *European Respiratory Journal*, **8**, 888–98.

Santa-Barbara, J., Woodward, C. A., Levin, S., Goodman, J. T., Streiner, D. L., Muzzin, L. *et al.* (1974). Variables related to outcome in family therapy: Some preliminary analyses. *Goal Attainment Review*, **1**, 5–12.

Schaeffer, N. C. (1991). Hardly ever or constantly? Group comparisons using vague quantifiers. *Public Opinion Quarterly*, **55**, 395–423.

Schuman, H. and Presser, S. (1981). *Questions and answers*. Academic Press, New York.

Schwarz, N. (1999). Self-reports: How the questions shape the answers. *American Psychologist*, **54**, 93–105.

Schwarz, N. and Hippler, H. J. (1995). Response alternatives: The impact of their choice and ordering. In *Measurement error in surveys* (ed. P. Biemer, R. Groves, N. Mathiowetz, and S. Sudman) pp. 41–56. Wiley, New York.

Schwarz, N., Hippler, H. J., Deutsch, B., and Strack, F. (1985). Response scales: Effects of category range on report behavior and subsequent judgments. *Public Opinion Quarterly*, **49**, 388–95.

Schwarz, N., Knauper, B., Hippler, H.-J., Noelle-Neumann, E., and Clark, L. (1991). Rating scales: Numeric values may change the meaning of scale labels. *Public Opinion Quarterly*, **55**, 570–82.

Scott, P. J. and Huskisson, E. C. (1978). Measurement of functional capacity with visual analog scales. *Rheumatology and Rehabilitation*, **16**, 257–9.

Scott, P. J. and Huskisson, E. C. (1979). Accuracy of subjective measurements made with and without previous scores: An important source of error in serial measurement of subjective states. *Annals of the Rheumatic Diseases*, **38**, 558–9.

Seymour, R. A., Simpson, J. M., Charlton, J. E., and Phillips, M. E. (1985). An evaluation of length and end-phrase of visual analog scales in dental pain. *Pain*, **21**, 177–85.

Shearman, J. K., Evans, C. E. E., Boyle, M. H., Cuddy, L. J., and Norman, G. R. (1983). Maternal and infant characteristics in abuse: A case control study. *Journal of Family Practice*, **16**, 289–93.

Spector, P. E. (1976). Choosing response categories for summated rating scales. *Journal of Applied Psychology*, **61**, 374–5.

Stolee, P., Rockwood, K., Fox, R. A., and Streiner, D. L. (1992). The use of goal attainment scaling in a geriatric care setting. *Journal of the American Geriatric Society*, **40**, 574–8.

Streiner, D. L. (1985). Global rating scales. In *Clinical competence* (ed. V. R. Neufeld and G. R. Norman), pp. 119–41. Springer, New York.

Suissa, S. (1991). Binary methods for continuous outcomes: A parametric alternative. *Journal of Clinical Epidemiology*, **44**, 241–8.

Torrance, G. (1976). Social preferences for health states: An empirical evaluation of three measurement techniques. *Socio-Economic Planning Sciences*, **10**, 129–36.

Torrance, G. W. (1987). Utility approach to measuring health-related quality of life. *Journal of Chronic Diseases*, **40**, 593–600.

Torrance, G., Thomas, W. H., and Sackett, D. L. (1972). A utility maximization model for evaluation of health care programs. *Health Services Research*, **7**, 118–33.

Townsend, J. T. and Ashby, F. G. (1984). Measurement scales and statistics: The misconception misconceived. *Psychological Bulletin*, **96**, 394–401.

van der Vleuten, C. P., Norman, G. R., and de Graaff, E. (1991). Pitfalls in the pursuit of objectivity: Issues of reliability. *Medical Education*, **25**, 110–18.

Von Neumann, J. and Morgenstern, O. (1953). *The theory of games and economic behavior.* Wiley, New York.

Weinberg, S. L. (1991). An introduction to multidimensional scaling. *Measurement and Evaluation in Counseling and Development,* 24, 12–36.

Wildt, A. R. and Mazis, A. B. (1978). Determinants of scale response: Label versus position. *Journal of Marketing Research,* 15, 261–7.

Wright, D. B., Gaskell, G. D., and O'Muircheartaigh, C. A. (1994). How much is 'Quite a bit'? Mapping between numerical values and vague quantifiers. *Applied Cognitive Psychology,* 8, 479–496.

Chapter 5

Selecting the items

In previous chapters, we have discussed how to develop items that would be included in the new scale. Obviously, not all of the items will work as intended; some may be confusing to the respondent, some may not tell us what we thought they would, and so on. Here we examine various criteria used in determining which ones to retain and which to discard.

Interpretability

The first criterion for selecting items is to eliminate any that are ambiguous or incomprehensible. Problems can arise from any one of a number of sources: the words are too difficult; they contain jargon terms that are used only by certain groups of people, such as health professionals; or they are 'double-barrelled'.

Reading level

Except for scales that are aimed at a selected group whose educational level is known, the usual rule of thumb is that the scale should not require reading skills beyond that of a 12-year-old. This may seem unduly low, but many people who are high-school graduates are unable to comprehend material much above this level. Many ways have been proposed to assess the reading level required to understand written material. Some methods, like the 'cloze' technique (Taylor 1957), eliminate every nth word to see at what point meaning disappears; the easier the material, the more words can be removed and accurately 'filled in' by the reader. Other methods are based on the number of syllables in each word or the number of words in each sentence (e.g. Flesch 1948; Fry 1968). However, these procedures can be laborious and time-consuming, and others may require up to 300 words of text (e.g. McLaughlin 1969). These are usually inappropriate for scales or questionnaires, where each item is an independent passage, and meaning may depend on one key word.

Within recent years, a number of computer packages have appeared that purport to check the grammar and style of one's writing. Some of these programs further provide one or more indices of reading level, and these have also been incorporated into various word processing packages. Since the procedures used in the programs are based on the techniques we just mentioned, their results should probably be interpreted with great caution when used to evaluate scales.

Another method is to use a list of words that are comprehensible at each grade level (e.g. Dale and Eichholz 1960). While it may be impractical (and even unnecessary) to check every word in the scale, those which appear to be difficult can be checked. Even glancing through one of these books can give the scale-developer a rough idea of the complexity of Grade 6 words. Approaching the problem from the other direction, Payne (1954) compiled a very useful list of 1000 common words, indicating whether each was unambiguous, problematic, or had multiple meanings.

Ambiguity

This same method is often used to determine if the items are ambiguous or poorly worded. Even a seemingly straightforward item such as 'I like my mother', can pose a problem if the respondent's mother is dead. Some people answer by assuming that the sentence can also be read in the past tense, while others may simply say 'no', reflecting the fact that they cannot like her now. On a questionnaire designed to assess patients' attitudes to their recent hospitalization, one item asked about information given to the patient by various people. A stem read 'I understand what was told to me by:', followed by a list of different health care professionals, with room to check either 'yes' or 'no'. Here, a 'no' response opposite 'social worker', for instance, could indicate that:

- the patient did not understand what the social worker said;
- she never saw a social worker;
- she does not remember whether she saw the social worker or not.

While these latter two possibilities were not what the test-developer intended, the ambiguity of the question and the response scheme forced the subject to respond with an ambiguous answer.

Ambiguity can also arise by the vagueness of the response alternatives. The answer to the question, 'Have you seen your doctor recently' depends on the subject's interpretation of 'recently'. One person may feel that it refers to the previous week, another to the past month, and a third person may believe it covers the previous year. Even if we rephrase the question to use a seemingly more specific term, ambiguity can remain. 'Have you seen your doctor during the past year?' can mean:

- during the last 12 months, more or less;
- since this date one year ago;
- since 1 January of this year.

The message is to avoid vague terms such as 'often', 'lately', or 'recently'. If a specific time-frame (or any other variable) is called for, it should be spelled out explicitly. We will return to the problems of recall in the next chapter.

Double-barrelled question

A 'double-barrelled' item is one that asks two or more questions at the same time, each of which can be answered differently. These are unfortunately quite common in questionnaires probing for physical or psychological symptoms, such as 'My eyes are red and teary'. How should one answer if one's eyes are red but not teary, or teary but not red? Since some people will say 'yes' only if both parts are true, while others will respond this way if either symptom was present, the final result may not reflect the actual state of affairs. A more subtle instance of a double-barrelled question would be, 'I do not smoke because of the fear of lung cancer'. This item has one part that measures the occurrence or non-occurrence of a behaviour ('I do not smoke'), and a second that taps motivation ('because of the fear of lung cancer'). People who do not smoke for other reasons, such as religious beliefs, concern about impaired lung functioning, fear of heart disease, dislike of the smell, and so forth, are in a quandary. They may be reluctant to answer 'False' because that might imply that they do smoke; yet they cannot answer 'True' because the rationale stated in the item does not correspond to their motivation for not smoking. Pre-testing on a large group, where it is likely that some people will fall into these grey areas, can reduce the risk of these types of items occurring.

Jargon

Jargon terms can slip into a scale or questionnaire quite insidiously. Since we use a technical vocabulary on a daily basis, and these terms are fully understood by our colleagues, it is easy to overlook the fact that these words are not part of the everyday vocabulary of others, or may have very different connotations. Terms like 'lesion', 'care-giver', or 'range of motion' may not be ones that the average person understands. Even more troublesome are words which *are* understood, but in a manner different from what the scale developer intended. 'Hypertension', for example, means 'being very tense' to some people; and asking some what colour their stool is may elicit the response that the problem is with their gut, not their furniture. Samora *et al.* (1961) compiled a list of 50 words which physicians said they used routinely with their patients, and then asked 125 patients to define them. Words that were erroneously defined at least 50 per cent of the time included 'nutrition', 'digestion', 'orally', and 'tissue'; words that most clinicians would assume their patients knew. The range of definitions given for *appendectomy* included a cut rectum, sickness, the stomach, a pain or disease, taking off an arm or leg, something contagious, or something to do with the bowels, in addition to surgical removal of the appendix. Patients and physicians differ even in terms of what should be called a disease. Campbell *et al.* (1979) state that 'the medically qualified were consistently more generous in their acceptance of disease connotation than the laymen' (p. 760). Over 90 per cent of general practitioners, for instance, called duodenal ulcers a disease, while only 50 per cent of lay people did. Boyle (1970) found the greatest disagreement between physicians and patients to be in the area of the location of internal organs. Nearly 58 per cent of patients had the heart occupying the entire thorax, or being adjacent to the left shoulder (almost 2 per cent had it near the right shoulder). Similarly, the majority of patients placed the stomach over the belly button, somewhat south of its actual location. Not surprisingly, knowledge of medical terms, and the etiology, treatment, and symptoms of various disorders, is strongly associated with educational level

(Seligman *et al.* 1957). Again, pre-testing is desirable, with the interviewer asking the people not whether they had the complaint, but rather what they think the term means.

Value-laden words

A final factor affecting the interpretation of the question is the use of value-laden terms. Items such as 'Do you often go to your doctor with trivial problems?' or 'Do physicians make too much money?' may prejudice the respondents, leading them to answer as much to the tenor of the question as to its content. (Both items also contain ambiguous terms, such as 'often', 'trivial', and 'too much'.) Perhaps the second-most egregious real example of value-laden words was found in a survey of physicians by a company flogging its product. The last question reads, 'Given that [the product] will provide substantial cost savings to your hospital, would you be willing to use [the product] for your cataract procedures?'. The most egregious was from a poll conducted by a conservative organization on behalf of an even more conservative politician who was in favour of limiting law suits against large companies. The question read, 'We should stop excessive legal claims, frivolous lawsuits and overzealous lawyers'. Can you guess how people responded? Naturally, such value-laden terms should be avoided.

Positive and negative wording

We design scales and questionnaires assuming highly motivated people, who read each item carefully, ponder the alternatives, and put down an answer reflecting their true beliefs or feelings. Unfortunately, not all respondents fit this ideal picture. As we discuss in more depth in the next chapter, some people, because of a lack of motivation or poor cognitive skills, take an easy way out; they may say 'Yes' to everything, or just go down the right-hand column of response alternatives. In order to minimize any such response set, some people have recommended balancing the items, so that some are worded positively and others negatively (e.g. Anastasi 1982; Likert 1932). However, research has shown that this is generally a bad idea. Negatively worded items—that is, those that use words such as 'not' or 'never,' or have words with negative prefixes (e.g. in-, im-, or un-)—should be avoided whenever possible for a number of reasons. First, simply reversing the polarity of an item does not necessarily reverse the meaning. Answering 'Yes' to the question 'I feel well' connotes a positive state; whereas saying 'No' to 'I do not feel well' reflects the absence of a negative one, which is not always the same thing. Second, children, and lower-functioning adults, have difficulty grasping the concept that they have to disagree with an item in order to indicate a positive answer, such as reporting being in good health by having to say 'No' to 'I feel unwell much of the time' (Benson and Hocevar 1985; Melnick and Gable 1990). Third, there is a tendency for respondents to endorse a negative item rather than reject a positive one (Campostrini and McQueen 1993; Reiser *et al.* 1986). Finally, negatively worded items have lower validity coefficients than positively worded ones (Holden *et al.* 1985; Schriesheim and Hill 1981); and scales that have stems with both positive and negative wording are less reliable than those where all the stems are worded in the same direction (Barnette 2000).

Length of items

Items on scales should be as short as possible, although not so short that comprehensibility is lost. Item validity coefficients tend to fall as the number of letters in the item increases. Holden *et al.* (1985) found that, on average, items with 70–80 letters had validity coefficients under 0.10, while items containing 10–20 characters had coefficients almost four times higher.

Testing the questions

Having obeyed all of these rules, there is still no guarantee that the questions will be interpreted by the subjects as they were intended to be. Belson (1981), for example, found that fewer than 30 per cent of survey questions were correctly interpreted by readers. Unfortunately, these results are typical of findings in this area.

Perhaps the best way to ensure that the items are understood, unambiguous, and jargon-free is to pre-test them on a group of people comparable to those who will be the ultimate targets. Following a technique introduced by Nuckols (1953), the people are asked to rephrase the question in their own words, trying to keep the meaning as close to the original as possible. The responses, which are written down verbatim, are later coded into one of four categories: fully correct; generally correct (no more than one part altered or omitted); partially wrong (but the person understood the intent); and completely wrong (Foddy 1993). Similarly, problem items are identified if the subject responds with statements such as 'I never heard of that' or 'Can you repeat the question?' (Schechter and Herrmann 1997). Other techniques that can be used to test the subjects' understanding of these items are the *double interview, asking people to think aloud*, and *verbal probing*. In the first method, the entire questionnaire is given. Then, for each subject, three or four questions are selected, and the interviewer asks questions such as, 'What led you to answer...' or 'Tell me exactly how you came to that answer' (Foddy 1993). In the second technique, the subjects are asked to think aloud as they formulate their responses. Verbal probing is somewhat more directive than thinking aloud, and asks the person directly, for example, 'What does the term *illness* (or *stomach*, or whatever) mean to you?'. These probes can be developed beforehand, or spurred by the respondent's answer to the item (Willis *et al.* 1991). Further, it is possible to identify problematic items if, while probing for accuracy, the person says, 'I didn't know that what was you meant,' or 'I didn't think of that' (Schechter and Hermann 1997). Naturally, all of these approaches can be used for the same items, with different groups of respondents.

In all cases, though, it is important that the subjects are representative of the people who will ultimately be completing the questionnaire. Using one's colleagues or samples of convenience, which may bear little resemblance to the final user population, will most likely result in underestimating any potential problems. If pre-testing does not uncover any difficulties with the wording of any the items, it is more likely a sign of problems with the pre-testing procedure, rather than an indication that everything is fine. It is difficult to say *a priori* on how many people the scale should be pre-tested. It is probably best to use the criterion used by qualitative researchers, that of 'sampling to redundancy'. That is, people are interviewed until no new problems are uncovered. In most cases, this occurs somewhere between eight and 15 interviews.

Rechecking

Even after all of the items have passed these checks and have been incorporated into the scale, it is worthwhile to check them over informally every year or so to see if any terms may have taken on new meanings. For example, liking to go to 'gay parties' has a very different connotation now than it did some years ago, when to most people the word 'gay' had no association with homosexuality.

Face validity

One issue that must be decided before the items are written or selected is whether or not they should have *face validity*. That is, do the items appear on the surface to be measuring what they actually are? As is often the case, there are two schools of thought on this issue, and the 'correct' answer often depends on the purpose that the measure will be used for.

Those who argue for face validity state, quite convincingly, that it serves at least five useful functions. It:

(1) increases motivation and cooperation among the respondents;

(2) may attract potential candidates;

(3) reduces dissatisfaction among users;

(4) makes it more likely that policy makers and others accept the results; and

(5) improves public relations, especially with the media and the courts (Nevo 1985).

If the item appears irrelevant, then the respondent may very well object to it or omit it, irrespective of its possibly superb psychometric properties. For example, it is commonly believed that some psychiatric patients manifest increased religiosity, especially during the acute phase of their illness. Capitalizing on this fact, the MMPI contains a few items tapping into this domain. Despite the fact that these items are psychometrically quite good, it has opened the test to much (perhaps unnecessary) criticism for delving into seemingly irrelevant, private matters.

On the other hand, it may be necessary in some circumstances to disguise the true nature of the question, lest the respondents try to 'fake' their answers, an issue we will return to in greater detail in Chapter 6. For example, patients may want to appear worse than they actually are in order to ensure that they will receive help; or better than they really feel in order to please the doctor. This is easy to do if the items have face validity—that is, their meaning and relevance are self-evident—and much harder if they do not. Thus, the ultimate decision depends on the nature and purpose of the instrument.

If it is decided that the scale should have face validity (which is usually the case), then the issues become:

(1) who should assess it; and

(2) how.

Because face validity pertains to how respondents and other users of the test perceive it, it should be judged by them, and not by experts in the field; and it is sufficient to ask them to simply rate it on a five-point scale, ranging from Extremely Suitable to Irrelevant (Nevo 1985).

Frequency of endorsement and discrimination

After the scale has been pre-tested for readability and absence of ambiguity, it is then given to a large group of subjects to test for other attributes, including the endorsement frequency. (The meaning of 'large' is variable, but usually 50 subjects would be an absolute minimum.) The frequency of endorsement is simply the proportion of people (p) who give each response alternative to an item. For dichotomous items, this reduces to simply the proportion saying 'yes' (or, conversely, 'no'). A multiple-choice item has a number of 'frequencies of endorsement'; the proportion choosing alternative A, one for alternative B, and so forth.

In achievement tests, the frequency of endorsement is a function of the *difficulty* of the item, with a specific response alternative reflecting the correct answer. For personality measures, the frequency of endorsement is the 'popularity' of that item; the proportion of people who choose the alternative which indicates more of the trait, attitude, or behavior (Allen and Yen 1979).

Usually, items where one alternative has a very high (or low) endorsement rates are eliminated. If p is over 0.95 (or under 0.05), then most people are responding in the same direction or with the same alternative. Since we can predict what the answer will be with greater than 95 per cent accuracy, we learn very little by knowing how a person actually responded. Such questions do not improve a scale's psychometric properties, and may actually detract from them while making the test longer. In practice, only items with endorsement rates between 0.20 and 0.80 are used.

Using this criterion, which is quite liberal, may result in items that are highly skewed, in that the responses bunch up at one end of the continuum or the other. However, this does not have a major deleterious effect on the psychometric properties of the scale (assuming, of course, that p is somewhere between 0.05 and 0.95). Especially when the mean inter-item correlation is high (at least 0.25 or so), we can live with highly skewed items (Bandalos and Enders 1996; Enders and Bandalos 1999; Feldt 1993). Thus, items should not be thrown out simply on the basis of the skewness of the distribution of responses.

There are some scales, though, which are deliberately made up of items with a high endorsement frequency. This is the case where there may be some question regarding the subject's ability or willingness to answer honestly. A person may not read the item accurately because of factors such as illiteracy, retardation, or difficulties in concentration; or may not answer honestly because of an attempt to 'fake' a response for some reason. Some tests, like the MMPI or the *Personality Research Form* (Jackson 1984), have special scales to detect these biases, comprised of a heterogeneous group of items which have only one thing in common: an endorsement frequency of 90–95 per cent. To get rates this high, the questions have to be either quite bizarre (e.g. 'I have touched money') or extremely banal ('I eat most days'). A significant number of questions answered in the 'wrong' direction is a flag that the person was not reading the items carefully and responding as would most people. This may temper the interpretation given to other scales that the person completes.

Another index of the utility of an item, closely related to endorsement frequency, is its *discrimination* ability. This tells us if a person who has a high total score is more likely to have endorsed the item; conversely, if the item discriminates between those who score high (and supposedly have more of the trait) and those who score low. It is related to endorsement frequency in that, from a psychometric viewpoint, items which discriminate best among people have values of p near the cut-point of the scale. It differs in that it looks at the item in relation to all of the other items on the scale, not just in isolation.

A simple item discrimination index is given by the formula:

$$d_i = \frac{U_i - L_i}{n_i},$$

where U_i is the number of people above the median who score positive on item i, L_i is the number of people below the median who score positive on item i, and n_i is the number of people above (or below) the median.

Homogeneity of the items

In most situations, whenever we are measuring a trait, behaviour, or symptom, we want the scale to be homogeneous. That is, all of the items should be tapping different aspects of the same attribute, and not different parts of different traits. (Later in this chapter we deal with the situation where we want the test to measure a variety of characteristics.) For example, if we were measuring the problem-solving ability of medical students, then each item should relate to problem-solving. A high degree of homogeneity is desirable in a scale, because it 'speaks directly to the ability of the clinician or the researcher to interpret the composite score as a reflection of the test's items' (Henson 2001). This has two implications:

(1) the items should be moderately correlated with each other;

(2) each should correlate with the total scale score.

Indeed, these two factors form the basis of the various tests of homogeneity or 'internal consistency' of the scale.

Before the mechanics of measuring internal consistency are discussed, some rationale and background are in order. In almost all areas we measure, a simple summing of the scores over the individual items is the most sensible index; this point will be returned to in Chapter 7. However, this 'linear model' approach (Nunnally 1970) works only if all items are measuring the same trait. If the items were measuring different attributes, it would not be logical to add them up to form one total score. On the other hand, if one item were highly correlated with a second one, then the latter question would add little additional information. Hence there is a need to derive some quantitative measure of the degree to which items are related to each other; i.e. the degree of 'homogeneity' of the scale.

Current thinking in test development holds that there should be a moderate correlation among the items in a scale. If the items were chosen without regard for homogeneity, then the resulting scale could possibly end up tapping a number of traits. If the correlations were too high, there would be much redundancy, and a possible loss of content validity.

It should be noted that this position of taking homogeneity into account, which is most closely identified with Jackson (1970) and Nunnally (1970), is not shared by all psychometricians. Another school of thought is that internal consistency and face validity make sense if the primary aim is to *describe* a trait, behaviour, or disorder, but not necessarily if the goal is to *discriminate* people who have an attribute from those who do not. That is, if we are trying to measure the degree of depression, for example, the scale should *appear* to be measuring it and all of the items should relate to this in a coherent manner. On the other hand, if our aim is to *discriminate* depressed patients from other groups, then it is sufficient to choose items which are answered differently by the depressed group, irrespective of their content. This in fact was the method used in constructing the MMPI, one of the most famous paper-and-pencil questionnaires for psychological assessment. An item was included in the Depression Scale (*D*) based on the criterion that depressed patients responded to it in one way significantly more often than did non-depressed people, and without regard for the correlation among the individual items. As a result, the *D* scale has some items which seem to be related to depression, but also many other items which do not. On the other hand, the more recent CES-D (Radloff 1977), which measures depressive symptomatology without diagnosing depression, was constructed following the philosophy of high internal consistency, and its items all appear to be tapping into this domain. If a trend can be detected, it is toward scales that are more grounded in theory and are more internally consistent, and away from the empiricism that led to the MMPI.

One last comment is in order before discussing the techniques of item selection. Many inventories, especially those in the realms of psychology and psychiatry, are multidimensional; that is, they are comprised of a number of different scales, with the items intermixed in a random manner. Measures of homogeneity should be applied to the individual scales, as it does not make sense to talk of homogeneity across different subscales.

Item–total correlation

One of the oldest, albeit still widely used, methods for checking the homogeneity of the scale is the *item–total correlation*. As the name implies, it is the correlation of the individual item with the scale total *omitting that item*. If we did not remove the item from the total score, the correlation would be artificially inflated, since it would be based in part on the item correlated with itself. The item can be eliminated in one of two ways: physically or statistically. We can physically remove the item by not including it when calculating the total score. So, for a five-item scale, Item 1 would be correlated with the sum of Items 2–5; Item 2 with the sum of 1 and 3–5; and so on. One problem with this approach is that, for a *k-item* scale, we have to calculate the total score *k* times; not a difficult problem, but a laborious one, especially if a computer program to do this is not readily available.

The second method is statistical; the item's contribution to the total score is removed using the formula given by Nunnally (1978):

$$r_{i(t-1)} = \frac{r_{it}\sigma_t - \sigma_i}{\sqrt{(\sigma_i^2 + \sigma_t^2 - 2\sigma_i\sigma_t r_{it})}},$$

where $r_{i(t-1)}$ is the correlation of item i with the total, removing the effect of item i; r_{it} is the correlation of item i with the total score; σ_i is the standard deviation of item i; and σ_t is the standard deviation of the total score.

The usual rule of thumb is that an item should correlate with the total score above 0.20. Items with lower correlations should be discarded (Kline 1986).

In almost all instances, the best coefficient to use is the *Pearson product-moment correlation* (Nunnally 1970). If the items are dichotomous, then the usually recommended point-biserial correlation yields identical results; if there are more than two response alternatives, the product-moment correlation is robust enough to produce relatively accurate results, even if the data are not normally distributed (see for example Havlicek and Peterson 1977).

Split-half reliability

Another approach to testing the homogeneity of a scale is called *split-half reliability*. Here, the items are randomly divided into two subscales, which are then correlated with each other. This is also referred to as 'odd–even' reliability, since the easiest split is to put all odd-numbered items in one half and even-numbered ones in the other. If the scale is internally consistent, then the two halves should correlate highly.

One problem is that the resulting correlation is an underestimate of the true reliability of the scale, since the reliability of a scale is directly proportional to the number of items in it. Since the subscales being correlated are only half the length of the version that will be used in practice, the resulting correlation will be too low. The Spearman–Brown 'prophesy' formula is used to correct for this occurrence.

The equation for this is:

$$r_{SB} = \frac{kr}{1 + (k - 1)r},$$

where k is the factor by which the scale is to be increased or decreased, and r is the original correlation.

In this case, we want to see the result when there are twice the number of items, so k is set at 2. For example, if we found that splitting a 40-item scale in half yields a correlation of 0.50, we would substitute into the equation as follows:

$$r_{SB} = \frac{2 \times 0.50}{1 + (2 - 1) \times 0.50}.$$

Thus, the estimate of the split-half reliability of this scale would be 0.67.

Since there are many ways to divide a test into two parts, there are in fact many possible split-half reliabilities; a 10-item test can be divided 126 ways, a 12-item test 462 different ways, and so on. (These numbers represent the combination of n items taken $n/2$ at a time. This is then divided by 2, since (assuming a 6-item scale) items 1, 2, and 3 in the first half, and 4, 5, and 6 in the second is the same as 4, 5, and 6 in the first part and the remaining items in the second.) These reliability coefficients may differ quite considerably from one split to another.

There are three situations when we should *not* divide a test randomly:

(1) where the score reflects how many items are completed within a certain span of time;

(2) if the items are given in order of increasing difficulty;

(3) when the items are either serially related or all refer to the same paragraph that must be read.

In the first case, where the major emphasis is on how quickly a person can work, most of the items are fairly easy, and failure is due to not reaching that question before the time limit. Thus, the answers up to the timed cut-off will almost all be correct, and those after it all incorrect. Any split-half reliability will yield a very high value, only marginally lower than 1.0.

The second situation, items presented in order of difficulty, is often found on individually-administered intelligence and achievement tests, as well as some activities of daily living scales. Here, items are presented until they surpass the person's level of ability. Similar to the previous case, the expected pattern of answers is all correct up to that level, and all wrong above it (or, if partial credits are given, then a number of items with full credit, followed by some with partial credit, and ending with a group given no credit). As with timed tests, it is assumed that people will differ only with regard to the number of items successfully completed, and that the pattern of responding will be the same from one person to the next. Again, the split-half reliability will be very close to 1.0.

With related or 'chained' items, failure on the second item could occur in two ways: not being able to answer it correctly; or being able to do it, but getting it wrong, because of an erroneous response to the previous item. For example, assume that the two (relatively simple) items were as follows:

A. The organ for pumping blood is:
    (1) the pineal gland
    (2) the heart
    (3) the stomach.

B. It is located in:
    (1) the chest
    (2) the gut
    (3) the skull.

If the answer to A were correct, then a wrong response to B would indicate that the person did not know where the heart is located. However, if A and B were wrong, then the person *may* have known that the heart is located in the chest, but went astray in believing that blood is pumped by the pineal gland. Whenever this can occur, it is best to keep both items in the same half of the scale.

Kuder-Richardson 20 and coefficient α

There are two problems in using split-half reliability to determine which items to retain. First, as we have just seen, there are many ways to divide a test; and second, it does not tell us which item(s) may be contributing to a low reliability. Both of these problems are addressed with two related techniques, *Kuder-Richardson formula 20* (KR-20; Kuder and Richardson 1937) and *coefficient α* (also called Cronbach's alpha; Cronbach 1951).

KR-20 is appropriate for scales with items which are answered dichotomously, such as 'true–false', 'yes–no', 'present–absent', and so forth. To compute it, the proportion of people answering positively to each of the questions and the standard deviation of the total score must be known, and then put into the formula:

$$ KR - 20 = \frac{n}{n-1}\left(1 - \frac{\Sigma\, p_i q_i}{\sigma_T^2}\right), $$

where n is the number of items; p_i is the proportion answering correctly to question i; $q_i = (1 - p)$ for each item; and σ_T is the standard deviation of the total score.

Cronbach's α (alpha) is an extension of KR-20, allowing it to be used when there are more than two response alternatives. If α were used with dichotomous items, the result would be identical to that obtained with KR-20. The formula for α is very similar to KR-20, except that the standard deviation for each item (σ_i) is substituted for $p_i q_i$:

$$ \alpha = \frac{n}{n-1}\left(1 - \frac{\Sigma\, \sigma_i^2}{\sigma_T^2}\right). $$

Conceptually, both equations give the average of all of the possible split-half reliabilities of a scale. Their advantage in terms of scale development is that, especially with the use of computers, it is possible to do them n times, each time omitting one item. If KR-20 or α increases significantly when a specific item is left out, this would indicate that its exclusion would increase the homogeneity of the scale.

It is nearly impossible these days to see a scale development paper that has not used α, and the implication is usually made that the higher the coefficient, the better. However, there are problems in uncritically accepting high values of α (or KR-20), and especially in interpreting them as reflecting simply internal consistency. The first problem is that α is dependent not only on the magnitude of the correlations among the items, but also on the number of items in the scale. A scale can be made to look more 'homogeneous' simply by doubling the number of items, even though the average correlation remains the same. This leads directly to the second problem. If we have two scales which each measure a distinct construct, and combine them to form one long scale, α will be high. Cortina (1993) concluded that, "if a scale has more than 14 items, then it will have an alpha of 0.70 or better even if it consists of two orthogonal dimensions with modest (i.e., 0.30) item correlations. If the dimensions are correlated with each other, as they usually are, then alpha is even greater" (p. 102). Third, if α is too high, then it may suggest a high level of item redundancy; that is, a number of items asking the same question in slightly different ways (Boyle 1991; Hattie 1985). This may indicate that some of the items are unnecessary, and that the scale as a whole may be too narrow in its scope to have much validity. Thus, α should be above 0.70 (Nunnally 1978), but probably not higher than 0.90.

Multifactor inventories

If the scale is one part of an inventory which has a number of other scales (usually called 'multifactor' or 'multidimensional' inventories), more sophisticated item analytic techniques are possible. The first is an extension of the item–total procedure, in which the item is correlated with its scale total, *and with the totals of all of the other scales*. The item should meet the criteria outlined above for a single index; additionally, this correlation should be higher than with any of the scales it is *not* included in.

The second technique is *factor analysis*. Very briefly, this statistic is predicated on the belief that a battery of tests can be described in terms of a smaller number of underlying factors. For example, assume students were given five tests: vocabulary, word fluency, verbal analogies, mechanical reasoning, and arithmetic. It might be expected that their scores on the first three tasks would be correlated with one another, that the last two would be correlated, but that the two sets of scores would not necessarily be related to each other. That is, high scores on the first three may or may not be associated with high scores on the latter two. We would postulate that the first group reflected a 'verbal' factor, and the second a 'reasoning' one. (A very basic introduction to factor analysis is given in Appendix C. For more details presented in a non-mathematical fashion, see Norman and Streiner 2003; if you are comfortable with introductory statistics, see Norman and Streiner 2000; and if you love matrix algebra, see Harman 1976.)

In an analogous manner, each item in a multifactorial test could be treated as an individual 'test'. Ideally, then, there should be as many factors as separate scales in the inventory. The item should 'load on' (i.e. be correlated with) the scale it belongs to, and not on any other one. If it loads on the 'wrong' factor, or on two or more factors, then it is likely that it may be tapping something other than what the developer intended, and should be either rewritten or discarded.

More recent developments in factor analysis allow the test-developer to specify beforehand what he or she thinks the final structure of the test should look like. The results show how closely the observed pattern corresponds to this hypothesized pattern (Darton 1980). Although factor analysis has been used quite often with dichotomous items, this practice is highly suspect, and can lead to quite anomalous results (Comrey 1978).

When homogeneity does not matter

Our discussion of homogeneity of the scale was based on classical test theory. The assumption is that there is a 'universe' of items that tap a given trait or behaviour, and the scale is composed of a random subset of them. Another way to think of this is that the underlying trait (variously called a *hypothetical construct* or just a *construct* in personality theory, or a *latent trait* in statistics; terms we will return to in Chapter 10) causes a number of observable manifestations, which are captured by the items. For example, anxiety may result in sweatiness, a feeling of impending doom, excessive worrying, irritability, sleep disturbance, difficulty concentrating, and a host of other symptoms, as shown in the left side of Fig. 5.1. Using the drawing conventions of

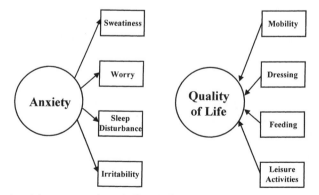

Fig. 5.1 A pictorial representation of effect indicators on the left, and causal indicators on the right.

structural equation modeling (Norman and Streiner 2000), the construct is shown as a circle, and the observed (or *measured*) variables as rectangles. The observed variables, in this case, are also called *effect indicators*, because they reflect the effect of the construct (Bollen and Lennox 1991).

There are a number of implications of this. First, the items should all be correlated with each other to varying degrees. This means that the average inter-item correlation should be in the moderate range; item–total correlations should be between 0.20 and 0.80; and coefficient α should be somewhere between 0.70 and 0.90. Second, in order to measure the construct, the specific items do not really matter. That is, it is of little concern if we do not have an item about irritability, or discard it because of wording or psychometric issues, because there are many other, correlated, items that are tapping anxiety. We may be unhappy that the scale does not have an item that measures an important aspect of anxiety (an issue of face validity), but from the viewpoint of constructing a scale, the absence of that specific item is of no import. Finally, if we run a factor analysis, we should find a strong first factor, on which all of the items load.

However, there are situations where none of this holds. In the right side of Fig. 5. 1, we again have a construct (in this case, quality of life, or QOL), but here the arrows point *to* it rather than *from* it. This reflects the fact that now the measured variables define the construct rather than being defined by it. In this case, the observed variables are referred to as *causal indicators* (Bollen and Lennox 1991). We encounter this situation in a number of other areas in addition to QOL indices. The most usual is a checklist of phenomena that are not causally related to each other. For example, Holmes and Rahe (1967) constructed a scale of recent stressful life events, including such items as the death of a spouse, receiving a driving ticket, and buying a house. There is no reason to believe that if one event occurred, the others will, too. As another example, Goldberg's General Health Questionnaire (1979) consists of a number of health concerns, drawn from a wide range of disorders. Not only would it not be expected that all of the symptoms would be related to each other, some, such as mania and lethargy, may be mutually exclusive.

The implications of this are almost diametrically opposite to the ones we just discussed. First, as the items are not expected to be correlated with each other, it is not appropriate to use the various indices of homogeneity, such as coefficient α, the mean inter–item correlation, and item–total correlations; nor to use statistics that are based on the assumption of homogeneity, such as factor analysis. Second, and perhaps more importantly, the specific items *do* matter. If the Holmes and Rahe scale omitted divorce, for example, the total score would therefore underestimate a recently divorced person's level of stress. Further, because that item is not expected to be correlated with other ones, its effect will be missed entirely.

Thus, we are concerned with the internal consistency of a scale only when the measured variables are effect indicators, reflecting the effects of an underlying construct; but not when they are causal indicators, that define the construct by their presence. (For more on when α does and does not matter, see Streiner 2003a, 2003b.).

Putting it all together

In outline form, these are the steps involved in the initial selection of items:

A. Pre-test the items to ensure that they:
   (1) are comprehensible to the target population;
   (2) are unambiguous; and
   (3) ask only a single question.

B. Eliminate or rewrite any items which do not meet these criteria, and pre-test again.

C. Discard items endorsed by very few (or very many) subjects.

D. Check for the internal consistency of the scale using:
   (1) item–total correlation:
      (a) correlate each item with the scale total omitting that item;
      (b) eliminate or rewrite any with Pearson r's less than 0.20;
      (c) rank order the remaining ones and select items starting with the highest correlation;
   or
   (2) coefficient α or KR-20
      (a) calculate a eliminating one item at a time;
      (b) discard any item where a significantly increases.

E. For multiscale questionnaires, check that the item is in the 'right' scale by:
   (1) correlating it with the totals of all the scales, eliminating items that correlate more highly on scales other than the one it belongs to; or
   (2) factor-analyzing the questionnaire, eliminating items which load more highly on other factors than the one it should belong to.

References

Alien, G. I., Breslow, L., Weissman, A., and Nisselson, H. (1954). Interviewing versus diary keeping in eliciting information in a morbidity survey. *American Journal of Public Health*, **44**, 919–27.

Allen, M. J. and Yen, W. M. (1979). *Introduction to measurement theory*. Brooks/Cole, Monterey, CA.

Anastasi, A. (1982). *Psychological testing* (5th edn). Macmillan, New York.

Bandalos, D. L. and Enders, C. K. (1996). The effects of non-normality and number of response categories on reliability. *Applied Measurement in Education*, **9**, 151–60.

Barnette J. J. (2000). Effects of stem and Likert response option reversals on survey internal consistency: If you feel the need, there is a better alternative to using those negatively worded stems. *Educational and Psychological Measurement*, **60**, 361–70.

Belson, W. A. (1981). *The design and understanding of survey questions*. Gower, Aldershot.

Benson, J. and Hocevar, D. (1985). The impact of item phrasing on the validity of attitude scales for elementary school children. *Journal of Educational Measurement*, **22**, 231–40.

Bollen, K. and Lennox, R. (1991). Conventional wisdom on measurement: A structural equation perspective. *Psychological Bulletin*, 110, 305–14.

Boyle, C. M. (1970). Differences between patients' and doctors' interpretation of some common medical terms. *British Medical Journal*, 2, 286–9.

Boyle, G. J. (1991). Does item homogeneity indicate internal consistency or item redundancy in psychometric scales? *Personality and Individual Differences*, 12, 291–4.

Campbell, E. J. M., Scadding, J. G., and Roberts, R. S. (1979). The concept of disease. *British Medical Journal*, ii, 757–62.

Campostrini, S. and McQueen, D. V. (1993). The wording of questions in a CATI-based lifestyle survey: Effects of reversing polarity of AIDS-related questions in continuous data. *Quality & Quantity*, 27, 157–70.

Comrey, A. L. (1978). Common methodological problems in factor analysis. *Journal of Consulting and Clinical Psychology*, 46, 648–59.

Cortina, J. M. (1993). What is coefficient alpha? An examination of theory and applications. *Journal of Applied Psychology*, 78, 98–104.

Cronbach, L. J. (1951). Coefficient alpha and the internal structure of tests. *Psychometrika*, 16, 297–334.

Dale, E. and Eichholz, G. (1960). *Children's knowledge of words*. Ohio State University, Columbus, OH.

Darton, R. A. (1980). Rotation in factor analysis. *The Statistician*, 29, 167–94.

Flesch, R. (1948). A new readability yardstick. *Journal of Applied Psychology*, 32, 221–33.

Enders, C. K. and Bandalos D. L. (1999). The effects of heterogeneous item distributions on reliability. *Applied Measurement in Education*, 12, 133–50.

Feldt, L. S. (1993). The relationship between the distribution of item difficulties and test reliability. *Applied Measurement in Education*, 6, 37–48.

Foddy, W. (1993). *Constructing questions for interviews and questionnaires*. Cambridge University Press, Cambridge.

Fry, E. A. (1968). A readability formula that saves time. *Journal of Reading*, 11, 513–16.

Goldberg, D. P. (1979). *Manual of the general health questionnaire*. NFER Publishing Co, Windsor.

Harman, H. H. (1976). *Modern factor analysis* (3rd edn). University of Chicago Press, Chicago.

Hattie, J. (1985). Methodology review: Assessing unidimensionality of tests and items. *Applied Psychological Measurement*, 9, 139–64.

Havlicek, L. L. and Peterson, N. L. (1977). Effect of the violation of assumptions upon significance levels of the Pearson r. *Psychological Bulletin*, 84, 373–7.

Henson, R. K. (2001). Understanding internal consistency reliability estimates: A conceptual primer on coefficient alpha. *Measurement and Evaluation in Counseling and Development*, 34, 177–89.

Holden, R. R., Fekken, G. C., and Jackson, D. N. (1985). Structured personality test item characteristics and validity. *Journal of Research in Personality*, 19, 386–94.

Holmes, T. H. and Rahe, R. H. (1967). The social readjustment rating scale. *Journal of Psychosomatic Research*, 11, 213–8.

Jackson, D. N. (1970). A sequential system for personality scale development. In *Current topics in clinical and community psychology*, Vol. 2 (ed. C. D. Spielberger) pp. 61–96. Academic Press, New York.

Jackson, D. N. (1984). *Personality Research Form manual.* Research Psychologists Press, Port Huron MI.

Kline, P. (1986). *A handbook of test construction.* Methuen, London.

Kuder, G. F. and Richardson, M. W. (1937). The theory of estimation of test reliability. *Psychometrika,* **2,** 151–60.

Likert, R. A. (1932). A technique for the measurement of attitudes. *Archives of Psychology,* **140,** 44–53.

Linton, M. (1975). Memory for real world events. In *Explorations in cognition* (ed. D. A. Norman and D. E. Rumelhart) pp. 376–404. Freeman, San Francisco.

McLaughlin, G. H. (1969). SMOG grading: A new readability formula. *Journal of Reading,* **12,** 639–46.

Means, B., Nigam, A., Zarrow, M., Loftus, E. F., and Donaldson, M. S. (1989). Autobiographical memory for health-related events. *Vital and health statistics,* Series 6: Cognition and Survey Measurement, No. 2. Public Health Service, Hyattsville, MD.

Melnick, S. A. and Gable, R. K. (1990). The use of negative stems: A cautionary note. *Educational Research Quarterly,* **14**(3), 31–6.

Neisser, U. (1986). Nested structure in autobiographical memory. In *Autobiographical memory* (ed. D. C. Rubin) pp. 71–81. Cambridge University Press, Cambridge.

Nevo, B. (1985). Face validity revisited. *Journal of Educational Measurement,* **22,** 287–93.

Norman, G. R. and Streiner, D. L. (1986). *PDQ statistics.* B. C. Decker, Toronto.

Norman, G. R. and Streiner, D. L. (2000). *Biostatistics: The bare essentials* (2nd edn). B. C. Decker, Toronto.

Nuckols, R. C. (1953). A note on pre-testing public opinion questions. *Journal of Applied Psychology,* **37,** 119–20.

Nunnally, J. C., Jr. (1970). *Introduction to psychological measurement.* McGraw-Hill, New York.

Nunnally, J. C., Jr. (1978). *Psychometric theory* (2nd edn). McGraw-Hill, New York.

Payne, S. L. (1954) *The art of asking questions.* Princeton University Press, Princeton NJ.

Radloff, L. S. (1977). The CES-D scale: A self-report depression scale for research in the general population. *Applied Psychological Measurement,* **1,** 385–401.

Reiser, M., Wallace, M., and Schuessler, K. (1986). Direction of wording effects in dichotomous social life feeling items. *Sociological Methodology,* **16,** 1–25.

Samora, J., Saunders, L., and Larson, R. F. (1961). Medical vocabulary knowledge among hospital patients. *Journal of Health and Human Behavior,* **2,** 83–92.

Schechter, S. and Hermann, D. (1997). The proper use of self-report questions in effective measurement of health outcomes. *Evaluation & the Health Professions,* **20,** 28–46.

Schriesheim, C. A. and Hill, K. D. (1981). Controlling acquiescence response bias by item reversals: The effect on questionnaire validity. *Educational and Psychological Measurement,* **41,** 1101–14.

Seligman, A. W., McGrath, N. E., and Pratt, L. (1957). Level of medical information among clinic patients. *Journal of Chronic Diseases,* **6,** 497–509.

Streiner, D. L. (2003a). Starting at the beginning: An introduction of coefficient alpha and internal consistency. *Journal of Personality Assessment,* **80,** 99–103.

Streiner, D. L. (2003b). Being inconsistent about consistency: When coefficient alpha does and does not matter. *Journal of Personality Assessment,* **80,** 217–22.

Taylor, W. L. (1957). 'Cloze' readability scores as indices of individual differences in comprehension and aptitude. *Journal of Applied Psychology,* **41,** 19–26.

United States National Health Survey (1965). *Reporting of hospitalization in the Health Interview Survey*. Health Statistics, Series 3, No. 6. Public Health Service, Hyattsville, MD.

Willis, G. B., Royston, P., and Bercini, D. (1991). The use of verbal report methods in the development and testing of survey questionnaires. *Applied Cognitive Psychology*, 5, 251–67.

Chapter 6

Biases in responding

When an item is included in a questionnaire or scale, it is usually under the assumption that the respondent will answer honestly. However, there has been considerable research, especially since the 1950s, showing that there are numerous factors which may influence a response, making it a less than totally accurate reflection of reality. The magnitude and seriousness of the problem depends very much on the nature of the instrument and the conditions under which it is used. At the extreme, questionnaires may end up over- or under-estimating the prevalence of a symptom or disease; or the validity of the scale may be seriously jeopardized.

Some scale developers bypass the entire problem of responder bias by asserting that their instruments are designed merely to differentiate between groups. In this situation, the truth or falsity of the answer is irrelevant, as long as one group responds in one direction more often than does another group. According to this position, responding 'yes' to an item such as 'I like sports magazines' would not be interpreted as accurately reflecting the person's reading preferences. The item's inclusion in the test is predicated solely on the fact that one group of people *says* it likes these magazines more often than do other groups. This purely empirical approach to scale development reached its zenith in the late 1940s and 1950s, but may still be found underlying the construction of some measures.

However, with the gradual trend toward instruments which are more grounded in theory, this approach to scale construction has become less appealing. The objective now is to reduce bias in responding as much as possible. In this chapter, we will examine some of the sources of error, what effects they may have on the scale, and how to minimize them.

The differing perspectives

The people who develop a scale, those who use it in their work, and the ones who are asked to fill it out, all approach scales from different perspectives, for different reasons, and with differing amounts of information about the instrument. For the person administering the instrument, a specific answer to a given question is often of little interest. That item may be just one of many on a scale, where the important information is the total score, and there is little regard for the individual items which have contributed to it. In other situations, the responses may be aggregated across dozens or hundreds of subjects, so that the individual person's answers are buried in a mass of those from other anonymous subjects. Further, what the questioner wants is 'truth'—did the person have this symptom or not, ever engage in this behaviour or not, and so forth. The clinician cannot help the patient, or the researcher discover important facts, unless honest answers are given. Moreover, the assessment session is perceived, at least in the assessors' minds, as non-judgemental and their attitude as disinterested. This may appear so obvious to scale-developers that it never occurs to them that the respondents may perceive the situation from another angle.

The respondents' perspectives, however, are often quite different. They are often unaware that the individual items are ignored in favour of the total score. Even when told that their responses will be scored by a computer, it is quite common to find marginal notes explaining or elaborating their answers. Thus, it appears that respondents treat each item as important in its own right, and often believe that their answers will be read and evaluated by another person.

Additionally, their motivation may include the very natural tendency to be seen in a good light; or to be done with this intrusion in their lives as quickly as possible; or to ensure that they receive the help they feel they need. As we will discuss, these and other factors may influence the response given.

Answering questions: the cognitive requirements

Asking a simple question, such as 'How strongly do you feel that you should never spank a child?', requires the respondent to undertake a fairly complex cognitive task. Depending on the theory, there are four (e.g. Tourangeau 1984) or five (Schwarz and Oyserman 2001) steps that people must go through, with an opportunity for bias to creep (or storm) in at each step.

1. *Understanding the question.* The issue here is whether the respondent's interpretation of the question is the same as the test designer's. In the previous chapter, we discussed some methods to try to minimize the difference: by avoiding ambiguous terms and double-barrelled questions, using simple language, and pre-testing in order to determine what the respondent thinks is being asked. Even so, other factors may influence the interpretation. For example, one person may interpret 'spank' to mean any physical action that causes the child to cry; while another may feel that it pertains only to punishment, and that slapping a child's hand if he puts it too near the stove is done for the child's protection and does not constitute spanking. The item format itself may affect how the person interprets the question (Schwarz 1999). For instance, if an item asks how often the person gets 'really irritated' and one response alternative is 'less than once a year', the respondent may infer that the question refers only to major annoyances, since it is highly unlikely that minor ones would occur that infrequently. This may or may not be what the questionnaire developer had in mind, though. Similarly, giving the person a long time-frame, such as 'over the past year', would lead the respondent to think the item is referring to more serious events than a shorter time frame of 'over the past week' (Winkielman *et al.* 1998).

2. *Recalling the relevant behaviour, attitude, or belief.* Once the respondents have read and understood (or even misunderstood) the item, they must recall how often they have done a specific action, or how they felt about something. Questionnaire developers vastly overestimate people's ability to recall past events. Surprising as it

may seem, the results of a major study showed that 42 per cent of people did not recall that they had been in hospital one year after the fact (Cannell *et al.* 1965). In another study, there was a 22 per cent false-positive rate and a 69 per cent false-negative rate in the recall of serious medical events after one year, and a 32 per cent false-positive and 53 per cent false-negative rate for minor events (Means *et al.* 1989). The problem is even more severe if the people did not receive medical help for their illness (Allen *et al.* 1954). Drawing on cognitive theory (e.g. Linton 1975; Neisser 1986), Means *et al.* (1989) hypothesize that, especially for chronic conditions which result in recurring events, people have a 'generic memory' for a group of events and medical contacts, and therefore have difficulty recalling specific instances. Further, autobiographical memory is not organized by events, such as being ill, drinking too much, or going to the gym. Rather, there is a hierarchy with *extended periods* at the top (e.g. 'when I worked at Company X' or 'during my first marriage'). Under this are *summarized events*, which reflect repeated behaviours (e.g. 'I worked out a lot during that time'), and *specific events* are at the bottom (Schwarz and Oyserman 2001). Thus, asking respondents how often they saw a physician in the last year, or to recall how they felt six months ago, does not correspond to the manner in which these behaviours are stored in memory, and answers to such questions should be viewed with some degree of scepticism. As Schwarz and Oyserman (2001) state, 'Many recall questions would never be asked if researchers first tried to answer them themselves' (p. 141).

3. *Inference and estimation.* Because questionnaires rarely ask for events to be recalled in the same way that they are stored in memory, respondents must use a number of inference and estimation strategies. One is called *decomposition and extrapolation* (Schwarz and Oyserman 2001). If a person is asked how many times in the last year she saw a dentist, she may remember that she went twice in the last three months. Then she would try to determine whether this was unusual or represented a typical pattern. If the latter, then she would multiply the number by four, and report than she went eight times. There are two possible sources of error; the recall over a shorter period, and the determination of how usual this was. Most people overestimate how often rare behaviours occur, and underestimate frequent actions (e.g. Sudman *et al.* 1996), and multiplying the two only compounds the error. Another manifestation of decomposition and extrapolation is that numerical answers are often given in multiples of 5 or 10; and estimates of elapsed time usually correspond to calendar divisions (i.e. multiples of seven days or four weeks). A beautiful example of this *end-digit bias* comes from an article by Norcross *et al.* (1997), which looked at, among other things, the publication record of clinical psychologists. The respondents' recall of the number of articles they published is shown in Fig. 6.1. There is a steep, relatively smooth decline until 9, and then peaks at multiples of 10, and secondary peaks at multiples of 5. By the same token, other end-digits are conspicuous by their absence; mainly 2, 3, and 7, which is fairly universal. Another inferential strategy, which bedevils researchers and clinicians trying to assess improvement or deterioration, is a person's *subjective theory of stability and change*. A very common question, both on questionnaires and in the clinical interview, is 'How are you feeling now compared to the last time I saw you?' (or '...the last time

you filled out this scale?'). The reality is that people do not remember how they felt three or six months ago. Rather, they use their implicit theory (Ross 1989) of whether or not they have changed or the treatment worked (Schwarz and Oyserman 2001, p. 144):

> [R]espondents may reconstruct their earlier behaviors as having been more problematic than they were, apparently confirming the intervention's success—provided they believe the intervention was likely to help them (a belief that entails a subject theory of change).... To assess actual change, we need to rely on before-after, or treatment-control comparisons, and if we have missed asking the right question before the intervention, little can be done after the fact to make up for the oversight.

4. *Mapping the answer onto the response alternatives.* Having arrived at some estimate of the frequency of a behaviour, or the strength of an attitude, the person now has to translate that to map onto the scale used in the questionnaire. Here we encounter the factors discussed in Chapter 4—how people interpret vague adjectives such as 'very often' or 'frequently', the effects of the numbers placed on the line, the number of response categories, and so forth. The issue is that the response format does not correspond to how respondents originally conceptualized their answer in their own minds. Their response, either orally or by a mark on an answer sheet, represents a 'translation' from their own words into the researcher's; and, as with any translation, something gets lost.

5. *'Editing' the answer.* What the respondent actually thinks, and what he or she is willing to tell the researcher, are not necessarily the same thing. As we outlined in the previous section, the researcher and the respondent have different perspectives

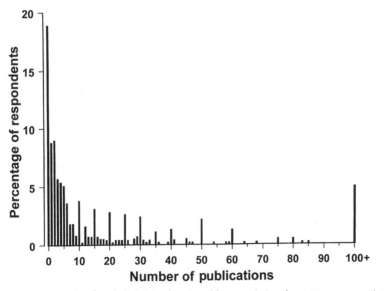

Fig. 6.1 Example of end-digit bias (reprinted by permission from Norcross *et al.* 1997).

and agendas. How and why respondents may edit their answers is the topic for the remainder of this chapter.

Optimizing and satisficing

The hope of the scale-developer is that all of the respondents will perform the five steps outlined above in a careful and comprehensive manner. Borrowing a term from economic decision-making (Simon 1957), Krosnick (1991) uses the term *optimizing* to describe this ideal way of answering. However, as we outlined in the previous section, the aims of the person who developed the scale and those of the person filling it out are not the same. Especially if the questionnaire is long, the items require considerable cognitive effort to answer them, and the purpose of filling it out is seemingly trivial or irrelevant to the respondents, they may adopt a strategy which allows them to complete the task without as much effort. Using another economic decision-making term, Krosnick calls this *satisficing*, giving an answer which is satisfactory (i.e. a box on the form is filled in), but not optimal. He describes six ways in which satisficing may occur. He refers to the first two as 'weak' forms, in that some cognitive effort is required; whereas the last four are 'strong' types of satisficing, since little or no thought is required.

First, the person may select the first response option that seems reasonable. If the options are presented in written form, the respondent will opt for the one that occurs first, and give only cursory attention to those which appear later. Conversely, if the options are given verbally, it is easier to remember those which came most recently; that is, those toward the end of the list. In either case, the choices in the middle get short shrift. Awareness of this phenomenon has led some organizations to minimize its effects in balloting. Recognizing that most voters do not know the people running for office, except for the long and often boring (and unread) position statements they write, and that the task of choosing among them is difficult and seemingly irrelevant for many voters, there is a danger that those whose names are closer to the top of the ballot will receive more votes. Consequently, organizations have adopted the strategy of using multiple forms of the ballot, with the names randomized differently on each version.

A second form of satisficing consists of simply agreeing with every statement, or answering 'true' or 'false' to each item. We will return to this bias later in this chapter, in the section on yea-saying and acquiescence.

Third, the person may endorse the status quo. This is not usually a problem when asking people about their physical or psychological state or about behaviours they may or may not do, but can be an issue when enquiring about their attitudes toward some policy. Having been asked their opinion about, for instance, whether certain procedures should be covered by universal health insurance or if we should allow *in vitro* fertilization of single women, it is easier to say 'keep things as they are' rather than considering the effects of change.

A fourth strategy is to select one answer for the first item, and then to use this response for all of the subsequent questions. This is a particular problem when the response options consist of visual analog or Likert scales keyed in the same direction, so that the person simply has to go down the page in a straight line, putting check marks on each line. The trade-off is that changing the options for each question may minimize this tendency (or at least make it more obvious to the scorer), but it places an additional cognitive demand on the subject, which further fosters satisficing.

Fifth, the person may simply say 'I do not know' or place a mark in a neutral point along a Likert scale. In some circumstances, it may be possible to eliminate these alternatives, such as by using a scale with an even number of boxes, as we described in Chapter 4. However, these may be valid options for some optimizing subjects, and their removal may make their responses less valid.

The last way a person may satisfice is to mentally flip a coin; that is, to choose a response at random. Krosnick (1991) believes that this is the 'method of last resort', and used only when the previous ones cannot be.

There are two general ways to minimize satisficing. First, the task should be kept as simple as possible. At the most superficial level, this means that the questions should be kept short and the words easy to understand; points covered in Chapter 5. Further, the mental processes required to answer the question should not be overly demanding. For example, it is easier to say how you currently feel about something than how you felt about it in the past; less difficult to remember what you did for the past month than over the past year; and how you feel about one thing rather than comparing two or more, since each requires its own retrieval and evaluation process. Last, the response options should not be overly complex, but must include all possibilities. If there are even a few questions which do not have appropriate answers for some subjects, they may stop trying to give the optimal answer and start satisficing.

The second way to decrease satisficing is to maintain the motivation of the respondents. One way is to include only individuals who are interested in the topic, rather than using samples of convenience. Second, recognize that motivation is usually higher at the start of a task, and begins to flag as it gets longer and more onerous. Consequently, instruments should be kept as short as possible. (However, as we will see in Chapter 13, 'short' can be up to 100 items or 10 pages.) A third way is to make the respondents accountable for their answers; that is, they feel that they may have to justify what they said. This can be accomplished by asking them to explain why they gave the answer which they did. Last, motivation can be provided externally, by rewarding them for their participation; we will also discuss this further in Chapter 13.

Social desirability and faking good

A person's answer to an item like, 'During an average day, how much alcohol do you consume?' or 'I am a shy person' may not correspond to what an outside observer would say about that individual. In many cases, people give a socially desirable answer; the drinker may minimize his daily intake, or the retiring person may deny it, believing it is better to be outgoing. As *social desirability* is commonly conceptualized, the subject is not deliberately trying to deceive or lie; he or she is unaware of this tendency to put the best foot forward (Edwards 1957). When the person *is* aware and is intentionally attempting to create a false-positive impression, it is called *faking good*. Although conceptually different, the two biases create similar problems for the scale developer, and have similar solutions.

Social desirability (SD) depends on many factors: the individual, the person's sex and cultural background, the specific question, and the context in which the item is asked; e.g. face-to-face interview versus an anonymous questionnaire. Sudman and Bradburn (1982) derived a list of threatening topics which are prone to SD bias. Among the 'socially desirable' ones apt to lead to over-reporting are being a good citizen (e.g. registering to vote and voting, knowing issues in public debates), being well-informed and cultured (e.g. reading newspapers and books, using the library, attending cultural activities), and having fulfilled moral and social responsibilities (e.g. giving to charity, helping friends and relatives). Conversely, there will be under-reporting of 'socially undesirable' topics, such as certain illnesses and disabilities (e.g. cancer, sexually transmitted diseases, mental disorders), illegal and non-normative behaviours (e.g. committing a crime, tax evasion, use of drugs and alcohol, non-marital sex), and financial status (income, savings, having expensive possessions).

Another aspect of SD bias is that, as Smith (cited in Berke 1998) quipped, 'The average person believes he is a better person than the average person'. This was said in the context of a poll conducted during the President Clinton sex scandal. People were asked how interested they were in the story, and how interested they felt others were. The results are shown in Fig. 6.2, and speak for themselves—others are much more déclassé than are the respondents.

A debate has raged for many years whether SD is a trait (whereby the person responds in the desirable direction irrespective of the context) or a state (dependent more on the question and the setting). While the jury is still out, two suggestions have

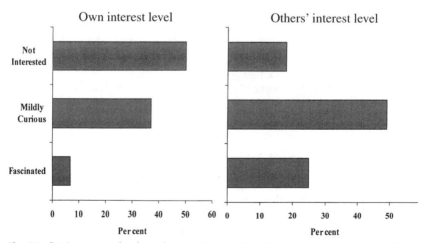

Fig. 6.2 One's own and others' interest in President Clinton's sex life (adapted from Berke 1998).

emerged: SD should be minimized whenever possible, and the person's propensity to respond in this manner should be assessed whenever it may affect how he or she answers (e.g. Anastasi 1982; Jackson 1984).

If answers are affected by social desirability, the validity of the scale may be jeopardized for two reasons. First, if the object of the questionnaire is to gather factual information, such as the prevalence of a disorder, behaviour, or feeling, then the results obtained may not reflect the true state of affairs. The prime example of this would be items tapping socially sanctioned acts, like drug taking, premarital sexual relations, or abortions; but SD may also affect responses to embarrassing, unpopular, or 'unacceptable' feelings, such as anger towards one's parents, or admitting to voting for the party which lost the last election (or won, depending on recent events). In a similar fashion, the occurrence of positive or socially desired behaviours may be overestimated.

The second problem, to which we will return in Chapter 10, involves what is called the 'discriminant validity' of a test. Very briefly, if a scale correlates highly with one factor (e.g. SD), then that limits how highly it can correlate with the factor which the scale was designed to assess. Further, the theoretical rationale of the scale is undermined, since the most parsimonious explanation of what the test is measuring would be 'social desirability', rather than anything else.

The social desirability of an item can be assessed in a number of ways. One method is to correlate each item on a new instrument with a scale specifically designed to measure this tendency. Jackson (1970) has developed an index called the *Differential Reliability Index* (DRI), defined as:

$$\text{DRI} = \sqrt{(r_{is}^2 - r_{id}^2)},$$

where r_{is} is the item-scale correlation, and r_{id} is the item–SD correlation.

The DRI in essence is the difference between the item-total correlation and the item–SD correlation. Any item which is more highly 'saturated' on SD than with its scale total will result in a DRI approaching zero (note that if r_{id} is ever larger than r_{is}, DRI is undefined). Such an item should either be rewritten or discarded.

A number of scales have been developed to specifically measure the tendency to give socially desirable answers. These include the Crowne and Marlow (1960) *Social Desirability Scale*, which is perhaps the most widely used such instrument; the *Desirability* (DY) scale on the *Personality Research Form* (Jackson 1984); one developed by Edwards (1957); and most recently, the *Balanced Inventory of Desirable Responding* (BIDR) of Paulhus (1994). These scales most often consist of items that are socially approved, but rarely occur in real life, such as 'I know everything about the candidates before I vote' or 'My manners are as good at home as when I eat out'. These are sometimes given in conjunction with other scales, not so much in order to develop a new instrument, as to see if SD is affecting the subject's responses. If it is not, then there is little to be concerned about; if so, though, there is little that can be done after the fact except to exercise caution in interpreting the results. Unfortunately, the correlations among the social desirability scales are low. Holden and Fekken (1989) found that the Jackson and Edwards scales correlated 0.71, but that the correlation between the Jackson and Crowne–Marlowe scales was only 0.27, and 0.26 between the Edwards and Crowne–Marlowe scales. They interpreted their factor analysis of these three scales to mean that the Jackson and Edwards scales measured 'a sense of own general capability', and the Crowne–Marlowe scale tapped 'interpersonal sensitivity'. Similar results were found by Paulhus (1983, 1984). He believes that his factor analysis of various scales indicates that the Edwards scale taps the more covert tendency of social desirability (what he calls 'self-deception'), while the Crowne–Marlowe scale comprises aspects of both self-deception and faking good (his term is 'impression management'). Despite the negative connotation of the term 'self-deception', there is some evidence that it is a characteristic of well-adjusted people, who are more apt to minimize failures, ignore minor criticisms, and believe they will be successful in undertaking new projects (Paulhus 1986). These findings would explain the relatively low correlation between the Crowne–Marlowe scale and the others.

This leaves the scale constructor in something of a quandary regarding which, if any, SD scale to use. Most people use the Crowne and Marlowe scale, probably more by habit and tradition than because of any superior psychometric qualities. Some have cautioned that, because of the content of its items, the Edwards scale is confounded with psychopathology, primarily neuroticism (Crowne and Marlow 1960; Mick 1996), so that it should be eliminated from the running altogether. The newest scale, the BIDR Version 6 (Paulhus 1994), appears to be the most carefully developed. Although Paulhus recommended scoring the items dichotomously, Stöber *et al.* (2002) found, not surprisingly, that using a continuous 5- or 7-point Likert scale yielded better results.

A second method to measure and reduce SD, used by McFarlane *et al.* (1981) in the development of their *Social Relations Scale*, is to administer the scale twice; once using the regular instructions to the subjects regarding its completion, and then asking them to fill it in as they would like things to be, or in the best of all possible worlds. This involved asking them first to list whom they talk to about issues that come up in their lives in various areas. A few weeks later (by which time they should have forgotten their original responses), they were asked to complete it 'according to what you consider to be good or ideal circumstances'. If the scores on any item did not change from the first to the second administration, it was assumed that its original answer was dictated more by SD than by the true state of affairs (or was at the 'ceiling' and could not detect any improvement). In either case, the item failed to satisfy at least one desired psychometric property, and was eliminated.

The term 'faking good' is most often applied to an intentional and deliberate approach by the person in responding to personality inventories. An analogous bias in responding to items on questionnaires is called 'prestige bias' (Oppenheim 1966). To judge from responses on questionnaires, nobody watches game shows or soap operas on TV, despite their obvious popularity; everyone watches only educational and cultural programs. Their only breaks from these activities are to attend concerts, visit museums, and brush their teeth four or five times each day. (One can only wonder why the concert halls are empty and dentists' waiting rooms are full.)

Whyte (1956, p. 197), only half in jest, gave some advice to business people who had to take personality tests in order for them to advance up the company ladder. He wrote that, in order to select the best reply to a question, the person should repeat to himself:

- I loved my father and my mother, but my father a little bit more.
- I like things pretty well the way they are.
- I never much worry about anything.
- I do not care for books or music much.
- I love my wife and children.
- I do not let them get in the way of company work.

Since faking good and the prestige bias are more volitional than social desirability, they are easier to modify through instructions and careful wording of the items. The success of these tactics, though, is still open to question.

Deviation and faking bad

The opposite of socially desirable responding and faking good are *deviation* and *faking bad*. These latter two phenomena have been less studied than their positive counterparts, and no scales to assess them are in wide use. Deviation is a concept introduced by Berg (1967) to explain (actually, simply to name) the tendency to respond to test items with deviant responses. As is the case for faking good, faking bad occurs primarily within the context of personality assessment, although this may happen any time a person feels he or she may avoid an unpleasant situation (such as the military draft) by looking bad.

Both SD (or perhaps faking good) and deviance (or faking bad) occur together in an interesting phenomenon called the 'hello–goodbye' effect. Before an intervention, a person may present himself in as bad a light as possible, thereby hoping to qualify for the program, and impressing the staff with the seriousness of his problems. At termination, he may want to 'please' the staff with his improvement, and so may minimize any problems. The result is to make it appear that there has been improvement when none has occurred, or to magnify any effects which did occur. This effect was originally described in psychotherapy research, but it may arise whenever a subject is assessed on two occasions, with some intervention between the administrations of the scale.

Three techniques have been proposed to minimize the effects of these different biases. One method is to try to disguise the intent of the test, so the subject does not know what is actually being looked for. Rotter's scale to measure locus of control (Rotter 1966), for example, is called the *Personal Reaction Inventory*, a vague title which conveys little about the purpose of the instrument. (But then again, neither does 'locus of control'.)

However, this deception is of little use if the content of the items themselves reveals the objective of the scale. Thus, the second method consists of using 'subtle' items, ones where the respondent is unaware of the specific trait or behaviour being tapped. The item may still have face validity, since the respondent could feel that the question is fair and relevant; however, its actual relevance may be to some trait other than that assumed by the answerer (Holden and Jackson 1979). For example, the item, 'I would enjoy racing motorcycles' may appear to measure preferences for spending one's leisure time, while in fact it may be on an index of risk-taking. The difficulty with this technique, though, is that the psychometric properties of subtle items are usually poorer than those of obvious ones, and often do not measure the traits for which they were originally intended (Burkhart *et al.* 1976; Jackson 1971).

The third method of minimizing social desirability bias, especially regarding illegal, immoral, or embarrassing behaviors, is called the *random response technique* (Warner 1965). In the most widely used of many variants of the technique, the respondent is handed a card containing two items; one neutral and one sensitive. For example, the statements can be:

A. I own a VCR.

B. I have used street drugs within the past six months.

The respondent is also given a device which randomly selects an A or a B. This can be as simple as a coin, or a spinner mounted on a card divided into two zones, each labeled with one of the letters. He or she is told to flip the coin (or spin the arrow), and truthfully answer whichever item is indicated; the interviewer is not to know *which* question has been selected, only the response.

In practice, only a portion of the respondents are given these items; the remaining subjects are asked the neutral question directly in order to determine the prevalence of 'True' responses to it in the sample. When two or more such items are used, half of the group will be given the random response technique on half of the questions, and asked about the neutral stems for the remaining items; while this would be reversed for the second half of the sample. An alternative is to use a neutral item where the true prevalence is well known, such as the proportion of families owning two cars or with three children. Of course, the scale-developer must be quite sure that the sample is representative of the population on which the prevalence figures were derived.

With this information, the proportion of people answering 'true' to the sensitive item (p_s) can be estimated using the equation:

$$p_s = [p_t - (1 - P) p_d]/P$$

where p_t is the proportion of people who answered 'true', p_d is the proportion saying 'true' to the neutral item on direct questioning, and P is the probability of selecting the sensitive item.

The variance of p_s is:

$$Var(p_s) = \frac{p_t(1 - p_t)}{nP^2}$$

and the estimated standard error is the square root of this.

The probability of selecting the sensitive item (P) is 50 per cent using a coin toss, but can be modified with other techniques. For example, the two zones on the spinner can be divided so that A covers only 30 per cent and B 70 per cent. Another modification uses two colours of balls drawn from an urn; here, the proportion of each colour (representing each stem) can be set at other than 50 per cent. The closer P is to 1.0, the smaller the sample size needed to get an accurate estimate of p_s, but the technique begins to resemble direct questioning, and anonymity becomes jeopardized.

One difficulty with this form of the technique is the necessity to think of neutral questions and estimate their prevalence. An alternative approach, proposed by Greenberg *et al.* (1969), is to divide the spinner into three zones, or use three colours of balls. The subject is required to:

(1) answer the sensitive question truthfully if the spinner lands in zone A (or colour A is chosen);

(2) say 'yes' if the spinner points to zone B; or

(3) say 'no' if it ends up in zone C.

The estimates of p_s and its variance are the same as in the previous case. Although this variant eliminates one problem, it leads to another; some people told to answer 'yes' actually respond 'no' in order to avoid appearing to have engaged in an illegal or embarrassing act.

Another difficulty with the original Warner technique and its variants is that they are limited to asking questions with only dichotomous answers; 'yes–no' or 'true–false'. Greenberg *et al.* (1971) modified this so that both the sensitive and the neutral questions ask for numerical answers, such as:

A. How many times during the past year have you slept with someone who is not your spouse?

B. How many children do you have?

In this case, the estimated mean of the sensitive item (μ_s) is:

$$\mu_s = \frac{(1 - P_1)\,\bar{z}_1 - (1 - P_2)\,\bar{z}_2}{P_1 - P_2}$$

with variance:

$$Var(\mu_s) = \frac{(1 - P_2)^2 \left(\frac{s_1^2}{n_1}\right) + (1 - P_1)^2 \left(\frac{s_2^2}{n_2}\right)}{(P_1 - P_2)^2}$$

where $\bar{z}_1$ is the mean for sample 1, n_1 is its sample size, s_1^2 the variance of $\bar{z}_1$ for sample 1, and P_l the probability of having chosen question A. The terms with the subscript '2' are for a second sample, which is needed to determine the mean value of question B. Other variations on this theme are discussed by Scheers (1992).

The advantage of the random response technique is that it gives a more accurate estimate of the true prevalence of these sensitive behaviours than does direct questioning. For example, nine times as many women reported having had an abortion when asked with the random response method as compared with traditional questioning (Shimizu and Bonham 1978). However, there are some penalties associated with this procedure. First, it is most easily done in face-to-face interviews, although it is possible over the telephone. Second, since it is not known which subjects responded to each stem, the answers cannot be linked to other information from the questionnaire. Third, the calculated prevalence depends upon three estimates: the proportion of subjects responding to the sensitive item; the proportion answering 'true'; and the proportion of people who respond 'true' to the neutral stem. Since each of these is measured with error, a much larger sample size is required to get stable estimates.

Yea-saying or acquiescence

Yea-saying, also called *acquiescence bias*, is the tendency to give positive responses, such as 'true', 'like', 'often', or 'yes', to a question (Couch and Keniston 1960). At its most extreme, the person responds in this way irrespective of the content of the item, so that even mutually contradictory statements are endorsed. Thus, the person may respond 'true' to two items like 'I always take my medication on time' and 'I often forget to take my pills'. At the opposite end of the spectrum are the 'nay-sayers'. It is believed that this tendency is more or less normally distributed, so that relatively few people are at the extremes, but that many people exhibit this trait to lesser degrees.

The amount that has been written about yea- and nay-saying can literally fill volumes. Despite this, there is still considerable controversy whether or not it actually exists. Rorer (1965), for example, acknowledges that some people are more prone to answer 'true' than 'false', but maintains that this tendency exists only on tests which tap a person's knowledge (what he calls 'examinations'), and when the person is ignorant of the correct answer. Insofar as personality tests are concerned, though, he states that his review of the extensive literature failed to show a content-free tendency to agree or disagree with any statement. Just as vehemently, Jackson (1967) and Messick (1967) argue that acquiescence (and its opposite) have been amply demonstrated, and pose real threats to test construction. The recent evidence tends to favour Jackson's and Messick's position. Krosnick (1999) reports that, across 40 studies, the correlation between mutually exclusive items (e.g. 'I enjoy sports' and 'I do not enjoy sports') is only -0.22, whereas the expected correlation is -1.00. He estimates that there is an average acquiescence effect of about 10 per cent in favour of answering True or Yes.

No specific scales have been developed to measure yea-saying or nay-saying. Rather, some people (see, for example, Phillips and Clancy 1970) simply count the number of items on a scale answered positively or negatively by each subject. The usual way to correct for this potential bias is to have an equal number of items keyed in the positive and negative directions. A scale for compliance with medication, then, would be randomly divided so that 'true' on half of the items would reflect compliance, as would 'false' on the remaining ones. As mentioned in Chapter 5, however, the items should be balanced with respect to how they are *keyed*, but negatively *worded* items should be avoided.

End-aversion, positive skew, and halo

In addition to the distortions already mentioned, scales which are scored on a continuum, such as visual analog and Likert scales, are prone to other types of biases. These include end-aversion bias, positive skew, and the halo effect.

End-aversion bias

End-aversion bias, which is also called the *central tendency bias*, refers to the reluctance of some people to use the extreme categories of a scale. It is based in part on people's difficulty in making absolute judgements, since situations without mitigating or extenuating circumstances rarely occur. The problem is similar to the one some people have in responding to 'true–false' items; they often want to say, 'It all depends' or 'Most of the time, but not always'. The effect of this bias is to reduce the range of possible responses. Thus, if the extremes of a five-point Likert scale are labeled 'always' and 'never', an end-aversion bias would render this a three-point scale, with the resulting loss of sensitivity and reliability.

There are two ways of dealing with the end-aversion bias. The first is to avoid absolute statements at the end-points; using 'almost never' and 'almost always' instead of 'never' and 'always'. The problem with this approach is that data may be thrown away; some people may *want* to respond with absolutes, but not allowing them to dilutes their answers with less extreme ones. The advantage is a greater probability that all categories will be used.

The second, and opposite, tack is to include 'throw away' categories at the ends. If the aim is to have a 7-point scale, then 9 alternatives are provided, with the understanding that the extreme boxes at the ends will rarely be checked, but are there primarily to serve as anchors. This more or less ensures that all seven categories of interest will be used, but may lead to the problem of devising more adjectives if each box is labeled.

Positive skew

It often happens, though, that the responses are not evenly distributed over the range of alternatives, but show a positive *skew* toward the favourable end. (Note that this definition of skew is opposite to that used in statistics.) This situation is most acute when a rating scale is used to evaluate students or staff. For example, Linn (1979) found that the mean score on a 5-point scale was 4.11 rather than 3.00, and the scores ranged between 3.30 and 4.56—the lower half of the scale was never used. Similarly, Cowles and Kubany (1959) asked raters to determine if a student was in the lower one-fifth, top one-fifth, or middle three-fifths of the class. Despite these explicit instructions, 31 per cent were assigned to the top fifth and only 5 per cent to the bottom one-fifth.

This may reflect the feeling that since these students survived the hurdles of admission into university and then into professional school, the 'average' student is really quite exceptional. It is then difficult to shift sets, so that 'average' is relative to the other people in the normative group, rather than the general population.

The effect of skew is to produce a *ceiling effect*; since most of the marks are clustered in only a few boxes at one extreme, the scores are very near the top of the scale.

This means that it is almost impossible to detect any improvement, or to distinguish among various grades of excellence.

A few methods have been proposed to counteract this bias, all based on the fact that 'average' need not be in the middle. Since no amount of instruction or training appears to be able to shake an evaluator's belief that the average person under his or her supervision is far above average, the aim of a scale is then to differentiate among degrees of excellence. Using a traditional Likert scale, like:

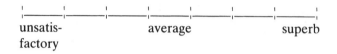

unsatis-   average   superb
factory

will result in most of the scores bunching in the three right-most boxes (or two, if an end-aversion is also present). However, we can shift the centre to look like this:

unsatis- average   superb
factory

This gives the evaluator five boxes above average, rather than just three.

Another strategy is to capitalize on the fact that the truly superb students or employees need little feedback, except to continue doing what they have been all along, while the unsatisfactory ones are readily apparent to all evaluators even without scales. Rather, we should use the scale to differentiate among the majority of people who fall between these extremes. In this situation, the middle is expanded, at the expense of the ends:

out!   below   average   above   much   excel-   great!
       average   average above   lent
                                   average

Note that this version clearly distinguishes the extremes, and offsets 'average'; many other variations on this theme are possible, reflecting the needs and philosophies of the program.

Halo

Halo is a phenomenon first recognized 80 years ago (Wells 1907), whereby judgements made on individual aspects of a person's performance are influenced by the rater's overall impression of the person. Thorndike (1920), who named this effect, gave what is still the best description of it (p. 447):

> The judge seems intent on reporting his final opinion of the strength, weakness, merit, or demerit of the personality as a whole, rather than on giving as discriminating a rating as possible for each separate characteristic.

For example, if a resident is well-regarded by a staff physician, then the resident will be evaluated highly in all areas. Conversely, a resident who is felt to be weak in clinical skills, for example, can do no right, and will receive low scores in all categories. To some degree, this reflects reality; people who are good at one thing tend to do well in related areas. Also, many of the individual categories are dependent upon similar traits or behaviours: the ability to establish rapport with patients likely is dependent on the same skills that are involved in working with nurses and other staff. Cooper (1981) refers to this real correlation among categories as 'true halo'.

However, the ubiquity of this phenomenon and the very high intercorrelations among many different categories indicate that more is going on: what Cooper calls 'illusory halo', and what we commonly refer to when we speak of the 'halo effect'. There have been many theories proposed to explain illusory halo, but many simply boil down to the fact that raters are unable to evaluate people along more than a few dimensions. Very often, one global, summary rating scale about the person conveys as much information as do the individual scales about each aspect of the person's performance.

Many of the techniques proposed to minimize illusory halo involve factors other than the scale itself, such as the training of raters, basing the evaluations on larger samples of behaviour, and using more than one evaluator (e.g. Cooper 1981). The major aspect of scale design, which may reduce this effect, is the use of behaviourally anchored ratings (BARs); instead of simply stating 'below average', for example, concrete examples are used, either as part of the descriptors themselves, or on a separate instruction page (e.g. Streiner 1985). This gives the raters concrete meaning for each level on the scale, reducing the subjective element and increasing agreement among raters.

Framing

Another bias, which particularly affects econometric scaling methods, is called *framing* (Kahneman and Tversky 1984). The name refers to the fact that the person's choice between two alternative states depends on how these states are framed. For example, consider the situation where an outbreak of influenza is expected to kill 600 people in the country. The subject must choose between two programs:

Program A: 200 people will be saved.

Program B: there is a one-third probability that 600 people will be saved, and two-thirds that nobody will be saved.

Nearly 75 per cent of subjects prefer Program A—assurance that 200 people will be saved—rather than the situation which offers the possibility that everyone could be saved, but at the risk of saving no one. Now consider presenting the same situation, but offering two different programs:

Program C: 400 people will die.

Program D: there is a one-third probability that nobody will die, and two-thirds that 600 will die.

Programs A and C are actually the same, as are B and D; all that differs is how the situations are presented (or 'framed'). In A, the number of survivors is explicitly stated, and the number who die (400) is implicit; this is reversed in C, where the number who die is given, but not the number who live. From a purely arithmetic point of view, the proportion of people opting for C, then, should be similar to those who choose A. In fact, over 75 per cent select Program D rather than C, the exact reverse of the first situation.

Kahneman and Tversky explain these seemingly contradictory results by postulating that people are 'risk averse' when gain is involved and 'risk takers' in loss situations. That is, when offered the possibility of a gain (saving lives, winning a bet, and so on), people tend to take the safer route of being sure they gain something, rather than the riskier alternative of perhaps getting much more but possibly losing everything. In loss situations, though, such as choosing between Programs C and D, people will gamble on minimizing their losses (although there is the risk that they can lose everything), rather than taking the certain situation that they will lose something.

The problem that this poses for the designer of questionnaires is that the manner in which a question is posed can affect the results that are obtained. For example, if the researchers were interested in physicians' attitudes toward a new operation or drug, they may get very different answers if they said that the incidence of morbidity was 0.1 per cent, as opposed to saying that there was a 99.9 per cent chance that nothing untoward would occur.

In conclusion, the safest strategy for the test developer is to assume that all of these biases are operative, and take the necessary steps to minimize them whenever possible.

Biases related to the measurement of change

Earlier in the chapter, we noted briefly that questions of the form, 'Compared to how you were a year ago...' should be viewed with considerable skepticism, since they require prodigious feats of memory. That is, in answering a question of this form, the respondents are required, self-evidently, to compare their present state to how they were a year ago, and subjectively estimate the amount of change that has occurred in the interim. As we indicated, people's memories for events over a period as long as one year is extremely fallible.

A moment's reflection will serve to indicate that some memories are fallible over time periods far shorter than one year. While you may be able to recall what you had for dinner on your last birthday, it is quite unlikely that you will be able to recall what you ate last Tuesday (unless it was your birthday). As a consequence, it is plausible that measures of change from a previous health state may be vulnerable to possible biases.

Despite these concerns, there has been considerable recent interest in so-called 'transition' measures, which ask the patient to estimate change from a previous state. As one example, a method used to determine the minimally important difference in quality of life on a standard questionnaire asks the patient to consider a four- to six-week time period and first state whether she is better, the same or worse, and then indicate on a 7-point scale how much she has changed, from *slightly better* to *a great deal better*.

A critical test of whether such estimates are biased is to examine the correlation between the subjective measure of change in health and (a) the present state, or (b) the initial state, as measured by, for example, a standard index of health-related quality of life. If the transition measure is unbiased, and the variances of the pre-test and post-test are equal, then the correlations with pre-test and post-test should be equal and opposite (Guyatt *et al.* 2002). That does not turn out to be the case; typically, the correlation with pre-test is much smaller than post-test (Guyatt *et al.* 2002; Norman *et al.* 1997).

It would appear, then, that transition measures are potentially biased in favour of the present state. But is this simply a reflection of fallible memory for the previous state? Here, the plot thickens. Two theories have emerged to explain this phenomenon— *Response Shift* and *Implicit Theories of Change*. Both specifically address the issue of assessment of a prior health state, which may have occurred days or months earlier. Both also attempt to reconcile the difference which arises between prospective measures, gathered at the time, and retrospective measures, looking back on the previous state. Interestingly, they arrive at opposite conclusions as to the relative validity of prospective and retrospective measures.

Estimates of the prior state—response shift

According to the theory of response shift, one's judgement of health may stay relatively stable despite large changes in objective measures of health, or alternatively, judgements of health may change in a situation where there is no objective change in health, because the criterion of good health has shifted in light of new information (Schwartz and Sprangers 1999). It has been invoked as an explanation for several paradoxes in the health literature, such as:

(1) patients with chronic diseases rate their quality of life similarly to non-patients;

(2) patients tend to rate their quality of life higher than do their providers; and

(3) discrepancies arise between objective measures of health and self-rated health.

Response shift rests on the assumption that a change in a retrospective rating of a prior health state, in comparison with the initial rating, results from new insights or new standards, hence represents a reasoned change, which is, in principle, knowable through sufficiently careful and rigorous inquiry regarding the cognitive variables underlying the judgement (although Schwartz and Sprangers allow that this may not always be the case). The changes resulting from response shift are unidirectional and enduring, resulting directly from stable changes in internal states. Hence, the retrospective judgement of a health state is more valid because more information is available on the second occasion.

Estimates of the prior state—implicit theory of change

An alternative view is that, in fact, people do not remember the previous state. Instead, their judgement is based on an 'implicit theory' of change beginning with their present state and working backwards (Ross 1989). People begin with 'How do I feel today?', then ask themselves, 'How do I think that things have been changing over the past weeks (months, years)?'. This implicit theory of change might imply that there has been steady improvement, deterioration, no change, improvement followed by leveling off, or several other possibilities. But it is based on an impression of the time course, not on analysis of health at specific time points. Finally, the respondents work back from their present state, using their 'implicit theory' to infer what their initial state must have been. From this position, the retrospective judgement of the initial state is viewed as biased, and the prospective judgement obtained at the time is more valid.

Reconciling the two positions

Interestingly, these two theories—response shift and implicit theory of change—can examine the same data showing a low correlation between a retrospective and a prospective judgement of a prior health state (or equivalently, a low correlation between a judgement of change and the pre-test) and arrive at opposite conclusions. For the response shift theorist, a retrospective judgement derives from additional information which was, by definition, not available at the time of the initial assessment; hence the retrospective judgement is more valid. The implicit theorist presumes that the discrepancy does not arise from a conscious adjustment of the initial state at all, but instead begins with the present state and invokes an implicit theory of change, which cannot be externally verified. From the perspective of implicit theory, the retrospective test is based on two information sources which are irrelevant to the initial judgement—the present state, and the theory of change. Hence, the prospective assessment is more valid.

At the time of writing, no critical comparative test of these theories has been conducted. Indeed, it is not at all straightforward to determine what might constitute a critical test (Norman 2003). Regardless, one clear conclusion is possible. Retrospective judgements of change based on recall of a previous state are not at all straightforward and unbiased. The uncritical application of 'transition' measures (which regrettably, is all too common) is fraught with potential problems of interpretation.

References

Allen, G. I., Breslow, L., Weissman, A., and Nisselson, H. (1954). Interviewing versus diary keeping in eliciting information in a morbidity survey. *American Journal of Public Health*, 44, 919–27.

Anastasi, A. (1982). *Psychological testing* (5th edn). Macmillan, New York.

Berg, I. A. (1967). The deviation hypothesis: A broad statement of its assumptions and postulates. In *Response set in personality assessment* (ed. I. A. Berg) pp. 146–90. Aldine, Chicago.

Berke, R. L. (1998). Clinton's O. K. in the polls, right? *New York Times*, February 15, pp. 1, 5.

Burkhart, B. R., Christian, W. L., and Gynther, M. D. (1976). Item subtlety and faking on the MMPI: A paradoxical relationship. *Journal of Personality Assessment*, 42, 76–80.

Cannell, C. F., Fisher, G., and Bakker, T. (1965). Reporting on hospitalization in the Health Interview Survey. *Vital and Health Statistics*. Series 3, No. 6. Public Health Service, Hyattsville, MD.

Cooper, W. H. (1981). Ubiquitous halo. *Psychological Bulletin*, **90**, 218–44.

Couch, A. and Keniston, K. (1960). Yeasayers and naysayers: Agreeing response set as a personality variable. *Journal of Abnormal and Social Psychology*, **60**, 151–74.

Cowles, J. T. and Kubany, A. J. (1959). Improving the measurement of clinical performance in medical students. *Journal of Clinical Psychology*, **15**, 139–42.

Crowne, D. P. and Marlowe, D. (1960). A new scale of social desirability independent of psychopathology. *Journal of Consulting Psychology*, **24**, 349–54.

Edwards, A. L. (1957). *The social desirability variable in personality assessments and research*. Dryden, New York.

Greenberg, B. C., Abul-Ela, A., Simmons, W., and Horvitz, D. (1969). The unrelated question randomized response model: Theoretical framework. *Journal of the American Statistical Association*, **64**, 520–39.

Greenberg, B. C., Kuebler, R. R., Abernathy, J. R., and Horvitz, D. G. (1971). Application of the randomized response technique in obtaining quantitative data. *Journal of the American Statistical Association*, **66**, 243–50.

Guyatt, G. H., Norman, G. R., and Juniper, E. F. (2002). A critical look at transition ratings. *Journal of Clinical Epidemiology*, **55**, 900–8.

Holden, R. R. and Fekken, G. C. (1989). Three common social desirability scales: Friends, acquaintances, or strangers? *Journal of Research in Personality*, **23**, 180–91.

Holden, R. R. and Jackson, D. N. (1979). Item subtlety and face validity in personality assessment. *Journal of Consulting and Clinical Psychology*, **47**, 459–68.

Jackson, D. N. (1967). Acquiescence response styles: Problems of identification and control. In *Response set in personality assessment* (ed. I. A. Berg) pp. 71–114. Aldine, Chicago.

Jackson, D. N. (1970). A sequential system for personality scale development. In *Current topics in clinical and community psychology*, Vol. 2 (ed. C. D. Spielberger) pp. 61–96. Academic Press, New York.

Jackson, D. N. (1971). The dynamics of structured personality tests: 1971. *Psychological Review*, **78**, 229–48.

Jackson, D. N. (1984). *Personality Research Form manual*. Research Psychologists Press, Port Huron, MI.

Kahneman, D. and Tversky, A. (1984). Choices, values, and frames. *American Psychologist*, **39**, 341–50.

Krosnick, J. A. (1991). Response strategies for coping with the cognitive demands of attitude measures in surveys. *Applied Cognitive Psychology*, **5**, 213–36.

Krosnick, J. A. (1999). Survey research. *Annual Review of Psychology*, **50**, 537–67.

Linn, L. (1979). Interns' attitudes and values as antecedents of clinical performance. *Journal of Medical Education*, **54**, 238–40.

Linton, M. (1975). Memory for real world events. In *Explorations in cognition* (ed. D. A. Norman and D. E. Rumelhart) pp. 376–404. Freeman, San Francisco.

McFarlane, A. H., Neale, K. A., Norman, G. R., Roy, R. G., and Streiner, D. L. (1981). Methodological issues in developing a scale to measure social support. *Schizophrenia Bulletin*, **1**, 90–100.

Means, B., Nigam, A., Zarrow, M., Loftus, E. F., and Donaldson, M. S. (1989). Autobiographical memory for health-related events. *Vital and Health Statistics*. Series 6, No. 2. Public Health Service, Hyattsville, MD.

Messick, S. J. (1967). The psychology of acquiescence: An interpretation of the research evidence. In *Response set in personality assessment* (ed. I. A. Berg) pp. 115–45. Aldine, Chicago.

Mick, D. G. (1996). Are studies of dark side variables confounded by socially desirable responding? The case of materialism. *Journal of Consumer Research,* **23,** 106–19.

Neisser, U. (1986). Nested structure in autobiographical memory. In *Autobiographical memory* (ed. D. C. Rubin) pp. 71–81. Cambridge University Press, Cambridge.

Norcross, J. C., Karg, R. S., and Prochaska, J. O. (1997). Clinical psychologist in the 1990s: II. *The Clinical Psychologist,* **5**(3), 4–11.

Norman, G. R. (2003). Hi! How are you? Response shift, implicit theories and differing epistemologies. *Quality of Life Research,* **12,** 239–49.

Norman, G. R., Regehr, G., and Stratford, P. S. (1997). Bias in the retrospective calculation of responsiveness to change: The lesson of Cronbach. *Journal of Clinical Epidemiology,* **8,** 869–79.

Oppenheim, A. N. (1966). *Questionnaire design and attitude measurement.* Heinemann, London.

Paulhus, D. L. (1983). Sphere-specific measures of perceived control. *Journal of Personality and Social Psychology,* **44,** 1253–65.

Paulhus, D. L. (1984). Two-component models of socially desirable responding. *Journal of Personality and Social Psychology,* **46,** 598–609.

Paulhus, D. L. (1986). Self deception and impression management in test responses. In *Personality assessment via questionnaire* (ed. A. Angleitner and J. S. Wiggins) pp. 143–65. Springer, New York.

Paulhus, D. L. (1994). *Balanced Inventory of Desirable Responding: Reference manual for BIDR Version 6.* Unpublished manuscript, University of British Columbia, Vancouver, BC.

Phillips, D. L. and Clancy, K. J. (1970). Response biases in field studies of mental illness. *American Sociological Review,* **35,** 503–15.

Rorer, L. G. (1965). The great response-style myth. *Psychological Bulletin,* **63,** 129–56.

Ross, M. (1989). Relation of implicit theories to the construction of personal histories. *Psychological Review,* **96,** 341–7.

Rotter, J. (1966). Generalized expectancies for internal versus external control of reinforcement. *Psychological Monographs: General and Applied,* **80** (1, Whole No. 609).

Scheers, N. J. (1992). A review of randomized response techniques. *Measurement and Evaluation in Counseling and Development,* **25,** 27–41.

Shimizu, I. M. and Bonham, G. S. (1978). Randomized response technique in a national survey. *Journal of the American Statistical Association,* **73,** 35–9.

Schwartz, C. E. and Sprangers, M. A. G. (1999). Methodological approaches for assessing response shift in longitudinal health related quality of life research. *Social Science and Medicine,* **48,** 1531–48.

Schwarz, N. (1999). Self-reports: How the questions shape the answers. *American Psychologist,* **54,** 93–105.

Schwarz, N. and Oyserman, D. (2001). Asking questions about behavior: Cognition, communication, and questionnaire construction. *American Journal of Education,* **22,** 127–60.

Simon, H. A. (1957). *Models of man.* Wiley, New York.

Stöber, J., Dette, D. E., and Musch, J. (2002). Comparing continuous and dichotomous scoring of the Balanced Inventory of Desirable Responding. *Journal of Personality Assessment,* **78,** 370–89.

Streiner, D. L. (1985). Global rating scales. In *Assessing clinical competence* (ed. V. R. Neufeld and G. R. Norman) pp. 119–41. Springer, New York.

Sudman, S. and Bradburn, N. M. (1982). *Asking questions: A practical guide to questionnaire design.* Jossey-Bass, San Francisco.

Sudman, S., Bradburn, N. M., and Schwarz, N. (1996). *Thinking about answers: The application of cognitive processes to survey methodology.* Jossey-Bass, San Francisco.

Thorndike, E. L. (1920). A constant error in psychological ratings. *Journal of Applied Psychology*, **4**, 25–9.

Tourangeau, R. (1984). Cognitive sciences and survey methods. In *Cognitive aspects of survey methodology: Building a bridge between disciplines* (ed. T. Jabine, M. Straf, J. Tanur, and R. Tourangeau) pp. 73–100. National Academy Press, Washington DC.

Warner, S. L. (1965). Randomized response: A survey technique for eliminating evasive answer bias. *Journal of the American Statistical Association*, **60**, 63–9.

Wells, F. L. (1907). A statistical study of literary merit. *Archives of Psychology*, **1**(7).

Whyte, W. H., Jr. (1956). *The organization man*. Simon and Schuster, New York.

Winkielman, P., Knäuper, B., and Schwarz, N. (1998). Looking back at anger: Reference periods change the interpretation of (emotion) frequency questions. *Journal of Personality and Social Psychology*, **75**, 719–28.

Chapter 7

From items to scales

Some scales consist of just one item, such as a visual analog scale, on which a person may rate his or her pain on a continuum from 'no pain at all' to 'the worst imaginable pain'. However, the more usual and desirable approach is to have a number of items to assess a single underlying characteristic. This then raises the issue of how we combine the individual items into a scale, and then express the final score in the most meaningful way.

By far the easiest solution is to simply add the scores on the individual items and leave it at that. In fact, this is the approach used by many scales. The *Beck Depression Inventory* (BDI; Beck *et al.* 1961), for instance, consists of 21 items, each scored on a 0–3 scale, so the final score can range between 0 and 63. This approach is conceptually and arithmetically simple, and makes few assumptions about the individual items; the only implicit assumption is that the items are equally important in contributing to the total score.

Since this approach is so simple, there must be something wrong with it. Actually, there are two potential problems. We say 'potential' because, as will be seen later, they may not be problems in certain situations. First, some items may be more important than others, and perhaps should make a larger contribution to the total score. Second, unlike the situation in measuring blood pressure, for example, where it is expected that each of the different methods should yield exactly the same answer, no one presumes that all scales tapping activities of daily living should give the same number at the end. Under these circumstances, it is difficult, if not impossible, to compare scores on different scales, since each uses a different metric. We shall examine both of these points in some more detail.

Weighting the items

Rather than simply adding up all of the items, a scale or index may be developed which 'weights' each item differently in its contribution to the total score. There are two general approaches to doing this, theoretical and empirical. In the former, a test constructor may feel that, based on his or her understanding of the field, there are some aspects of a trait that are crucial, and others which are still interesting, but perhaps less germane. It would make at least intuitive sense for the former to be weighted more heavily than the latter. For example, in assessing the recovery of a cardiac patient, his or her ability to return to work may be seen as more important than resumption of leisure-time activities. In this case, the scale-developer may multiply, or weight, the score on items relating to the first set of activities by a factor which would reflect its greater importance. (Perhaps we should mention here that the term 'weight' is preferred by statisticians to the more commonly used 'weigh'.)

The empirical approach comes from the statistical theory of multiple regression. Very briefly, in multiple regression we try to predict a score (Y) from a number of independent items *(Xs)*, and takes the form:

$$Y = \beta_0 + \beta_1 X_1 + \beta_2 X_2 + \ldots + \beta_k X_k$$

where β_0 is a constant, and $\beta_1 \ldots \beta_k$ are the 'beta weights' for the k items.

We choose the βs to maximize the predictive accuracy of the equation. There is one optimal set, and any other set of values will result in less accuracy. In the case of a scale, Y is the trait or behaviour we are trying to predict, and the Xs are the individual items. This would indicate that a weighting scheme for each item, empirically derived, would improve the accuracy of the total score (leaving aside for the moment the question of what we mean by 'accuracy').

One obvious penalty for this greater sophistication introduced by weighting is increased computation. Each item's score must be multiplied by a constant, and these then added together; a process which is more time-consuming and prone to error than treating all items equally (i.e. giving them all weights of 1).

The question then is whether the benefits outweigh the costs. The answer is that it all depends. Wainer's (1976) conclusion was that if we eliminate items with very small β weights (that is, those that contribute little to the overall accuracy anyway), then 'it don't make no nevermind' whether the other items are weighted or not.

This was demonstrated empirically by Lei and Skinner (1980), using the Holmes and Rahe (1967) *Social Readjustment Rating Scale* (SRRS). This checklist consists of events that may have occurred in the past six months, and weighted to reflect how much adjustment would be required to adapt to it. Lei and Skinner looked at four versions of the SRRS:

(1) using the original weights assigned by Holmes and Rahe;

(2) using simply a count of the number of items endorsed, which is the same as using weights of 1 for all items;

(3) using 'perturbed' weights, where they were randomly shuffled from one item to another; and

(4) using randomly assigned weights, ranging between 1 and 100.

The life events scale would appear to be an ideal situation for using weights, since there is a 100-fold difference between the lowest and highest. On the surface, at least, this differential weighting makes sense, since it seems ridiculous to assign the same weight to the death of a spouse as to receiving a parking ticket. However, they found that the correlations among these four versions was 0.97. In other words, it did not matter whether original weights, random weights, or no weights were used; people who scored high on one variant scored high on all of the others, and similarly for people who scored at the low end. Similar results with the SRRS were found by Streiner *et al.* (1981).

Moreover, this finding is not peculiar to the SRRS; it has been demonstrated with a wide variety of personality and health status measures (e.g. Jenkinson 1991; Streiner *et al.* 1993). Indeed, Gulliksen (1950) derived an equation to predict how much (or rather, how little) item weighting will affect a scale's correlation with other measures, and hence its validity. The correlation (*R*) between the weighted and unweighted versions of a test is:

$$R = 1 - \left(\frac{1}{2\,K\bar{r}}\right)\left(\frac{s}{M}\right)^2$$

where *K* is the number of items in the scale; $\bar{r}$ is the average correlation among the *K* items; *M* is the average of the weights; and *s* is the standard deviation of the weights.

What this equation shows is that the correlation between the weighted and unweighted versions of the test is higher when:

(1) there are more items;

(2) the average inter-item correlation is higher; and

(3) the standard deviation of the weights is lower relative to their mean value.

Empirical testing has shown that actual values are quite close to those predicted by the formula (Retzlaff *et al.* 1990; Streiner and Miller 1989).

To complicate matters, though, a very different conclusion was reached by Perloff and Persons (1988). They indicated that weighting can significantly increase the predictive ability of an index, and criticize Wainer's work because he limited his discussion to situations where the β weights were evenly distributed over the interval from 0.25 to 0.75, which they feel is an improbable situation.

So, what conclusion can we draw from this argument? The answer is far from clear. It would seem that when there are at least 40 items in a scale, differential weighting contributes relatively little, except added complexity for the scorer. With fewer than 40 items (20, according to Nunnally, 1970), weighting *may* have some effect. The other consideration is that if the scale is comprised of relatively homogeneous items, where the β weights will all be within a fairly narrow range, the effect of weighting may be minimal. However, if an index consists of unrelated items, as is sometimes the case with functional status measures, then it may be worthwhile to run a multiple regression analysis and determine empirically if this improves the predictive ability of the scale.

There are two forms of weighting that are more subtle than multiplying each item by a number, and are often unintended. The first is having a different number of items for various aspects of the trait being measured, and the second is including items which are highly correlated with one another. To illustrate the first point, assume we are devising a scale to assess childhood difficulties. In this instrument, we have one item tapping into problems associated with going to bed, and five items looking at disciplinary problems. This implicitly assigns more weight to the latter category, since its potential contribution to the total score can be five times as great as the first area. Even if the parents feel that putting the child to bed is more troublesome to them than the child's lack of discipline, the scale would be weighted in the opposite direction.

There are a few ways around this problem. First, the number of items tapping each component can be equal (which assumes that all aspects contribute equally) or proportional to the importance of that area. An item-by-item matrix can be used to verify this, as was discussed in Chapter 3. A second solution is to have subscales, each comprised of items in one area. The total for the sub-scale would be the number of items endorsed divided by the total number of items within the sub-scale (and perhaps multiplied by 10 or 100 to eliminate decimals). The scale total is then derived by adding up these transformed sub-scale scores. In this way, each sub-scale contributes equally to the total score, even though each sub-scale may consist of a different number of items.

The second form of implicit weighting is through correlated items. Using the same example of a scale for childhood problems, assume that the section on school-related difficulties includes the following items:

1. Is often late for school.

2. Talks back to the teacher.

3. Often gets into fights.

4. Does not obey instructions.

5. Ignores the teacher.

If items 2, 4, and 5 are highly correlated, then getting a score on any one of them almost automatically leads to scores on the other two. Thus, these three items are likely measuring the same thing and, as such, constitute a sub-sub-scale, and lead to problems analogous to those found with the first form of subtle weighting. The same solutions can be used, as well as a third solution: eliminating two of the items. This problem is almost universal, since we expect items tapping the same trait to be correlated; just not *too* correlated.

Unlike explicit weighting, these two forms are often unintentional. If the effects are unwanted (as they often are), special care and pre-testing the instrument are necessary to ensure that they do not occur.

Multiplicative composite scores

The previous section focused on the situation in which each item was given the same weight, and the conclusion was that it is hardly ever worth the effort. In this section, we will discuss a seemingly similar case—where each item is given a different weight by different subjects—and come to a similar recommendation: do not do it unless it is unavoidable or you are prepared to pay the price in terms of increased sample size and complexity in analysing the results.

Multiplicative composite scores are those in which two values are multiplied together to yield one number. At first glance, this would seem to be a very useful maneuver with few drawbacks. Imagine, for example, that supervisors must rate interns on a form which lists a number of components, such as clinical skills, interpersonal skills, self-directed learning, and knowledge base. In any one rotation, the supervisor may have had ample opportunity to observe how the student performs in some of these areas, but may have had a more limited chance to see others. It would seem to make sense that we should ask the supervisor a second question for each component, 'How confident are you in this rating?'. Then, when the rating is multiplied by the confidence level, those areas in which the supervisor was more confident would make a greater contribution to the total score, and areas where the supervisor was not as confident would add less. Similarly, if you were devising a quality of life scale, it would seem sensible to multiply people's rating of how well or poorly they could perform some task by some other index, which reflects the importance of that task for them. In that way, a person would not be penalized by being unable to do tasks that are done rarely or not at all (e.g. males are not too concerned about their inability to reach behind their back to do up their bra, nor females by the fact that they have difficulty shaving their faces each morning). Conversely, the total score on the scale would be greatly affected by the important tasks, thus making it easier to detect any changes in quality of life due to some intervention or over time.

The problem arises because multiplying two numbers together (i.e. creating a composite measure) affects the resulting total's correlation with another score. More importantly, even if the ratings are kept the same, but simply transformed from one weighting scheme to another (e.g. changed from a -3 to $+3$ system to a 1- to 7-point scheme), *the scale's correlation with another scale can alter dramatically.*

To illustrate this, imagine that we have an instrument with five items, where each item is scored along a 7-point Likert scale. These are then summed, to form a score (X) for each of five subjects. The items, and their sums, are shown in the second column of Table 7.1, the one labeled Item Score (X). If we correlate these five totals with some other measure, labeled Y in Table 7.1, we find that the correlation is 0.927.

Next assume that each item is weighted for importance on a 7-point scale, with 1 indicating not at all important, and 7 extremely important (column 3 in Table 7.1). These scores are then multiplied by X, and the result, along with each subject's total, are shown in column 4. If we correlate these totals with the Ys, we find that the result is 0.681. Now comes the interesting part. Let us keep exactly the same weights for each person but score them on a 7-point scale, where not at all important is -3, and extremely important is $+3$; that is, we have done nothing more than subtract four points from each weight. The results of this are shown in the last two columns.

Has this changed anything? Amazingly, the results are drastically different. Instead of a correlation of $+0.681$, we now find that the correlation is -0.501. That is, by keeping the weights the same, and simply modifying the numbers assigned to each point on the scale, we have transformed a relatively high positive correlation into an almost equally high negative one. Other linear transformations of the weights can make the correlation almost any value in between (or even more extreme).

Why should this be? The mathematics of it are beyond the scope of this book (the interested reader should look at Evans (1991) for a complete explanation). A brief summary is that the correlation between X and Y, where X is a composite score,

Table 7.1 The effects of changing weighting schemes

Subject	Item score		+l to +7 Weighting		−3 to +3 Weighting	
	(X)	Y	Weight	Total	Weight	Total
1	7		1	7	−3	−21
	5		2	10	−2	−10
	7		3	21	−1	−7
	6		4	24	0	0
	3		5	15	1	3
Total	28	25		77		−35
2	1		6	6	2	2
	3		7	21	3	9
	1		1	1	−3	−3
	2		2	4	−2	−4
	4		3	12	−1	−4
Total	11	13		44		0
3	3		4	12	0	0
	4		5	20	1	4
	5		6	30	2	10
	4		7	28	3	12
	3		1	3	−3	−3
Total	19	18		93		23
4	5		2	10	−2	−10
	7		3	21	−1	−7
	6		4	24	0	0
	3		5	15	1	3
	2		6	12	2	4
Total	23	26		82		−10
5	2		7	14	3	6
	3		1	3	−3	−9
	2		2	4	−2	−4
	4		3	12	−1	−4
	5		4	20	0	0
Total	16	15		53		−11

depends in part on the variance of the weight, the covariance between X and the weight, and the mean of the weight. Thus, a change which affects any of these factors, but especially the weight's mean, can drastically affect the magnitude and the sign of the correlation.

There is a way to overcome the problem, but it is a costly one in terms of sample size. The method is to use hierarchical regression; that is, where the predictor variables are put into the regression equation in stages, under the control of the investigator (see Norman and Streiner (2000) for a fuller explanation). In the first step, any covariates are forced into the model. In step two, the X variable and the weights are added as two additional variables. In the third step, the interaction (i.e. the multiplication) of X and the weight is forced in. Any significant increase in the multiple correlation from step 1 to step 2 would indicate that the variables add something to the prediction of Y. Then, the real test of the hypothesis is to see if the multiple correlation increases significantly between the second and third steps; if so, it would show that the interaction between X and the weight adds something over and above what the variables tell us separately. Of course, we can also break step 2 down, to see if the weights themselves increase the predictive power of the equation.

The cost is that, rather than having one predictor and one dependent variable (ignoring any covariates), we now have three predictors: X, the weighting factor, and the interaction between the two. If we want to maintain a ratio of at least 10 subjects for every predictor variable (Norman and Streiner 2000), this triples the required sample size. In the end, unless one's theory demands an interaction term, multiplicative composites should be avoided.

Transforming the final score

The second drawback with simply adding up the items to derive a total score is that each new scale is reported on a different metric, making comparisons among scales difficult. This may not pose a problem if you are working in a brand new area, and do not foresee comparing the results to any other test. However, few such areas exist, and in most cases it is desirable to see how a person did on two different instruments. For example, the *BDI*, as we have said, ranges between a minimum score of 0 and a maximum of 63; while a similar test, the *Self-Rating Depression Scale* (SRDS; Zung 1965), yields a total score between 25 and 100. How can we compare a score of 23 on the former with one of 68 on the latter? It is not easy when the scores are expressed as they are.

The problem is even more evident when a test is comprised of many subscales, each with a different number of items. Many personality tests, like the *16PF* (Cattell *et al.* 1970) or the *Personality Research Form* (Jackson 1984) are constructed in such a manner, as are intelligence tests like those developed by Wechsler (1981). The resulting 'profile' of scale scores, comparing their relative elevations, would be uninterpretable if each scale were measured on a different yardstick.

The solution to this problem involves *transforming* the raw score in some way in order to facilitate interpretation. In this section, we discuss three different methods: percentiles, standard and standardized scores, and normalized scores.

Percentiles

A *percentile* is the percentage of people who score below a certain value; the lowest score is at the 0th percentile, since nobody has a lower one, while the top score is at the 99th percentile. Nobody can be at the 100th percentile, since that implies that everyone, including that person, has a lower score, an obvious impossibility. In medicine, perhaps the most widely used example of scales expressed in percentiles are developmental height and weight charts. After a child has been measured, his height is plotted on a table for children the same age. If he is at the 50th percentile, that means that he is exactly average for his age; half of all children are taller and half are shorter.

To show how these are calculated, assume a new test has been given to a large, representative sample, which is called a 'normative' or 'reference' group. If the test is destined to be used commercially, 'large' often means 1000 or more carefully selected people; for more modest aims, 'large' can mean about 100 or so. The group should be chosen so that their scores span the range you would expect to find when you finally use the test. The next step is to put the scores in *rank order*, ranging from the highest to the lowest. For illustrative purposes, suppose the normative group consists of (a ridiculously small number) 20 people. The results would look something like Table 7.2.

Starting with the highest score, a 37 for Subject 5, 19 of the 20 scores are lower, so a raw score of 37 corresponds to the 95th percentile. Subject 3 has a raw score of 21; since 12 of the 20 scores are lower, he is at the 60th percentile (i.e. 12/20). A slight problem arises when there are ties, as with Subjects 17 and 8, or 19 and 14. If there are an odd number of ties, as exists for a score of 16, we take the middle person

Table 7.2 Raw scores for 20 subjects on a hypothetical test

Subject	Score	Subject	Score
5	37	19	17
13	32	14	17
2	31	1	16
15	29	20	16
17	26	7	16
8	23	6	15
10	23	11	13
3	21	16	12
12	20	4	10
18	19	9	8

Table 7.3 The raw scores converted to percentiles

Subject	Score	Percentile	Subject	Score	Percentile
5	37	95	19	17	42.5
13	32	90	14	17	42.5
2	31	85	1	16	35
15	29	80	20	16	35
17	26	75	7	16	35
8	23	67.5	6	15	25
10	23	67.5	11	13	20
3	21	60	16	12	10
12	20	55	4	10	5
18	18	50	9	8	0

(Subject 20 in this case), and count the number of people below. Since there are six of them, a raw score of 16 is at the 30th percentile, and all three people then get this value. If there are an even number of ties, then you will be dealing with 'halves' of a person. Thus, 8.5 people have scores lower than 17, so it corresponds to the 42.5th percentile. We continue doing this for all scores, and then rewrite the table, putting in the percentiles corresponding to each score, as in Table 7.3.

The major advantage of percentiles is that most people, even those without any training in statistics or scale development, can readily understand them. However, there are a number of difficulties with this approach. One problem is readily apparent in Table 7.3; unless you have many scores, there can be fairly large jumps between the percentile values of adjacent scores. Also, it is possible that in a new sample, some people may have scores higher or lower than those in the normative group, especially if it was small and not carefully chosen. This makes interpretation of these more extreme scores problematic at best. Third, since percentiles are ordinal data, they should not be analyzed using parametric statistics; means and standard deviations derived from percentiles are not legitimate.

A fourth difficulty with percentiles is a bit more subtle, but just as insidious. The distribution of percentile scores is rectangular. However, the distribution of raw test scores usually resembles a normal, or bell-shaped, curve, with most of the values clustered around the mean, and progressively fewer ones as we move out to the extremes. As a result, small differences in the middle range become exaggerated, and large differences in the tails are truncated. For example, a score of 16 corresponds to the 35th percentile, while a score just two points higher is at the 50th percentile. By contrast, a five-point difference, from 32 to 37, results in just a five-point spread in the percentiles.

Standard and standardized scores

To get around these problems with percentiles, a more common approach is to use *standard scores*. The formula to transform raw scores to standard scores is:

$$z = \frac{X - \overline{X}}{\text{SD}}$$

where X is the total score for an individual, $\overline{X}$ is the mean score of the sample, and SD is the sample's standard deviation.

This 'transforms' the scale to have a mean of 0 and a standard deviation of 1, so the individual scores are expressed in standard deviation units. Moreover, since the transformation is linear, the distribution of the raw scores (ideally normal) is preserved. For example, the mean of the 20 scores in the table is 20.0, and the standard deviation is 7.75. We can convert Subject 5's score of 37 into a z-score by putting these numbers into the formula. When we do this, we find:

$$z = \frac{37 - 20}{7.75} = 2.19.$$

That is, his score of 37 is slightly more than two standard deviations above the mean on this scale. Similarly, a raw score of 12 yields a z-score of -1.55, showing that this person's score is about one and a half standard deviations below the group mean.

If all test scores were expressed in this way, then we could compare results across them quite easily. Indeed, we can use this technique on raw scores from different tests, as long as we have the means and standard deviations of the tests. Then, if we received scores on two tests given to a patient at two different times, and purportedly measuring the same thing, we can see if there has been any change by transforming both of them to z-scores. As an example, we can now answer the question, how does a score of 23 on the *BDI* compare with 68 on the *SRDS*? The mean and SD of the Beck are 11.3 and 7.7, and they are 52.1 and 10.5 for the Zung. Putting the raw scores into the equation with their respective means and SDs, we find that 23 on the Beck corresponds to a z-score of 1.52, and 65 on the Zung yields a z-score of 1.51. So, although the raw scores are very different, they probably reflect similar degrees of depression.

In real life, though, we are not used to seeing scores ranging from about -3.0 to $+3.0$; we are more accustomed to positive numbers only, and whole ones at that. Very often, then, we take a second step and transform the z-score into what is called a *standardized* or *T-score*, by using the formula:

$$T = \overline{X}' + z(\text{SD}')$$

where $\overline{X}'$ is the new mean that we want the test to have, SD' is the desired standard deviation, and z is the original z-score.

We can also go directly from the raw scores to the T-scores by combining this equation with that for the z-score transformation, in which case we get:

$$T = \bar{X}' + \frac{(\text{SD}')(X - \bar{X})}{\text{SD}}$$

A standardized or T-score is simply a z-score with a new mean and standard deviation, chosen relatively arbitrarily, and depending on custom, tradition, or just whim. For example, many personality tests use a mean of 50 and a standard deviation of 10 by convention; while the national tests for admission to university, graduate school, or professional programs use a mean of 500 and an SD of 100. Intelligence tests, for the most part, have a mean of 100 and an SD of 15. If we were developing a new IQ test, we would give it to a large normative sample and then transform each possible total raw score into a z-score. Then, setting $\bar{X}'$ to be 100 and SD$'$ to be 15, we would translate each z-score into its equivalent T-score. The result would be a new test, whose scores are directly comparable to those from older IQ tests.

The z- and T-scores do more than simply compare the results on two different tests. Like percentiles, they allow us to see where a person stands in relation to everybody else. If we assume that the scores on the test are fairly normally distributed, then we use the normal curve to determine what proportion of people score higher and lower. As a brief review, a normal curve looks like Fig. 7.1. Most of the scores are clustered around the mean of the test, with progressively fewer scores as we move out to the tails. By definition, 50 per cent of the scores fall below the mean, and 50 per cent above; while 68 per cent are between -1 and $+1$ SD. That means that 84 per cent of scores fall below 1 SD—the 50 per cent below the mean plus 34 per cent

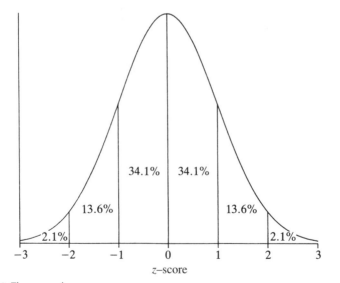

Fig. 7.1 The normal curve.

between the mean and $+1$ SD. To use a concrete example, the *MCAT* has a mean of 500 and a standard deviation of 100. So, 68 per cent of the people have scores between 400 and 600, and 84 per cent have scores lower than 600 (meaning that 16 per cent have higher scores). We can look up other values in a table of the normal distribution, which can be found in most statistics books. This is an extremely useful property of z- and T-scores, which is why many widely-used tests report their final scores in this way. Another advantage of these scores is that, since they are based on the normal curve, they often more closely meet the assumptions of parametric statistics than do either raw scores or percentiles, although it is not safe to automatically assume that standardized scores *are* normally distributed.

Any clinician who has undergone the painful process of having to relearn normal values of laboratory tests using the SI system must wonder why standard scores are not used in the laboratory. Indeed, the problem is twofold: switching from one measurement system to another; and different values of 'normal' within each system. For example, the normal range for fasting plasma glucose used to be between 70 and 110 mg per cent, and was 1.1–$4.1\,\mathrm{ng\,ml^{-1}\,h^{-1}}$ for plasma renin. In SI units, these same values are 3.9–$6.1\,\mathrm{mmol\,l^{-1}}$ for glucose, and 0.30–$1.14\,\mathrm{ng\,l^{-1}\,s^{-1}}$ for renin. Think how much easier life would be if the results of all these diverse tests could be expressed in a common way, such as standard or standardized scores.

Normalized scores

In order to ensure that standard and standardized scores are normally distributed, we can use other transformations which normalize the raw scores. One of the most widely used ones is the *normalized standard score*. Returning to Table 7.3, we take one further step, transforming the percentiles into standard scores from a table of the normal curve. For example, the 95th percentile corresponds to a normalized standard score of 1.65; the 90th percentile to a score of 1.29, and so on. As with non-normalized standard scores, we can, if we wish, convert these to *standardized*, normalized scores, with any desired mean and standard deviation. In Table 7.4, we have added two more columns; the first showing the transformation from percentiles to normalized standard (z) scores, and then to normalized standardized (T) scores, using a mean of 100 and a standard deviation of 10.

Age and sex norms

Some attributes, especially those assessed in adults like cardiac output, show relatively little change with age and do not differ between males and females. Other factors, such as measures of lung capacity like FVC, show considerable variation with age or gender. It is well known, for example, that females are more prone to admit to depressive symptomatology than are men. The psychometric solution to this problem is relatively easy: separate norms can be developed for each sex, as was done for the Depression scale and some others on the MMPI. However, this may mask a more important and fundamental difficulty; do the sexes differ only in terms of their willingness to endorse depressive items, or does this reflect more actual depression in

Table 7.4 Percentiles transformed into normalized standard standardized scores

Subject	Score	Percentile	Normalized standard score (z)	Normalized standardized score (T)
5	37	95	1.65	116.5
13	32	90	1.29	112.9
2	31	85	1.04	110.4
15	29	80	0.84	108.4
17	26	75	0.67	106.7
8	23	67.5	0.45	104.5
10	23	67.5	0.45	104.5
3	21	60	0.25	102.5
12	20	55	0.13	101.3
18	18	50	0.00	100.0
19	17	42.5	−0.19	98.1
14	17	42.5	−0.19	98.1
1	16	35	−0.39	96.1
20	16	35	−0.39	96.1
7	16	35	−0.39	96.1
6	15	25	−0.67	93.3
11	13	20	−0.84	91.6
16	12	10	−1.29	87.1
4	10	5	−1.65	83.5
9	8	0	−3.00	70.0

women? Separate norms assume that the distribution of depression is equivalent for males and females, and it is only the reporting that is different.

The opposite approach was taken by Wechsler (1958) in constructing his intelligence tests. He began with the explicit assumption that males and females do not differ on any of the dimensions that his instruments tap. During the process of developing the tests, he therefore discarded any tasks, such as spatial relations, which did show a systematic bias between the sexes.

These decisions were *theoretically founded* ones, not psychometric ones, based on the developer's conception of how these attributes exist in reality. Deciding whether sex norms should be used (as with the MMPI) or whether more endorsed items means more underlying depression (as in the Beck or Zung scales), or if the sexes *should* differ on some trait such as intelligence reflects a theoretical model. Since these are crucial in interpreting the results, they should be spelled out explicitly in any manual or paper about the instrument.

Age norms are less contentious, as developmental changes are more objective and verifiable. Some of the many examples of age-related differences are height, weight, or vocabulary. When these exist, separate norms are developed for each age group, and often age-sex group, as boys and girls develop at different rates. The major question facing the test constructor is how large the age span should be in each normative group. The answer depends to a large degree on the speed of maturation of the trait; a child should not change in his or her percentile level too much in crossing from the upper limit of one age group to the beginning of the next. If this does occur, then it is probable that the age span is too great.

Establishing cut points

Although we have argued throughout this book that continuous measures are preferable to categorical ones, there are times when it is necessary to use a continuous scale in order to predict a dichotomous outcome. For example, we may want to determine for which patients their score on a depression scale is high enough that we will presume they are clinically depressed; or which students have a score on a final exam so low that we could call them failures. Another reason for dichotomizing is that we may want to determine whether the benefit derived from a new treatment is sufficiently large to justify a change in management.

This latter decision has been a preoccupation of measurement in the health sciences, particularly in the assessment of health-related quality of life (HRQL). The goal is laudable, and rests on two points. The first is an explicit recognition that statistical significance reveals nothing about clinical importance, a fact drummed home *ad nauseam* in statistics books, but promptly forgotten when it comes to publication (e.g. the difference was *highly* significant ($p < 0.0001$)). There are many examples from clinical trials of results that achieved statistical significance, but were of no practical importance, such as streptokinase vs t-PA in the treatment of acute MI, where the differences amounted to 7.3 per cent versus 6.3 per cent (Van de Werf 1993). The second point is that, while it is easy to recognize that a difference in mortality of 1 per cent is of little consequence, a difference of 3.1 points on some HRQL instrument is much less comprehensible. Consequently, a literature has emerged that attempts to establish minimum standards for clinically important change (however defined). Conceptually, this is can be seen as an issue of establishing cut points; in this case, between those changes or treatment effects which are beneficial and those which are not.

A number of methods have been worked out in both the educational and clinical domains to approach the problem, and all can be classified roughly as based either on characteristics of the distribution, or on subjective judgements of the cut-point, which is more or less independent of the distribution. In education, the distinction is usually referred to as the difference between *norm-referenced* and *criterion-referenced* tests; while in some health measurement areas, such as assessing quality of life, the two broad strategies are called *distribution-based* and *anchor-based*. As we will see, the distinction ultimately blurs, but it remains a useful starting point.

We will begin by giving a simple (and simplistic) example from each of the approaches:

1. Many lab tests have an established range of normal beyond which the test result is declared to be abnormal (high or low). Not infrequently, the range of normal comes about by simply testing a large number of apparently normal individuals and then establishing a statistical range from the 2.5th to the 97.5th percentile (± 2 standard deviations). The problem, of course, is that this strategy ensures that, in any 'normal' population, 5 per cent will always be deemed abnormal. Even if the entire population improves (e.g. everyone starts watching their diet and the mean level of LDL cholesterol drops), by definition 5 per cent will still be abnormal, now including some people who were previously deemed healthy.

2. Most of us went through school and college facing an endless array of final exams, where the pass mark was set at 50 per cent (in Canada) or 65 per cent (in the US) or some other value, regardless of the actual exam. Occasionally, the results were so bad that the professor was embarrassed into 'bell-curving' the scores, but this was only used in exceptional circumstances. Somehow it never dawned on anyone that 50 per cent, 60 per cent or whatever the decreed 'pass-mark' was arbitrary, at best. Indeed, the whole necessity of 'bell-curving' comes about because the instructor was presumably unable to anticipate in advance how difficult the test would turn out to be. Such a criterion, however time-honoured, is indefensible, and only withstands assault because individual instructors learn, over time, what kinds of questions can be used in a test to ensure that an acceptable number of students pass and fail around this fixed cut-point.

We will now examine the formalized approaches to setting cut points, derived from education and health measurement.

Methods based on characteristics of the distribution

From educational measurement

Perhaps the oldest distribution-based method is the approach called *norm-referenced*. In this method, a fixed percentage of the distribution is set in advance to be below the cut point (i.e. to 'fail'). As one example, for many years, from about 1960 to 1990, the national licensing examinations for medical students in the US and Canada were norm-referenced. In Canada, the standard was that the failure rate for first-time Canadian graduates would be 4.5 per cent. This criterion, although seemingly as arbitrary as a fixed pass mark of 50 per cent, is actually a bit more rational. When the licensing body went to a multiple choice format from orals and essays, they could no longer rely on examiner judgement for calibration. Consequently, they looked at prior examinations, and found that year by year, about 4–5 per cent of candidates failed. They assumed that this indicated that of all candidates, on average, 4.5 per cent were incompetent (at least, as defined by test performance), and each year the scores were 'bell-curved' to ensure that the failure rate was 4.5 per cent.

The approach is usually assaulted on grounds that 'How can you assume that 5 per cent of the candidates are incompetent? Maybe they're all competent. But you arbitrarily fail some of them. How unfair!'. Actually, in the situation where it is used, at a national level, with large numbers of candidates (2000 to 20 000) and relatively smaller numbers of questions, it is statistically plausible that the candidate pool changes less from year to year than the question pool. (As a check, examination boards frequently will reuse a small number of questions each year to ensure that there is no drift.)

From health measurement

Historically, the first of distribution-based methods which is usually considered in the quality of life literature is Cohen's effect size[1] (ES; Cohen 1988), defined as the difference between the two means expressed in standard deviation (SD) units (mean difference/SD at baseline). He stated that, in the context of comparing group averages, a small ES is 0.2 (i.e. a difference between the means equal to one-fifth of the SD); a medium ES is 0.5; and a large ES is 0.8. His intent in doing so was simply to provide some basis for sample size calculations, not to provide any form of benchmark of clinical importance. However, these criteria have frequently been referred to in the context of deciding on important or unimportant changes.

A second class of distribution-based methods uses a variant on the ES, which divides by the standard error of measurement (SEM), and then establishes cutpoints based on statistics. There is clearly a relation between the two classes, since, as we showed earlier, the SEM is related to the test reliability and the baseline SD through the formula:

$$\text{SEM} = \sqrt{(1 - R)} \times \text{SD}_{Baseline}$$

Wyrwich *et al.* (1999) suggests using a value of 1 SEM, while McHorney and Tarlov (1995) recommend a value of 1.96 SEM, which amounts to a criterion of statistical significance.

Methods based on judgement

From education

Contrasting and borderline groups

The *contrasting groups* and *borderline groups* methods used to set pass/fail standards for examinations are almost completely analogous to the 'minimally important difference' (MID) approach discussed later in this section. The contrasting groups method asks judges to review examinee performance globally (e.g. by reading a whole

---

[1] An interesting paradox, since Jacob Cohen was an educational statistician, and his methods were originally developed for computing sample size for behavioural and educational interventions.

essay exam, or, in the case of candidates known to the judges, based on ongoing performance), and arrive at a consensus about who should pass or fail. The distributions of scores on the exam for passers and failers are plotted, and the cut score decided subjectively to minimize false-positives or negatives. (The ROC approach, described later in this section, would be a more objective way to go about this.)

The borderline groups method has been used in Canada to set standards for a national OSCE examination (Dauphinee *et al.* 1997; see Chapter 9 for a description of the OSCE). In this method, the examiner at each station completes a checklist indicating which of the actions that were supposed to occur were done by the candidate, so that the sum of these actions performed becomes the score for the station. The examiner also completes a global 7-point scale indicating whether the candidate is a clear fail, borderline fail, borderline pass, clear pass, and so on. The average checklist score for the two 'borderline' groups the becomes the pass mark for the station, and the sum across all stations becomes the overall pass mark.

Absolute methods

Another very complex and time-consuming method has been used almost exclusively for setting standards for multiple choice tests. Indeed, this family of methods is so time-consuming that it is rarely used in contexts other than national, high-stakes, examinations. In the three common approaches, the panel of judges reviews each question and its alternative answers, from the perspective of a borderline candidate and, depending on the method, decides:

1. What proportion of the borderline candidates would get it right (Angoff 1971)?
2. Which of the wrong answers a borderline candidate might choose (Nedelsky 1954)?
3. After grouping all the questions into homogeneous groups based on difficulty, what proportion of the questions in a group would a borderline group answer correctly (Ebel 1972)?

The pass mark then results from summing up these judgements with a method-specific algorithm.

While these methods appear to be fairer than those based on an arbitrary proportion of failures, in fact, unless actual performance data are available, the criterion may be wildly off the mark. A far better approach, and one that is most commonly applied, is to use a judgement approach conducted with performance data on each question, based on previous administrations of the test, available to the judge panel (Shepard 1984).

These absolute methods appear highly specific to multiple choice written examinations, but with some adaptation, might be useful in measuring health. For example, a clinician panel might review a depression inventory, and decide which of the items (e.g. 'I am tired all the time', 'I have lost my appetite') would be endorsed by a 'borderline' patient, at the margin of clinical depression. The sum of these items might become a cut score between normal and depressed.

From health measurement

Although there are a number of anchor-based methods (e.g. Lydick and Epstein 1993), far and away the most common is the Minimally Important Difference (MID; Jaeschke *et al.* 1989), defined as 'the smallest difference in score in the domain of interest which patients perceive as beneficial and which would mandate in the absence of troublesome side-effects and excessive cost, a change in the patient's management' (p. 408). The approach is directed at determining the difference on a HRQL scale corresponding to a self-reported small but important change on a global scale. To determine this, patients are followed for a period of time, and then asked whether they had got better, stayed about the same, or got worse. If they have improved or worsened, they rate the degree of change from 1 to 7 with 1 to 3 being a small improvement or worsening, to 6 to 7 reflecting being very much improved or worsened. The MID is then taken as the mean change on the HRQL scale of the patients who score 1 to 3.

One serious problem with this approach relates to the reliance on a single item global measure of change, which we have discussed extensively in Chapter 4. Such measures tend to be strongly influenced by the present state and only weakly by the initial state; hence, it is unclear what is meant by a 'small' change.

Summary

This has been a very brief and incomplete review of methods used for standard setting. For some comprehensive reviews of standard setting in education, see Norcini and Guelle (2002) and Berk (1986). For discussion of methods to ascertain the minimal difference, see Lydick and Epstein (1993).

However different these classes of methods appear at first glance, the differences may be more illusory than real. In applying the criterion-referenced educational strategies, these yield reliable results only when actual performance data on the test are available, so are hardly as independent of student performance as might be believed. Indeed, it seems that the main indicator of validity of any criterion-referenced approach is the extent to which it yields failure rates similar to the norm-referenced approach it replaced.

Receiver operating characteristic curves

Another, more objective, approach is used when there is some independent classification dividing people into two groups (as in several of the methods described above).

The technique for establishing the optimal cut point is derived from the early days of radar and sonar detection in the Second World War (Peterson *et al.* 1954), and the name still reflects that—Receiver Operating Characteristic (ROC) curve. As we increase the sensitivity of the radio, we pick up both the sound we want to hear as well as background static. Initially, the signal increases faster than the noise. After some point, though, a cross-over is reached, where the noise grows faster than the signal. The optimal setting is where we detect the largest ratio of signal to noise. This technique was later applied to the psychological area of the ability of humans to detect the presence or absence of signals (Tanner and Swets 1954), and then to the ability of tests to detect the presence or absence of a state or disease.

In the assessment arena, the 'signal' is the number of actual cases of hypertension or depression detected by our scale; the 'noise' is the number of non-cases erroneously labeled as cases; and the analog of amplification is the cut point of our new scale. If we use something like a quality of life scale, where lower scores indicate more problems, a very low cut-off score (Line A in Fig. 7.2) will pick up few true cases, and also make few false-positive errors. As we increase the cutting score (Line B), we hope we will pick up true cases faster than false ones. Above some optimal value, though, we will continue to detect more true cases, but at the cost of mislabelling many non-cases as cases (Line C). The task is to find this optimal value on our scale.

We begin by constructing a 2×2 table, as in Table 7.5. Cell A contains the number of actual cases (as determined by the dichotomous gold standard) who are labeled as cases by our new scale (the 'true positives'), while in Cell B are the non-cases erroneously labeled as cases by the test ('false-positives'). Similarly, Cell C has the false-negatives, and Cell D the true negatives. From this table, we can derive two necessary statistics: the *sensitivity* and the *specificity* of the test. Sensitivity (which is also called the *true positive rate*) is defined as $A/(A + C)$; that is, is the test 'sensitive' in detecting a disorder when it is actually present? Specificity (or the *true negative rate*) is $D/(B + D)$; is the test specific to this disorder, or is it elevated by other ones too?

To construct an ROC curve, we determine these two values for each possible cut-point. Let us assume that we test 500 cases and 500 controls (non-cases) with our

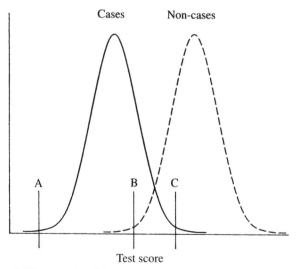

Fig. 7.2 Effects of different cut points.

Table 7.5 A 2 × 2 table for calculating sensitivity and specificity

		Gold Standard	
		Case	Non-case
New test	**Case**	A	B
	Non-case	C	D

Table 7.6 Calculations for an ROC curve

Cut-Off	Case	Non-case	Cut-Off	Case	Non-case	Cut-Off	Case	Non-case
10	49	0	11	136	5	10–12	228	9
11–20	441	500	12–20	364	495	13–20	272	491

Cut-Point	True Positives	False Positives	Sensitivity	1 – Specificity
< 10	0	0	0.000	0.000
10	49	0	0.098	0.000
11	136	5	0.272	0.010
12	228	9	0.456	0.018
13	311	18	0.622	0.036
14	369	48	0.738	0.096
15	437	118	0.874	0.236
16	466	179	0.932	0.358
17	491	235	0.982	0.470
18	495	361	0.990	0.722
19	500	474	1.000	0.948
20	500	500	1.000	1.000

new test, which has a total score that could range from 10 to 20. The first row of our first table would contain all the people who had scores of 10, and the second row scores of 11 through 20; the first row of the second table would have scores of 10 and 11, and the second row 12 and higher; and so on, until the last table, where the top row would have all people with scores up to 19, and the bottom row those with a score of 20. (In order to make the graph start and end at one of the axes, we usually add two other tables; one in which everyone has a score above the cut-point, and one where they all have scores below it.) The first few tables are shown in the top part of Table 7.6, and a summary of all 12 tables in the lower half. We then make a graph where the X-axis is 1 *minus* the specificity (i.e. the false-positive rate), and the Y-axis is the sensitivity (also called the true positive rate), as in Fig. 7.3.

The diagonal line which runs from point $(0,0)$ in the lower left-hand corner to $(1,1)$ in the upper right reflects the characteristics of a test with no discriminating ability. The better a test is in dividing cases from non-cases, the closer it will approach the upper left hand corner. So, Test A in Fig. 7.3 (which is based on the data in Table 7.6) is a better discriminator than Test B. The cut-point, which minimizes the overall number of errors (false-positive and false-negative), is the score that is closest to that corner. An index of the 'goodness' of the test is the area under the curve, which is usually abbreviated as D'. A non-discriminating test (one which falls on the diagonal) has an area of 0.5, and a perfect test has an area of 1.0. (If a test falls below the line, and has an area less than 0.5, then it is performing worse than chance; you would do better to simply go with the prevalence of the disorder in labelling people, rather than using the test results.) It is difficult to calculate D' by hand, but a number of computer programs are available (e.g. Center and Schwartz 1985; Dorfman and Alf 1969). The standard error of the ROC is given by Hanley and McNeil (1982) as:

$$SE = \left[\frac{D'(1-D') + (N_c - 1)(Q_1 - D'^2) + (N_n - 1)(Q_2 - D'^2)}{N_c N_n} \right]^{\frac{1}{2}}$$

where $Q_1 = D'/(2 - D')$, $Q_2 = 2D'^2/(1 - D')$, $N_c =$ number of cases, and $N_n =$ number of non-cases.

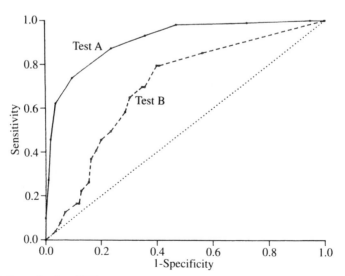

Fig. 7.3 Example of an ROC curve.

We mentioned previously that the cut-point nearest the upper left corner resulted in the smallest overall error rate. There may be some circumstances, though, where it may be preferable to move this point, either up or down, even though the number of false-positives or false-negatives may increase faster than the number of true positives. For example, if the consequences of missing a case can be tragic, and second-level tests exist which can weed out the false-positives (as with HIV sero-conversion), then the cut-off point may be lowered. Conversely, if there are more good applicants than positions, as is the case in admission requests for graduate or professional school, then it makes sense to raise the cut-off. The cost will be an increased number of false-negatives (i.e. potentially good students who are denied admission), but relatively few false-positives.

Summary

We have covered four points in this chapter. First, differential weighting of items rarely is worth the trouble. Second, if a test is being developed for local use only, it would probably suffice to use simply the sum of the items. However, for more general use, and to be able to compare the results with other instruments, it is better to transform the scores into percentiles, and best to transform them into z-scores or T-scores. Third, for attributes which differ between males and females, or which show development changes, separate age or age-sex norms can be developed. Fourth, we reviewed a variety of methods for setting cut scores or pass marks.

References

Angoff, W. H. (1971). Scales, norms and equivalent scores. In *Educational measurement* (ed. R. L. Thornkike) pp. 508–600. American Council on Education, Washington, DC.

Beck, A. T., Ward, C. H., Mendelson, M., Mock, J., and Erbaugh, J. (1961). An inventory for measuring depression. *Archives of General Psychiatry*, **4**, 561–71.

Berk, R. A. (1986). A consumer's guide to setting performance standards on criterion-referenced tests. *Review of Educational Research*, **56**, 137–72.

Cattell, R. B., Eber, H. W., and Tatsuoka, M. M. (1970). *Handbook for the Sixteen Personality Factor Questionnaire (16PF)*. Institute for Personality and Ability Testing, Champaign, IL.

Centor, R. M. and Schwartz, J. S. (1985). An evaluation of methods for estimating the error under the receiver operating characteristic (ROC) curve. *Medical Decision Making*, **5**, 149–56.

Cohen, J. (1988). *Statistical power analysis for the behavioral sciences* (2nd edn). Lawrence Erlbaum, Hillsdale, NJ.

Dauphinee, W. D., Blackmore, D. E., Smee, S., Rothman, A. I., and Reznick, R. (1997). Using the judgments of physician examiners in setting the standards for a national multi-center high stakes OSCE. *Advances in Health Sciences Education: Theory and Practice*, **2**, 201–11.

Dorfman, D. D. and Alf, E. (1969). Maximum likelihood estimation of parameters of signal detection theory and determination of confidence intervals-rating-method data. *Journal of Mathematical Psychology*, **6**, 487–96.

Ebel, R. L. (1972). *Essentials of educational measurement*. Prentice-Hall, Englewood Cliffs, NJ.

Evans, M. G. (1991). The problem of analyzing multiplicative composites: Interactions revisited. *American Psychologist*, **46**, 6–15.

Gulliksen, H. O. (1950). *Theory of mental tests*. Wiley, New York.

Hanley, J. A. and McNeil, B. J. (1982). The meaning and use of the area under a receiver operating characteristics (ROC) curve. *Radiology*, **143**, 29–36.

Holmes, T. H. and Rahe, R. H. (1967). The social readjustment rating scale. *Journal of Psychosomatic Research*, **11**, 213–18.

Jackson, D. N. (1984). *Personality Research Form manual*. Research Psychologists Press, Port Huron, MI.

Jacobson, N. S. and Truax, P. (1991). Clinical significance: A statistical approach to defining meaningful change in psychotherapy research. *Journal of Consulting and Clinical Psychology*, **59**, 12–9.

Jaeschke, R., Singer, J., and Guyatt, G. H. (1989). Measurement of health status. Ascertaining the minimally important difference. *Controlled Clinical Trials*, **10**, 407–15.

Jenkinson, C. (1991). Why are we weighting? A critical examination of the use of item weights in a health status measure. *Social Science and Medicine*, **32**, 1413–16.

Lei, H. and Skinner, H. A. (1980). A psychometric study of life events and social readjustment. *Journal of Psychosomatic Research*, **24**, 57–65.

Lydick, E. and Epstein, R. S. (1993). Interpretation of quality of life changes. *Quality of Life Research*, **2**, 221–6.

McHorney, C. and Tarlov, A. (1995). Individual-patient monitoring in clinical practice: Are available health status measures adequate? *Quality of Life Research*, **4**, 293–307.

Nedelsky, L. (1954). Absolute grading standards for objective tests. *Educational and Psychological Measurement*, **14**, 3–19.

Norcini, J. J. and Guille, R. (2002). Combining tests and setting standards. In *International handbook of research in medical education* (ed. G. Norman, C. P. M. van der Vleuten, and D. I. Newble) pp. 810–34. Kluwer, Dordrecht.

Norman, G. R. and Streiner, D. L. (2000). *Biostatistics: The bare essentials* (2nd edn). B. C. Decker, Toronto.

Nunnally, J. C., Jr. (1970). *Introduction to psychological measurement*. McGraw-Hill, New York.

Perloff, J. M. and Persons, J. B. (1988). Biases resulting from the use of indexes: An application to attributional style and depression. *Psychological Bulletin*, **103**, 95–104.

Peterson, W. W., Birdshall, T. G., and Fox, W. C. (1954). The theory of signal detectability. *IRE Transactions: Professional Group on Information Theory*, **4**, 171–212.

Retzlaff, P. D., Sheehan, E. P., and Lorr, M. (1990). MCMI-II scoring: Weighted and unweighted algorithms. *Journal of Personality Assessment*, **55**, 219–23.

Shepard, L. A. (1984). Setting performance standards. In *A guide to criterion referenced test construction* (ed. R. A. Berk), pp. 169–98. Johns Hopkins Press, Baltimore.

Streiner, D. L., Goldberg, J. O., and Miller, H. R. (1993). MCMI-II weights: Their lack of effectiveness. *Journal of Personality Assessment*, **60**, 471–6.

Streiner, D. L. and Miller, H. R. (1989). The MCMI-II: How much better than the MCMI? *Journal of Personality Assessment*, **53**, 81–4.

Streiner, D. L., Norman, G. R., McFarlane, A. H., and Roy, R. G. (1981). Quality of life events and their relationship to strain. *Schizophrenia Bulletin*, **7**, 34–42.

Tanner, W. P., Jr. and Swets, J. A. (1954). A decision-making theory of visual detection. *Psychological Review*, **61**, 401–9.

Van de Werf, F. (1993). Mortality results in GUSTO. *Australian and New Zealand Journal of Medicine*, **23**, 732–4.

Wainer, H. (1976). Estimating coefficients in linear models: It don't make no nevermind. *Psychological Bulletin*, **83**, 213–17.

Wechsler, D. (1958). *The measurement and appraisal of adult human intelligence* (4th ed.). Williams and Wilkins, Baltimore.

Wechsler, D. (1981). *WAIS-R manual: Wechsler Adult Intelligence Scale-Revised.* Psychological Corporation, New York.

Wyrwich, K. W., Nienaber, N. A., Tierney, W. M., and Wolinsky, F. D. (1999). Linking clinical relevance and statistical significance in evaluating intra-individual changes in health-related quality of life. *Medical Care* **37**, 469–78.

Zung, W. K. (1965). A self-rating depression scale. *Archives of General Psychiatry*, **12**, 63–70.

Chapter 8

Reliability

The concept of *reliability* is a fundamental way to reflect the amount of error, both random and systematic, inherent in any measurement. Yet despite its essential role in judgements of the adequacy of any measurement process, it is devilishly difficult to achieve a real understanding of the psychometric approach to reliability. Some health science researchers also tend to cloud the issue by invoking a long list of possible synonyms, such as 'objectivity', 'reproducibility', 'stability', 'agreement', 'association', 'sensitivity', and 'precision'. Since few of these terms have a formal definition, we will not attempt to show how each differs from the other. Instead, we will concern ourselves with a detailed explanation of the concept of reliability. While some of the terms will be singled out for special treatment later in the chapter, primarily to emphasize their shortcomings, others will be ignored.

Our reasons for this apparently single-minded viewpoint are simple. The technology of reliability assessment was worked out very early in the history of psychological assessment. We once traced its roots back to a textbook written in the 1930s, and the basic definitions were given without reference, indicating that, even seven decades ago, the classical definition was viewed as uncontroversial. There is complete consensus within the educational and psychological communities regarding the meaning of the term, and disagreement and debate are confined to a small cadre of biomedical researchers. Moreover, once one understands the basic concept it appears, in our view, to reflect perfectly the particular requirements of any measurement situation. Although there are some more recent theories in education and psychology, such as generalizability theory (see Chapter 9), these represent extensions of the basic approach. Other conflicting views which have arisen in the biomedical research community, such as the treatment of Bland and Altman (1986), offer, in our view, no advantage. This latter method, because of its recent popularity, will be discussed separately.

Basic concepts

What is this elusive concept, and why is it apparently so hard to understand? In order to explore it, we will begin with some commonsense notions of measurement error, and eventually link them to the more formal definitions of reliability.

Daily experience constantly reminds us of measurement error. We leap or crawl out of bed in the morning, and step on the scales. We know to disregard any changes less than about 2 lb or 1 kg, since bathroom scales are typically accurate to no better than ± 2 lb (± 1 kg). If our children are ill, we may measure their temperature with a home thermometer, accurate to about $\pm 0.2\,°C$. Baby's weight gain or loss is measured on a different scale, at home or at the doctor's surgery, accurate to about ± 20 gm. As we eat breakfast, we note the time on the wall, and implicitly recognize that if the clock has hands, there is a likely measurement error of about 5 minutes; if it displays numbers, the error is probably a fraction of a minute. Before donning our coat to leave the house, we check the outside thermometer ($\pm 2°F$; $\pm 1°C$). We leap into our cars and accelerate rapidly up to the speed limit, at least as assessed by our car's speedometer (± 5 km/h; ± 3 mph), and check the time again as we arrive at work, by looking at our wrist-watches (probably quartz, ± 15 s). We settle at our desks, pick up the first cup of coffee or tea of the day, and read a new paper on observer error which begins by stating that 'the reliability was calculated with an intraclass correlation, and equalled 0.86'.

Why, for goodness sake, do we have to create some arcane statistic, with no dimension and a range from zero to one, regardless of the measurement situation, in order to express measurement error? To explain, let us review the measurements of the previous paragraph. We begin by assuming that the reader will accept that the measurement errors we cited, while not precisely correct, were at least approximately consistent with our common experience. In the brief 'Day in the Life of…', we indicated two measurements of time, weight, and temperature, each with an approximate error. We are completely comfortable with a bathroom scale accurate to ± 1 kg, since we know that individual weights vary over far greater ranges than this, and typical changes from day to day are about the same order of magnitude. Conversely, we recognize that this error of measurement is unacceptable for weighing infants, because it exceeds important changes in weight. Similarly, an error of time measurement of several minutes is usually small compared with the anticipated tolerances in daily life (except for European trains). Indeed, many people have now reverted back to quartz analog watches, since they find the extreme accuracy of the digital readouts unnecessary and annoying. Finally, we tolerate an error of measurement of several degrees Celsius for outside air temperature, since we know that it may range from $-40°$ to $+40°$ Celsius (in the UK, from -5 to $+15$), so the measurement error is a small fraction of the true range. The same measurement error is, however, hopeless in a clinical situation since body temperature is restricted to a range of only a few degrees.

In all of these situations, our comfort resides in the knowledge that the error of measurement is a relatively small fraction of the range in the observations. Further, the reason that the measurement error alone provides useful information in the everyday world is that we share a common perception of the expected differences we will encounter. However, such everyday information is conspicuously absent for many measurement scales. To report that the error of measurement on a new depression scale is ± 3 is of little value since we do not know the degree of difference among patients, or between patients and non-patients. In order to provide useful information about measurement error, it must be contrasted with the expected variation amongst the individuals we may be assessing.

One way to include the information about expected variability between patients would be to cite the ratio of measurement error to total variability between patients. Since the total variability between patients includes both any systematic variation between patients and measurement error, this would result in a number between zero and one, with zero representing a 'perfect' instrument. Such a ratio would then indicate the ability of the instrument to differentiate among patients. In practice, the ratio is turned around, and researchers calculate the ratio of variability *between* patients to the *total* variability (the sum of patient variability and measurement error), so that zero indicates no reliability, and one indicates no measurement error and perfect reliability. Thus the formal definition of reliability is:

$$Reliability = \frac{Subject\ Variability}{Subject\ Variability + Measurement\ Error}$$

Since one statistical measure of variability is *variance*, this can be expressed more formally as:

$$Reliability = \frac{\sigma_s^2}{\sigma_s^2 + \sigma_e^2}$$

where the '*s*' subscript stands for 'Subjects', and the '*e*' for Error.

Thus the reliability coefficient expresses the proportion of the total variance in the measurements ($\sigma_s^2 + \sigma_e^2$) which is due to 'true' differences between subjects (σ_s^2). As we shall see, 'true' is defined in a very particular way, but this awaits a detailed discussion of the methods of calculation.

This definition of reliability has a very long history. Formally, it is derived from what is commonly referred to as *Classical Test Theory*, which goes back to the turn of the last century and the work of Karl Pearson, of Pearson's correlation fame. Classical test theory simply states that any observation, O_{ij} (the *j*th observation on object *i*) is composed of two components—a true score T_i (for object *i*) and error associated with the observation, e_{ij}. The formal calculation of the reliability formula, called an *intraclass correlation*, appears in Fisher's 1925 statistics book (Fisher 1925).

Philosophical implications

This formulation of reliability has profound consequences for the logic of measurement. At its root, the reliability coefficient reflects the extent to which a measurement instrument can differentiate among individuals, i.e. how well it can tell people apart, since the magnitude of the coefficient is directly related to the variability between subjects. The concept seems restrictively Darwinian and even feudal. But this interpretation is a political not a scientific one, and perhaps reflects a focus on the potentially negative use to which the measurement may be put, rather than the measurement itself.

Reflect back again on the everyday use of measurement. The only reason to apply a particular instrument to a situation is because the act of measurement is providing information about the object of observation. We look at the thermometer outside only because it tells us something about how this day differs from all other days. If the thermometer always gave the same reading because every day was the same temperature as every other day, we would soon stop reading it. We suspect, although we lack direct experience, that because of this people living in tropical climates pay little attention to the temperature, and that other factors, such as rain or humidity, are more important.

This intuition applies equally well to clinical and other professional situations. A laboratory measurement is useful only to the extent that it reflects true differences among individuals; in particular diseased and normal individuals. Chromosome count is not a useful genetic property (despite the fact that we can get perfect agreement among observers) because we all have 46 chromosomes. Similarly, most clinical supervisors question the value of global rating scales (the bit of paper routinely filled out by the supervisor at the end of an educational experience rating everything from knowledge to responsibility) precisely because everybody, from the best to the worst, gets rated 'above average'.

Again, this view flies in the face of some further intuitions. Reliability is not necessarily related to agreement, and in some cases can be inversely related to it. We have just demonstrated one example, where if all students on all occasions are rated above average, the agreement among raters is perfect but the reliability, by definition, is zero. This is also relevant to the 'number of boxes' issue discussed in Chapter 4. As we decrease the number of boxes on a rating scale, the information value of any observation is reduced, and the reliability drops, although the agreement among observers will increase. As an everyday example, Canadians now uniformly talk about the weather in degrees Celsius, but still refer to room temperature in degrees Fahrenheit. We think one reason for this phenomenon is that within the range of acceptable room temperature, from say 68° to 72° Fahrenheit or 20° to 21° Celsius (except the United Kingdom where the lower limit, particularly in bathrooms, is more like 32°F or 0°C), the Celsius scale has only two divisions compared to four for the Fahrenheit one, thus introducing a degree of measurement error, even though two thermometers would agree (within one degree) more often in Celsius.

Experimentalists, and many statisticians, have difficulty with the concept of reliability as well. To the experimentalist, the goal of science is to detect the effects of experimental interventions. This 'main effect', in a comparison between treatment and control groups, for example, is always confounded, to greater or lesser degree, by differences in individual subjects' responses. Nearly all statistical tests make this contrast explicit; the numerator of the test is the experimental effect, assessed as differences between means, differences in proportions cured or dead, and so on, and the denominator is the expected magnitude of the difference by chance *arising from differences among individuals*. Thus, it is precisely true that the psychometrician's (and arguably, the clinician's) *signal* is the experimentalist's and statistician's *noise*.

This paradox was first recognized by Cronbach, the inventor of the alpha coefficient (Chapter 5) and generalizability theory (Chapter 9), in a classic paper written in 1957, called 'The two disciplines of scientific psychology'. Perhaps because of the title, few readers outside psychology (and regrettably, few inside as well) are aware of it. The paradox rears its ugly head in many areas of research.

As one example, clinical researchers often go to great lengths to create inclusion and exclusion criteria in order to enrol just the right kind of (homogeneous) patients in their studies. Sometimes they go to extreme lengths, such as one trial of a cholesterol-lowering drug, which screened 300 000 men in order to find 4000 who fit the criteria. It is often forgotten that the reason for these extreme measures is because the small treatment effects common in cardiovascular research would be obscured by individual differences if all kinds of patients were enrolled.

On the analysis side, although we use standard statistical packages to develop reliability coefficients, it is literally true that every line in the ANOVA table of concern in these calculations is labeled 'ERROR' by most of the standard packages. Conversely, the 'main effects', or differences between means, which are of interest to the statisticians, are frequently (but not always) ignored in the calculations of reliability.

There is one last important consequence of this formulation. The reliability of a measure is intimately linked to the population to which one wants to apply the measure. There is literally no such thing as the reliability of a test, unqualified; the coefficient has meaning only when applied to specific populations. Reliability is relative, just as Einstein said about time. Although some researchers (Bland and Altman 1986) have decried this as a failure of conventional methods for assessing reliability, we believe that this is a realistic view of the act of measurement, and not a limitation of reliability. In fact, all of the formulae for reliability make this inevitable. The denominator always has a term reflecting the total variance of the scores. Naturally, the variance of, say, a quality of life scale will be very different in a homogeneous group of rheumatoid patients than in a group consisting of them, plus disease-free people, and those with ankylosing spondylitis; and therefore the reliability of the scale will be very different in the two groups. Although this may seem undesirable, it is an accurate reflection of the measurement situation. It *is* more difficult to tell people apart if they are relatively similar (i.e. homogeneous) than if they are very different. Reasonably, the reliability coefficient reflects this. Returning to the introduction, it makes no sense to speak of the error of measurement of a thermometer without knowledge of the range of temperature to be assessed. Small differences amongst the objects of measurement are more difficult to detect than large differences. The reliability coefficient explicitly recognizes this important characteristic.

Defining the reliability of a test

So far, we have described the idea of reliability in general terms. The time has come to define how to calculate reliability; that is, how to determine the different variance components which enter into the coefficient. Perhaps not surprisingly, the analytical approach is based on the statistical technique of Analysis of Variance (ANOVA). Specifically, because we have repeated observations on each subject or patient derived from different observers, times, or versions of the test, we use a method called repeated measures ANOVA.

Suppose, for example, that three observers assess a total of 10 patients for some attribute (e.g. sadness) on a 10-point scale. The scores are shown in Table 8.1.

Table 8.1 Degree of sadness on 10 patients rated by 3 observers

Patient	Observer 1	Observer 2	Observer 3	Mean
1	6	7	8	7.0
2	4	5	6	5.0
3	2	2	2	2.0
4	3	4	5	4.0
5	5	4	6	5.0
6	8	9	10	9.0
7	5	7	9	7.0
8	6	7	8	7.0
9	4	6	8	6.0
10	7	9	8	8.0
Mean	5.0	6.0	7.0	6.0

It is evident that there is some variability in the scores. Those assigned by the three observers to individual patients range from 2 to 10 units on the scale, with mean scores ranging from 2 to 9. The variability among the mean scores of the observers (5.0 vs. 6.0 vs. 7.0) suggests that there may be some systematic difference among them. Finally, there is as much as two units of disagreement in scores assigned to the same patient by different observers.

These three sources of variance—patients, observers, and error—are represented in different ways in the table: the patients, by the differences within the column on the right (their means); the observers, by the differences among their three column means; and 'random', or unsystematic variation, by the difference between an individual score within the table and its 'expected' value. Thus we have adopted a technical estimate of the 'true' score; it is simply the average of all the observed scores, whether applied to the true score of a patient (i.e. each patient's mean) or of an observer (their means). 'True' clearly has a technical definition which is somewhat more limited than the common definition. In fact, 'true' is a poor choice of words, but one that we are stuck with. Strictly speaking, it is the average score that would be obtained if the scale were given an infinite number of times (an obviously difficult task). Moreover, it refers only to the *consistency* of the score, not to its *accuracy*. For example, a person being evaluated for an executive position may deliberately understate the degree to which he mistrusts others. If he completed the scale 20 times, each time with the same bias in place, the average would be a good approximation of his true score, but a bad estimate of his actual feelings. Also, a person's true score will change (we hope) if the underlying characteristic changes. If a depressed person, who has a true score of 18 on some test, benefits from therapy, then both her depression and her true score should move closer to the normal range.

Bearing in mind what is meant by a 'true' score, we can quantify these sources of variance in sums of squares, calculated as below:

Sum of squares (observers) $= 10[(5.0 - 6.0)^2 + (6.0 - 6.0)^2 + (7.0 - 6.0)^2] = 20.0$.

The factor of 10 is there because 10 patients enter into each sum. Similarly:

Sum of squares (patients) $= 3[7.0 - 6.0)^2 + (5.0 - 6.0)^2 + (2.0 - 6.0)^2 + \cdots$
$$+ (8.0 - 6.0)^2] = 114.0$$

Again, there is a factor of 3 in the equation because there are three observers contributing to each value.

Finally, the sum of squares (Error) is based on the difference between each individual value and its expected value calculated from the row and column means. We will not go into detail about how these expected values are arrived at; any introductory text book in statistics, such as Norman and Streiner (2000), will explain it. For the first three patients and Observer 1, the expected scores are 6.0, 4.0, and 1.0. The sum of squares is then:

Sum of squares (error) $= (6.0 - 6.0)^2 + (4.0 - 4.0)^2 + (2.0 - 1.0)^2 + \cdots$
$$+ (8.0 - 9.0)^2 = 10.0$$

An ANOVA table can then be developed from the sums of squares, as in Table 8.2.

The next step is to break down the total variance in the scores into components of variance due to patients, observers, and error. It would seem that each mean square is a variance, and no further work is required, but such is not the case. Both the calculated mean square due to patients and that due to observers contain some contribution due to error variance. The easiest way to understand this concept is to imagine a situation where all patients had the same degree of sadness, as defined by some external gold standard. Would the patients all then obtain the same scores on our sadness scale? Not at all. There would be variability in the obtained scores directly related to the amount of random error present in the measurements. The relevant equations relating the mean square (MSs) to variances are below:

- Mean square (error) $= \sigma_{err}^2$
- Mean square (patients) $= 3\sigma_{pat}^2 + \sigma_{err}^2$
- Mean square (observers) $= 10\sigma_{obs}^2 + \sigma_{err}^2$

Table 8.2 Analysis of variance summary table

Source of variation	Sum of squares	Degrees of freedom	Mean square	F	Tail probability
Patients	114.00	9	12.67	22.80	0.0001
Observers	20.00	2	10.00	18.00	0.0001
Error	10.00	18	0.56		
Total	144.00	29			

From these we can show, by some algebraic manipulations, that:

- $\sigma^2(\text{error}) = MS_{err} = 0.56$
- $\sigma^2(\text{patients}) = (MS_{pat} - MS_{err})/3 = (12.67 - 0.56)/3 = 4.04$
- $\sigma^2(\text{observers}) = (MS_{obs} - MS_{err})/10 = (10.00 - 0.56)/10 = 0.94.$

Finally, we are in a position to define the reliability coefficient as the ratio of variance between patients to error variance:

$$r = \frac{\sigma^2_{patients}}{\sigma^2_{patients} + \sigma^2_{error}} = \frac{4.04}{4.04 + 0.56} = 0.88.$$

An alternative way of writing this formula, which does not involve first calculating the variances, is:

$$r = \frac{MS_{patients} - MS_{error}}{MS_{patients} + (k - 1)MS_{error}}$$

where k is the number of raters. This is the 'classical' definition of reliability. The interpretation is that 88 per cent of the variance in the scores results from 'true' variance among patients. It is important to note that when we are discussing reliability, it is the reliability coefficient, r, and not r^2, which is interpreted as the percentage of score variance attributable to different sources.

This coefficient is called an *Intraclass Correlation Coefficient* or ICC. It is not *the* ICC, but only one form of it. As we shall see, there are different versions, depending on various assumptions we make and what we want to look at. A bit of terminology—Fisher (1925) called it the 'intraclass correlation' because it is computed as the relationship among multiple observations of the *same* variable (that is, within a class of variable), to distinguish it from Pearson's correlation, which is usually between different variables, and hence is an *inter*class correlation. We will revisit this distinction a bit later.

Combining Shrout and Fleiss's (1979) and McGraw and Wong's (1996) terminology, we can refer to this version of the ICC as ICC2(C, 1); the 2 reflecting a 'class 2' ICC in which all patients are evaluated by all raters; C because we are looking at *consistency* among the raters rather than *absolute agreement* (a distinction we will discuss in the next section), and 1 because it is the reliability of a single rater.

Other considerations in calculating the reliability of a test
Measuring consistency or absolute agreement

What happened to the variance due to the raters or observers? Although it was calculated in the ANOVA table, and found to be highly significant, there was no further mention of it. Conventional treatments of reliability omitted the main effect of the rater, until the classic paper by Shrout and Fleiss (1979) re-introduced it into the calculation of different forms of the ICC.

Whether or not to include Observer is a decision dependent on whether we want to measure *consistency* or *agreement*. We can illustrate the difference with two examples. In the first, three raters (observers) independently evaluate the dossiers of 300 applicants for 50 openings for professional school, rating each applicant on a 100-point scale. The first rater is particularly harsh in his evaluations, while the third is far more lenient than the other two. In other words, none of the observers ever assign the same value to a student. However, since their job is, in essence, to rank order the applicants in order to choose the top 50, this lack of agreement is of no consequence. What is important is the consistency of their scores—is the rank ordering the same among them (i.e. is the Pearson or Spearman correlation high)? This is also the situation that obtains when tests are *norm referenced*; that is, when passing or failing is judged in relation to how others did (operationalized by the students' question on the first day of class, 'Will we be marked on a curve?').

In the second example, the raters must determine whether or not the applicants pass a licensing examination in which the examinees must attain a score of at least 65. This is referred to as a *criterion referenced* test, because there is an external criterion against which people are judged. In this case, numerical differences among the raters *are* important; they should agree not only with respect to the rank ordering of the students, but also with regard to their absolute value. A similar situation exists when students are tested to see how accurately they can measure a patient's blood pressure, where the criterion is the value obtained by an expert. Again, they must not only rank the patients in the same order, but also not deviate from the criterion.

Another way of thinking of the distinction between measuring only consistency as opposed to the more stringent measuring of absolute agreement is whether the raters can be considered a *fixed* or a *random* factor; terms that have been borrowed from ANOVA. Again, two examples will illustrate the difference, and their relationship to consistency and absolute agreement. If we did a study in which two raters estimated the degree of pain experienced by infants, we would want to know how reliable the ratings were. Our interest is not the reliability of raters in general, but only those who participated in the study. If there was any systematic bias between the raters, such that one tended to give higher values than the other, we could easily compensate for this by adding a constant to the lower rater's scores (or subtracting it from the higher rater's numbers, or using their mean). In this case, the raters are considered to be a *fixed* factor, and this would correspond to measuring *consistency*.

On the other hand, if we were developing the pain scale, and were interested in how reliably any two raters were in using it, then the raters in our study would be considered to be a random sample of all possible raters. Consequently, we would treat observers as a *random* factor. Because we cannot compensate for the difference between raters, they must also have similar *absolute* values.

We presented the formulae for the ICC for consistency in the previous section. The corresponding equations absolute agreement for a single score are:

$$ICC2(A,1) = \frac{\sigma^2_{patients}}{\sigma^2_{patients} + \sigma^2_{observers} + \sigma^2_{error}}$$

or

$$ICC2(A,1) = \frac{MS_{patients} - MS_{error}}{MS_{patients} + \frac{k}{n}(MS_{observer} - MS_{error}) + (k-1)MS_{error}}$$

where n is the number of subjects. If we put the numbers from Table 8. 2 into the equation, we will get a value of 0.73. This is lower than the value for ICC2(C, 1), which was 0.88. This is an almost universal truth; reliability based on absolute agreement is always lower than for agreement; on a conceptual level because we have a more stringent criterion, and on a mathematical level because we have added the variance due to observers to the denominator.

The observer nested within subject

One common situation arises when each subject is rated by several different observers, but no observers are common to more than one subject. Some examples would be: students on a course in different tutorial groups rate their tutors' teaching skills; junior residents on different teaching units are rated by chief residents, head nurses, and staff; and patients undergoing physiotherapy are rated by their own and another therapist, but treatment is given by different therapists at different hospitals. Common to these situations is that:

(1) all subjects receive more than one observation; but

(2) no observer rates more than one subject.

At first glance, it would seem impossible to extract a reliability coefficient from these data, since there seems to be no opportunity to actually compare observations. Certainly in the extreme case, where each subject is rated by only one observer, there is no way to separate subject variance, observer variance, and error. But in the situations above, at least a partial separation can be achieved.

The approach is to recognize that the variance of the mean values of the scores of each subject permits an estimate of subject variance, in the usual way. Conversely, variability of the observations around the mean of each subject is a result of within-subject variation, contributed by both systematic differences between observers and error variance. We cannot separate these two sources of variance but we do not really need to, since the denominator of the reliability coefficient contains contributions from both.

To analyze data of this form, we conduct a one-way ANOVA with the subject as a grouping factor, and the multiple observations within each subject cell as a 'within-subject' factor. We need not have the same number of observers for each subject, as long as the number of observations per subject exceeds one.

The one-way ANOVA results, eventually, in estimated mean squares between groups and within groups. The former is used to calculate subject variance, using the previous formula, and the mean square (within) estimates the error variance. The reliability coefficient can then be calculated with these variance estimates, using the formula for $ICC2(C,1)$. In this case, though, the formula would be referred to as $ICC1(C,1)$, because this is Shrout and Fleiss's 'class 1' ICC, in which the subjects are evaluated by different raters. All that is lost is the ability to separate the random error component from observer bias; but since observers are a random effect (using the concepts described in the previous subsection), this is of no consequence.

Even in those situations where there is partial overlap (for example, 15 interview teams of three interviewers conduct 10 interviews each), the analysis can be approached assuming no overlap of raters, and still yield an unbiased estimate of reliability.

Multiple observations

Finally, let us re-examine the issue of multiple observations. If each patient is assessed by multiple observers, or completes some inventory with a number of items, or fills out a pain scale on several occasions, it is intuitively obvious that the average of these observations should have a higher reliability than any single item, since the errors are random, and those associated with each observation are averaged out. In turn, this should be reflected in the reliability coefficient.

The approach is the essence of simplicity: we simply divide the error variance by the number of observations. The equations for the consistency version are:

$$ICC2(C,k) = \frac{\sigma^2_{subjects}}{\sigma^2_{subjects} + \sigma^2_{error} / k}$$

and

$$ICC2(C,k) = \frac{MS_{subjects} - MS_{error}}{MS_{subjects}}$$

and for the absolute agreement are:

$$ICC2(A,k) = \frac{\sigma^2_{subjects}}{\sigma^2_{subjects} + (\sigma^2_{observers} + \sigma_{error}) / k}$$

and

$$ICC2(A,k) = \frac{MS_{subjects} - MS_{error}}{MS_{subjects} + (MS_{observers} - MS_{error}) / n}$$

Note that if we set $k = 1$, this equation is the same as the one for $ICC2(A,1)$. We can use this fact to take the results from our actual study and estimate what the realiability would be if we were to use fewer or more raters. With $k =$ the actual number of observers in the study, $m =$ the number of raters we're interested in, and

$p = (k - m)$, we can then modify the equation for $ICC2(A,1)$ slightly to read:

$$ICC2(A,k,m) = \frac{MS_{subjects} - MS_{error}}{MS_{subjects} + \dfrac{p + 1}{n}\,(MS_{observer} - MS_{error}) + p\,(MS_{error})}$$

Other types of reliability

Up to this point, we have concerned ourselves with reliability as a measure of association, examining the effect of different observers on scores. The example we have worked through included only one source of error, that which resulted from different observers' perceptions of the same behaviour. Upon reflection, we can see that there may be other sources of error or contamination in an observation of an individual patient's 'sadness'. For instance, each observer may apply slightly different standards from day to day. This could be tested experimentally by videotaping a group of patients and having the observer do two ratings of the tapes a week or two apart. The resulting reliability is called an *intra-observer reliability* coefficient, since it measures variation that occurs within an observer as a result of multiple exposures to the same stimulus, as opposed to the *inter-observer* reliability we have already calculated.

Note that although many investigators maintain that the demonstration of both inter- and intra-observer reliability is a minimum requirement of a good test, this may be unnecessary. If we recognize that inter-observer reliability contains all the sources of error contributing to intra-observer reliability, plus any differences that may arise between observers, then it is evident that a demonstration of high inter-observer reliability is sufficient; the intra-observer reliability is bound to be higher. However, if the inter-observer reliability is low, we cannot be sure whether this arises from differences within or between observers (or both), and it may then be necessary to continue to an intra-observer reliability study in order to locate the source of unreliability.

Often there are no observers involved in the measurement, as with the many self-rated tests of psychological function, pain, or disease severity. Although there are no observers, we are still concerned about the reliability of the scale. The usual approach is to administer it on two occasions separated by a time interval sufficiently short that we can assume that the underlying process is unlikely to have changed. This approach is called *test–retest reliability*. Of course, the trick is to select an appropriate time interval: too long, and things may have changed; too short, and patients may remember their first response and put it down, rather than answering the question *de novo*. Expert opinions regarding the appropriate interval vary from an hour to a year depending on the task, but generally speaking, a retest interval of 2 to 14 days is usual. (The section on *Empirical data on retest reliability*, later in this chapter, shows the magnitude of the coefficient expected for various types of tests after different intervals.)

Frequently, measures of internal consistency, as described in Chapter 5, are reported as the reliability of a test. However, since they are based on performance observed in a single sitting, there are many sources of variance, which occur from day to day or between observers, which do not enter into the calculation. Because they can be computed from routine administration of a measure, without the special requirement for two or more administrations, they appear very commonly in the literature but should be interpreted with great caution.

Different forms of the reliability coefficient

There has been considerable debate in the literature regarding the most appropriate choice of the reliability coefficient. The coefficients we have derived to now are all forms of 'intraclass correlation coefficients'. However, other measures, in particular the Pearson product-moment correlation and Cohen's kappa (Cohen 1960), are frequently used. Altman and Bland (1983; Bland and Altman 1986) have also identified apparent weaknesses in the conventional approach and recommended an alternative. Accordingly, we will discuss these alternatives, and attempt to reconcile the differences among the measures.

Pearson correlation

The Pearson correlation is based on regression analysis, and is a measure of the extent to which the relationship between two variables can be described by a straight (regression) line. In the present context, this is a measure of the extent to which two observations on a group of subjects can be fitted by a straight line. One such relationship is shown in Fig. 8.1. Note that a perfect fit is obtained, resulting in a Pearson correlation of 1.0, despite the fact that the intercept is non-zero and the slope is not equal to 1.0. By contrast, the intraclass correlation will yield a value of 1.0 only if all the observations on each subject are identical, which dictates a slope of 1.0 and an intercept of 0.0. This suggests that the Pearson correlation is an inappropriate and liberal measure of reliability; that is to say, the Pearson coefficient will usually be higher than the true reliability. In practice, however, the predominant source of error is usually due to random variation, and under these circumstances, the Pearson and intraclass correlations will be very close.

There is a second reason to prefer the intraclass correlation over the Pearson correlation. We began this chapter with an example that used three observers, and proceeded to calculate a single ICC. If we had used the Pearson correlation, we must use the data pairwise, and would create one correlation for Observer 1 vs. Observer 2, another for Observer 1 vs. Observer 3, and a third for Observer 2 vs. Observer 3. With 10 observers, we would still have one ICC but we must now contend with 45 Pearson correlations, and there is no agreed way to average or combine them.

Although the pairwise correlation may be of use in identifying particular outlier examiners for further training, in general we presume that the observers are a random sample of all possible observers, and we have no particular interest in individuals. In these circumstances, it is of considerable value to use all the data to estimate a single ICC representing the average correlation between any two observers.

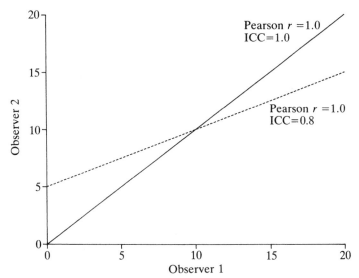

Fig. 8.1 Typical graph of inter-observer scores, showing difference between Pearson correlation and intraclass correlation.

Kappa coefficient

Although this chapter (and most of this book) has dealt at length with situations where there is a supposed underlying continuum, there are many situations in medicine which have only two levels—presence or absence, positive or negative, abnormal or normal, dead or alive (although with cardiac and electroencephalic monitoring, disagreement is rare in the latter instance). A straightforward approach is to calculate simple agreement: the proportion of responses in which the two observations agreed. Although straightforward, this measure is very strongly influenced by the distribution of positives and negatives. If there is a preponderance of either normal or abnormal cases, there will be a high agreement by chance alone. The kappa coefficient (Cohen 1960) explicitly deals with this situation by examining the proportion of responses in the two agreement cells (yes/yes, no/no) in relation to the proportion of responses in these cells which would be expected by chance, given the marginal distributions.

For example, suppose we were to consider a judgement by two observers of the presence or absence of a Babinski sign (an upgoing toe following scratching of the bottom of the foot) on a series of neurological patients. The data might be displayed in a contingency table like Table 8.3.

The overall agreement is simply $(20 + 55)/100 = 75$ per cent. However, we would expect that a certain number of agreements would arise by chance alone. Specifically, we can calculate the expected agreement from the marginals; the top left cell would have $(35 \times 30)/100 = 10.5$ expected observations, and the bottom right cell would

Table 8.3 Contingency Table for two observers

		Observer 2		
		Present	Absent	Total
	Present	20	15	35
Observer 1	Absent	10	55	65
	Total	30	70	100

have $(70 \times 65)/100 = 45.5$ expected ones. Kappa corrects for chance agreement in the following manner:

$$\kappa = \frac{P_o - P_e}{1.0 - P_e}$$

where P_o is the observed proportion of agreements, and P_e is the proportion expected by chance. In this case:

$$\kappa = \frac{\left(\dfrac{75}{100}\right) - \left(\dfrac{10.5 + 45.5}{100}\right)}{1.0 - \left(\dfrac{10.5 + 45.5}{100}\right)} = 0.43.$$

For a 2×2 table, we can also calculate the standard error of the kappa:

$$SE(\kappa) = \sqrt{\frac{P_o(1 - P_o)}{N(1.0 - P_e)^2}}$$

which in this case equals:

$$\sqrt{\frac{0.75\,(1 - 0.75)}{100\,(1.0 - 0.56)^2}} = 0.098.$$

Therefore, instead of a raw agreement of 0.75, we end up with a chance-corrected agreement of 0.43, with a standard error of about 0.10. In circumstances where the frequency of positive results is very low or very high, it is very easy to obtain impressive figures for agreement although agreement beyond chance is virtually absent.

In the example we have chosen, the approach to assessment of observer agreement appears to have little in common with our previous examples, where we used ANOVA methods. However, if we considered judgements which differ only slightly from Babinski signs, the parallel may become more obvious. For example, suppose the same observers were assessing muscle strength, which is conventionally done on a 6-point scale from $0 =$ flaccid to $5 =$ normal strength. In this case, a display of agreement would involve a 6×6 contingency table.

Since the coefficient we calculated previously considers only total agreement and does not provide partial credit for responses that differ by only one or two categories, it would be inappropriate for scaled responses as in the present example. However, an extension of the approach, called *weighted kappa* (Cohen 1968), does consider partial agreement.

Weighted kappa actually focuses on disagreement, so that the cells of total agreement on the top-left to bottom-right diagonal have weights of zero and two opposite corners have the maximum weights. Weighted kappa is then a sum of the weighted frequencies corrected for chance. The actual formula is:

$$\kappa_w = 1.0 - \frac{\sum w_{ij} \times P_{o_{ij}}}{\sum w_{ij} \times P_{e_{ij}}}$$

where w_{ij} is the weight assigned to the i, j cell, and $P_{o_{ij}}$ and $P_{e_{ij}}$ are the observed and expected proportions in the i, j cell.

As originally formulated, the weights could be assigned arbitrary values between 0 and 1. However, the problem with using your own weights, however sensible they may seem, is that you can no longer compare your kappa with anyone else's. Unless there are strong prior reasons the most commonly used weighting scheme, called *quadratic weights*, which bases disagreement weights on the square of the amount of discrepancy, should be used. *If this weighting scheme is used, then the weighted kappa is exactly identical to the intraclass correlation coefficient* (Fleiss and Cohen 1973). That is, if, in the second example, we simply took the numbers from 0 to 5 and did a repeated measures ANOVA on them with two observations, and then computed the ICC, it would turn out to be identical to the weighted kappa. Further, in the first example, with the Babinski sign, if we turned the 100 observations into 100 data points so that each positive sign is coded 1 and each negative sign coded 0, then everyone in the top-left cell would have numbers 1 and 1 assigned; in the bottom-left cell the numbers 0 and 1; in the top-right cell 1 and 0; and in the bottom-right cell, 0 and 0. Now, if we went ahead and did a repeated measures ANOVA treating these as two observations, and calculated the ICC, it would equal the unweighted kappa of 0.43.

The method of Bland and Altman

An alternative method of examining agreement was proposed by Altman and Bland (1983; Bland and Altman 1986), which has the apparent virtue of independence of the true variability in the observations. We have discussed earlier in this chapter why we would view this independence as a liability, not an asset. However, because this method has achieved considerable prominence in the British clinical literature, we will review it in detail.

The method is designed as an absolute measure of agreement between two measuring instruments, which are on the same scale of measurement. As such, it retains the virtue of the intraclass correlation, in contrast to the Pearson correlation, in explicitly separating the bias (or main effect) of the instrument from random error. The approach is used for pairs of observations, and begins with a plot of the difference between the two observations against the mean of the pairs of observations. One then calculates the average difference in the observations, and the standard deviation of the differences. The mean difference is analytically related to the observer variance calculated in the ICC (actually, it equals $\sqrt{(2/n) \cdot MS_{obs}}$). The standard deviation of the differences is similarly related to the error variance $\sqrt{MS_{err}}$. A statistical test of the observer bias can be performed, and would yield the same significance level as the test in the ANOVA. Finally, one calculates the *limits of agreement*, equal to the mean difference ± twice the standard error.

While, as we have seen, the parameters of the Altman and Bland method can be derived from the calculated values that go into the ICC, it has the small advantage that these values are reported directly. Further, the graph (which is rarely presented) can potentially alert the researcher to other systematic differences, such as a monotonic drift in the agreement related to the value of the measurement, or a systematic increase in error related to the value of the measurement.

Issues of interpretation
Reliability, the standard error of measurement, and the standard error of estimate

One difficulty with expressing the reliability coefficient as a dimensionless ratio of variances instead of an error of measurement is that it is difficult to interpret a reliability coefficient of 0.7 in terms of an individual score. However, since the reliability coefficient involves two quantities—the error variance and the variance between subjects—it is straightforward to work backwards and express the error of measurement in terms of the other two quantities. The *standard error of measurement* (SEM) is defined in terms of the standard deviation (σ) and the reliability (R) as:

$$SEM = \sigma\sqrt{1 - R}$$

This relationship is plotted for some values of reliability in Fig. 8.2. The interpretation of this graph is that if we begin with a sample of known standard deviation and, for example, a reliability of 0.8, the error of measurement associated with any individual score is 45 per cent of the standard deviation. With a reliability of 0.5, the standard error is 70 per cent of a standard deviation, so we have improved the precision of measurement by only 30 per cent over the information we would have prior to doing any assessment of the individual at all.

One reason for calculating the SEM is to allow us to draw a confidence interval (CI) around a score. A problem, though, is which score to use—the observed score

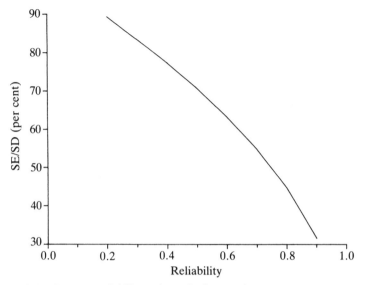

Fig. 8.2 Relation between reliability and standard error of measurement.

or the true score? The issue is that, except for scales that have a reliability of 1.0 (and we do not know of any), observed scores will always be further from the mean than the estimated true score (Charter 1996). What is called the 'traditional' approach (Charter and Feldt 2000, 2001) centres the CI around the observed score:

$$X_0 \pm Z(SEM)$$

where X_0 is the observed score, and Z is the value from the normal curve associated with the desired CI (1. 64 for the 90 per cent CI; 1. 96 for the 95 per cent CI). If we had a scale with a mean of 50, a standard deviation of 10, and a reliability of 0.8; and a person obtained a score of 65, then the 95 per cent CI would be:

$$SEM = 10\sqrt{1 - 0.8} = 4.47$$
$$CI_{95} = 65 \pm 1.96 \times 4.47 = 56.24 - 73.76.$$

Charter and Feldt (2001) state that this formula applies at the level of the *individual*— if we tested 1000 people and used a 95 per cent CI, then 95 per cent of the CIs would capture the true scores.

The second, or 'regression-based,' approach (Charter and Feldt 2000) centres the interval on the Estimated True Score (ETS), which is found by:

$$ETS = M + r(X_0 - M)$$

where M is the mean of the test, X_0 the observed score, and r the reliability. Rather than using the SEM to calculate the CIs, we use the Standard Error of Estimate

(SEE), which is:

$$SEE = \sigma\sqrt{r(1-r)}.$$

In this case, the CI is:

$$ETS \pm Z(SEE).$$

For the same individual discussed above:

$$SEE = 10\sqrt{0.8(1-0.8)} = 4.00$$

and

$$ETS = 50.0 + 0.8(65-50) = 62.0$$
$$CI_{95} = 62.0 \pm 1.96 \times 4.00 = 54.2 - 69.8.$$

The interpretation of this CI is slightly different. It focuses on the 'population' of people who, on this test, have obtained scores of 65; and 95 per cent of them have true scores within the interval of 54.2 − 69.8 (Charter and Feldt 2001). Note that the CI is not symmetric around the observed score, except when it is equal to the mean of the test; it is always larger on the side closer to the scale's mean. (This ties in with the concept of *regression toward the mean*, which we will discuss further in Chapter 11.)

Both approaches to calculating the CI are correct. Which one to use depends on the reason we want to know the CI—for use with an individual person (in which case we use the CI centered around observed score) or for all people with a given obtained score (where we would centre the CI around the ETS).

Expected difference in scores on retesting

If a person takes the same test on two occasions, how big a difference in test scores can be expected? The standard deviation of the difference between two scores is $\sqrt{2} \times$ SEM. Modifying the previous example slightly, imagine we have a test where the person's *observed* score was 15 and the SEM was 3. From the normal distribution, the probability is 68 per cent that the true score is between 12 and 18. If the person takes the test a second time, then the probability is 68 per cent that the second score will be somewhere within the interval of $15 - (\sqrt{2} \times 3)$ and $15 + (\sqrt{2} \times 3)$, or between 10.8 and 19. 2. The interval is larger because there will be some error in both the first and the second observed scores, whereas in determining the interval in which the true score lies, there is error involved only for the observed score, but not for the true one (Green 1981).

Empirical data on retest reliability

One way of evaluating the adequacy of reliability coefficients obtained from a new instrument is to compare them against tests which are generally assumed to have acceptable levels. Schuerger *et al.* (1982, 1989) compiled data from a number of personality questionnaires, re-administered over intervals ranging from 2 days to 20 years. Scales which tap relatively stable traits, such as extraversion, have test–retest coefficients in the high 0.70s to low 0.80s when readministered within the same year, dropping to the mid-0.60s over a 20-year span. Measures of mild and presumably variable pathological states, such as anxiety, have coefficients about 0.10 lower than trait measures. Conversely, IQ tests, especially when administered to adults, have retest reliabilities about 0.10 higher (Schuerger and Witt 1989). Some measures of competence, specifically specialty certification examinations, have been shown to have similar correlations of about 0.70 over a 7- to 10-year interval (Ramsey *et al.* 1989).

Standards for the magnitude of the reliability coefficient

From the previous sections, it should be evident that reliability cannot be conceived of as a property that a particular instrument does or does not possess; rather, any measure will have a certain degree of reliability when applied to certain populations under certain conditions. The issue which must be addressed is how much reliability is 'good enough'. Authors of textbooks on psychometric theory often make brief recommendations, usually without justification or reference to other recommendations. In fact, there can be no sound basis for such a recommendation, any more than there can be a sound basis for the decision that a certain percentage of candidates sitting an examination will fail.

For what it is worth, here are two authors' opinions for acceptable reliability for tests used to make a decision about individuals: Kelley (1927) recommended a minimum of 0.94, while Weiner and Stewart (1984) suggested 0.85. These standards may be too high, though, to be practical. Only two of the eight subscales of the well-validated SF-36 have reliabilities over 0.90 (Ware and Sherbourne 1992); and the 1-day test–retest reliability of automated systolic blood pressure readings in one study was 0.87, and 0.67 for diastolic blood pressure (Prisant *et al.* 1992).

Fortunately, some authors avoid any such arbitrary judgement. However, the majority of textbooks then make a further distinction: namely, that a test used for individual judgement should be more reliable than one used for group decisions or research purposes. Nunnally (1978), for example, recommended a minimum reliability of 0.70 when the scale is used in research, and 0.90 when it is used clinically. There are two possible justifications for this distinction. First, the research will draw conclusions from a mean score averaged across many individuals, and the sample size will serve to reduce the error of measurement in comparison to group differences. Second, rarely will decisions about research findings be made on the basis of a single study; conclusions are usually drawn from a series of replicated studies. But a recommendation of reliability, such as attempted by Weiner and Stewart (1984), remains tenuous since a sample of 1000 can tolerate a much less reliable instrument than a sample of 10, so that the acceptable reliability is dependent on the sample size used in the research.

Reliability and the probability of misclassification

An additional problem of interpretation arising from the reliability coefficient is that it does not, of itself, indicate just how many wrong decisions (false-positives or false-negatives) will result from a measure with a particular reliability. There is no straightforward answer to this problem, since the probability of misclassification, when the underlying measure is continuous, relates both to the property of the instrument and to the decision of the location of the cut point. For example, if we had people trained to assess hemoglobin using an office hemoglobinometer and classify patients as normal or anemic on the basis of a single random blood sample, the number of false-positives and false-negatives will be dependent on the reliability of the reading of a single sample, but will also depend on two other variables: where we decide to set the boundary between normal and anemic, and the base rate of anemia in the population under study.

Clearly there must be some relationship between the reliability of the scores and the likelihood that the decision will result in a misclassification. Some indication of the relationship between reliability and the probability of misclassification was given by Thorndike and Hagen (1969), who avoided the 'cut-point' problem by examining the ranking of individuals. Imagine 100 people who have been tested and ranked. Consider one individual ranked 25th from the top, and another ranked 50th. If the reliability is 0, there is a 50 per cent chance that the two will reverse order on repeated testing, since the measure conveys no information and the ordering, as a result, is arbitrary. With a reliability of 0.5, there is still a 37 per cent chance of reversal; a reliability of 0.8 will result in 20 per cent reversals; and 0.95 will result in their reversing order 2. 2 per cent of the time. From this example, it is evident that reliability of 0.75 is a fairly minimal requirement for a useful instrument.

Reliability and sample size

If a scale is used as an outcome measure, its reliability has a direct impact on the sample size required to show a statistically significant effect. The reason is that unreliability inflates the variance of the observed scores. More specifically, the observed score variance is σ^2/R, where σ^2 is the variance of the true score, and R the reliability of the scale. If we need N subjects in order to achieve significance with a perfectly reliable test, then we would need approximately N/R subjects if the reliability coefficient were actually R (Kraemer 1979). A test with a reliability of 0.80 would require a 25 per cent increase in sample size; we would need 43 per cent more subjects with a reliability of 0.70; and a reliability of 0.50 would require a doubling of the sample size. Obviously, the message is to use a scale with a high reliability.

Improving reliability

If we return to the basic definition of reliability as a ratio of subject variance to subject + error variance, we can improve reliability only by increasing the magnitude of the variance between subjects relative to the error variance. This can be accomplished in a number of ways, both legitimate and otherwise.

There are several approaches to reducing error variance. Many authors recommend observer training, although the specific strategies to be used in training raters are usually unspecified. Alternatively, Newble et al. (1980) have suggested that observers have difficulty acquiring new skills. They recommend, as a result, that if consistently extreme observers are discovered, they simply be eliminated from further use. The strategies for improving scale design discussed in Chapter 4 may also contribute to reducing error variance.

Similarly, there are a number of ways of enhancing the true variance. If the majority of individual scores are either very high or very low, so that the average score is approaching the maximum or minimum possible (the 'ceiling' or 'floor'), then many of the items are being wasted. The solution is to introduce items that will result in performance nearer the middle of the scale, effectively increasing true variance. One could also modify the descriptions on the scale; for example, by changing 'poor–fair–good–excellent' to 'fair–good–very good–excellent'.

An alternative approach, which is *not* legitimate, is to administer the test to a more heterogeneous group of subjects for the purpose of determining reliability. For example, if a measure of function in arthritis does not reliably discriminate among ambulatory arthritics, administering the test to both normal subjects and to bedridden hospitalized arthritics will almost certainly improve reliability. Of course, the resulting reliability no longer yields any information about the ability of the instrument to discriminate among ambulatory patients.

By contrast, it is sometimes the case that a reliability coefficient derived from a homogeneous population is to be applied to a population that is more heterogeneous. It is clear from the above discussion that the reliability in the application envisioned will be larger than that determined in the homogeneous study population. If the standard deviations of the two samples are known, it is possible to calculate a new reliability coefficient, or to *correct for attenuation*, using the following formula:

$$R_{revised} = \frac{R \times \sigma_{new}^2}{R \times \sigma_{new}^2 + (1 - R) \times \sigma_{old}^2}$$

where σ_{new}^2 and σ_{old}^2 are the variances of the new and original samples, respectively, and R is the original reliability.

Perhaps the simplest way to improve reliability is to increase the number of items on the test. It is not self-evident why this should help, but the answer lies in statistical theory. As long as the test items are not perfectly correlated, the true variance will increase as the square of the number of items, whereas the error variance will increase only as the number of items. So, if the test length is tripled, true variance will be nine times as large, and error variance three times as large as the original test, as long as the new items are similar psychometrically to the old ones. From the Spearman–Brown formula, which we discussed in Chapter 5, the new reliability will be:

$$R_{SB} = \frac{3 \times R}{1 + 2 \times R}$$

If the original reliability was 0.7, the tripled test will have a reliability of 0.875. The relationship between the number of items and test length is shown in Fig. 8.3.

In practice, the equation tends to overestimate the new reliability, since we tend to think up (or 'borrow') the easier, more obvious items first. When we have to devise new items, they often are not as good as the original ones.

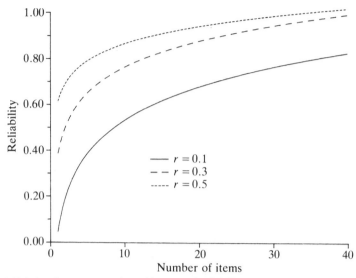

Fig. 8.3 Relation between number of items and reliability.

The Spearman–Brown formula can be used in another way. If we know the reliability of a test of a particular length is r and we wish to achieve a reliability of R, then the formula can be modified to indicate the factor by which we must increase the test length, k:

$$k = \frac{R(1-r)}{r(1-R)}$$

To improve measures of stability, such as test–retest reliability, one can always shorten the retest interval. However, if the instrument is intended to measure states of duration of weeks or months, the demonstration of retest reliability over hours or days is not useful.

Finally, it is evident from the foregoing discussion that there is not a single reliability associated with a measure. A more useful approach to the issue of reliability is to critically examine the components of variance due to each source of variation in turn, and then focus efforts on reducing the larger sources of error variance. This approach, called *generalizability theory*, is covered in the next chapter.

Standard error of the reliability coefficient and sample size

In conducting a reliability study, we are attempting to estimate the reliability coefficient with as much accuracy as possible; that is, we want to be certain that the true reliability coefficient is reasonably close to the estimate we have determined. This is one form of the *confidence interval* (for further discussion consult one of the recommended statistics books). As we might expect, the larger the sample size, the smaller will be the confidence interval, so that for a given estimate of the confidence interval, we can (in theory) compute the required sample size.

To do so, we need to first determine the standard error of the reliability coefficient (which is not the same as the standard error of measurement derived *from* the reliability coefficient, as we did a few pages ago). As it turns out, this is quite complex. It leans heavily on the Fisher z_R transformation of the intraclass correlation, given in Fisher's book (1925), which removes skewness in the standard error:

$$z_R = \frac{1}{2}\log_e\left[\frac{1 + (k - 1)R}{1 - R}\right]$$

where R is the value of the intraclass correlation and k is the number of observations per subject. From this, Fisher derived the formula of the standard error of the z_R transform:

$$SE(z_R) = \sqrt{\frac{k}{2(k - 1)(n - 2)}}$$

where n is the number of subjects.

So for any calculated reliability, R, and a given sample size, we can determine the standard error of the reliability coefficient. For example, if we had conducted a study with 102 observations, and five raters, and the reliability had turned out to be 0.75, we can then compute the standard error as follows:

(1) the z transformed reliability is:

$$z_R = \frac{1}{2}\log_e\left[\frac{1 + (4 \times 0.75)}{1 - 0.75}\right] = \frac{1}{2}\log_e(16) = 1.386;$$

(2) the standard error of the z transformed R is:

$$SE = \sqrt{\frac{5}{2(4)(100)}} = 0.079;$$

(3) so the upper and lower limits of the z transformed R is now:

$$1.386 \pm .079 = 1.307 \rightarrow 1.465;$$

(4) next, working backwards, the upper and lower limits of R, ± 1 SE (R_U and R_L, respectively), are:

$$R_U = \frac{1 + (k - 1)R_U}{1 - R_U} = e^{(2z_U)} = e^{(2.930)} = 0.780$$

and

$$R_L = \frac{1 + (k - 1)R_L}{1 - R_L} = e^{(2z_L)} = e^{(2.614)} = 0.717;$$

(5) so finally, we can say that the estimated reliability is 0.75, with a range ($\pm$SE) of 0.717 to 0.780. Because of the properties of the distribution, this is not quite symmetrical about the estimate.

To compute the required sample size, we begin with an estimate of the likely intraclass correlation, R. We then estimate the likely certainty we want in this estimate (± 1 SE). For example, if we think that the reliability computed from the study is 0.80, and we want to have sufficient sample size to be 95 per cent certain that it is definitely above 0.70, this amounts to setting the 95 per cent confidence interval around the reliability of 0.10 (0.80 minus 0.70). The SE, then, is half this confidence interval, or 0.05. We also have to know in advance the number of observations we are going to use in the study; for example, five. The derivation of sample size proceeds as follows:

First, compute $R^- = R - SE$. (We use $R - SE$ rather than $R + SE$ because it is more conservative, resulting in a somewhat larger sample size). Then from the formula above:

$$z_R = \frac{1}{2}\log_e\left[\frac{1 + (k-1)R}{1 - R}\right] \quad \text{and} \quad z_{R^-} = \frac{1}{2}\log_e\left[\frac{1 + (k-1)R^-}{1 - R^-}\right].$$

We can now compute the SE of the z scores as:

$$SE = z_R - z_{R^-}$$

but, from the previous equation:

$$SE(z_R) = \sqrt{\frac{k}{2(k-1)(n-2)}}.$$

Finally, squaring and cross-multiplying we get:

$$n = 2 + \frac{k}{2(k-1)(z_R - z_{R^-})^2}.$$

In our previous example, then, we began with a hypothesized reliability, R, of 0.80, a standard error of 0.05, and five observations per subject:
(1) the log transformed values of R and R^- are:

$$z_R = \frac{1}{2}\log_e(4.2/.2) = 0.661$$

and

$$z_{R^-} = \frac{1}{2}\log_e(3.0/.25) = 0.539;$$

(2) so the SE is:

$$z_R - z_{R^-} = 0.661 - 0.539 = 0.122;$$

(3) then the sample size, n, is:

$$n = 2 + 5/[(2)(4)(0.122)2] = 42.$$

It is possible to determine all this graphically, but, since the sample size depends on three estimates—R, k and the confidence interval—multiple graphs are required to display the results. Two such graphs, for $R = 0.75$ and 0.90, are shown in Fig. 8.4.

This approach differs from that taken by other authors (e.g. Donner and Eliasziw 1987), who base the calculation on the number of subjects needed to determine if the coefficient is significantly different from some arbitrary value. In most instances, this is not the question we are asking; we are usually more interested in estimating the magnitude of the reliability coefficient, rather than seeing if it is statistically significantly different from some other value.

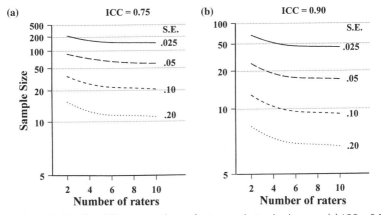

Fig. 8.4 Sample sizes for different numbers of raters and standard errors: (a) ICC = 0.75; and (b) ICC = 0.90.

Still another approach to estimating the sample size is to use a fixed number. Thus, Nunnally (1978) recommends that the study involve at least 300 subjects, while Guilford (1956) and Kline (1986) are a little less demanding and recommend 200 subjects. However, these suggestions do not take into account the fact that for a confidence interval of a given width, the sample size varies with the magnitude of the coefficient. So, for a CI of 0.10 (with $\alpha = 0.05$), Nunnally's recommendation would result in 'statistical overkill' for any coefficient greater than 0.18; and Guilford's and Kline's for any greater than 0.58. If we expected that the reliability coefficient would be 0.70, for example, the equation would yield a sample size requirement of only 130 subjects.

Summary

The discussion regarding appropriate measures of reliability is easily resolved. The Pearson correlation is theoretically incorrect but usually fairly close. The method of Altman and Bland is analogous (actually isomorphic) to the calculation of error variance in the ICC, and does not explicitly relate this to the range of observations. Thus we are left with kappa and the intraclass correlation, which yield identical results, so the choice can be dictated by ease of calculation, nothing else.

References

Altman, D. G. and Bland, J. M. (1983). Measurement in medicine: The analysis of method comparison studies. *Statistician*, 32, 307–17.

Bland, J. M. and Altman, D. G. (1986). Statistical methods for assessing agreement between two methods of clinical measurement. *Lancet*, i, 307–10.

Charter, R. A. (1996). Revisiting the standard errors of measurement, estimate, and prediction and their application to test scores. *Perceptual and Motor Skills*, 82, 1139–44.

Charter, R. A. and Feldt, L. S. (2000). The relationship between two methods of evaluating an examinee's difference scores. *Journal of Psychoeducational Assessment*, **18**, 125–42.

Charter, R. A. and Feldt, L. S. (2001). Confidence intervals for true scores: Is there a correct approach? *Journal of Psychoeducational Assessment*, **19**, 350–64.

Cohen, J. (1960). A coefficient of agreement for nominal scales. *Educational and Psychological Measurement*, **20**, 37–46.

Cohen, J. (1968). Weighted kappa: Nominal scale agreement with provision for scaled disagreement or partial credit. *Psychological Bulletin*, **70**, 213–20.

Cronbach, L. J. (1957). The two disciplines of scientific psychology. *American Psychologist*, **12**, 671–84.

Donner, A. and Eliasziw, M. (1987). Sample size requirements for reliability studies. *Statistics in Medicine*, **6**, 441–8.

Fisher, R. A. (1925). *Statistical methods for research workers*. Oliver and Boyd, Edinburgh.

Fleiss, J. L. and Cohen, J. (1973). The equivalence of weighted kappa and the intraclass correlation coefficient as measures of reliability. *Educational and Psychological Measurement*, **33**, 613–19.

Green, B. F. (1981). A primer of testing. *American Psychologist*, **36**, 1001–11.

Guilford, J. P. (1956). *Psychometric methods* (2nd edn). McGraw Hill, New York.

Kraemer, H. C. (1979). Ramifications of a population model for k as a coefficient of reliability. *Psychometrika*, **44**, 461–72.

Kelley, T. L. (1927). *Interpretation of educational measurements*. World Books, Yonkers.

Kline, P. (1986). *A handbook of test construction*. Methuen, London.

McGraw, K. O. and Wong, S. P. (1996). Forming inferences about some intraclass correlation coefficients. *Psychological Methods*, **1**, 30–46.

Newble, D. I., Hoare, J., and Sheldrake, P. F. (1980). The selection and training of examiners for clinical examinations. *Medical Education*, **4**, 345–9.

Norman, G. R. and Streiner, D. L. (2000). *Biostatistics: The bare essentials* (2nd edn). B. C. Decker, Toronto.

Nunnally, J. C. (1978). *Psychometric theory*. McGraw-Hill, New York.

Prisant, L. M., Carr, A. A., Bottini, P. B., Thompson, W. O., and Rhoades, R. B. (1992). Repeatability of automated ambulatory blood pressure measurements. *Journal of Family Practice*, **34**, 569–74.

Ramsey, P. G., Carline, J. D., Inui, T. S., Larson, E. B., LoGerfo, J. P., and Weinrich, M. D. (1989). Predictive validity of certification by the American Board of Internal Medicine. *Annals of Internal Medicine*, **110**, 719–26.

Schuerger, J. M. Tait, E., and Tavernelli, M. (1982). Temporal stability of personality by questionnaire. *Journal of Personality and Social Psychology*, **43**, 176–82.

Schuerger, J. M., and Witt, A. C. (1989). The temporal stability of individually tested intelligence. *Journal of Clinical Psychology*, **45**, 294–302.

Schuerger, J. M., Zarella, K. L., and Hotz, A. S. (1989). Factors that influence the temporal stability of personality by questionnaire. *Journal of Personality and Social Psychology*, **56**, 777–83.

Shrout, P. E. and Fleiss, J. L. (1979). Intraclass correlations: Uses in assessing rater reliability. *Psychological Bulletin*, **86**, 420–8.

Thorndike, R. L. and Hagen, E. (1969). *Measurement and evaluation in education and psychology*. Wiley, New York.

Ware, J. E. and Sherbourne, C. D. (1992). The MOS 36-Item Short-Form Survey (SF-36): I. Conceptual framework and item selection. *Medical Care*, **30**, 473–83.

Weiner, E. A. and Stewart, B. J. (1984). *Assessing individuals*. Little Brown, Boston.

Chapter 9

Generalizability theory

Classical test theory, upon which the reliability coefficient is based, begins with a simple assumption—that an observed test score can be decomposed into two parts: a 'true' score (which no one really knows) and an 'error' score (i.e. $\text{Score}_{\text{Observed}} = \text{Score}_{\text{True}} + \text{error}$). As we discussed in the previous chapter, this assumption then leads directly to the formulation of the reliability coefficient as the ratio of true variance to (true + error) variance.

We saw that there are many approaches to estimating reliability, each of which generates a different coefficient. One can examine scores from the same observer on two viewings of the same stimulus (intra-observer), different observers of the same stimulus (inter-observer), different occasions separated by a short time interval (test–retest), different items (internal consistency), different forms of the scale (parallel forms), and so on. Further, these standard measures do not exhaust the possible sources of variance. For example, some measures, such as bone density or tenderness, might be expected to be equal on both sides of the body (left–right reliability?), and skin color might be expected to be the same on the soles of hands and feet (top–bottom reliability?).

Clearly, the assumption that all variance in scores can be neatly divided into true and error variance is simplistic. Instead, for each person we have measured there are, in addition to the 'true' score of that individual, multiple potential sources of error. Our goal is to obtain the most precise estimate we can of the score that person should have if there were no sources of error contaminating our results; each of the multiple forms of reliability that we have mentioned identifies and quantifies only one source of error variance.

This may not, of itself, be problematic. Conceptually at least, we could consider a long series of studies, each of which determined one source of error variance. We could, perhaps, then put all of these error variances together to arrive at the appropriate reliability coefficients.

Unfortunately, in addition to the semi-infinite research agenda this would generate (those eager for tenure and promotion may view this as an advantage rather than a handicap), there are other flies in the ointment. Remember that we estimate the true score optimistically as the average across all the allowed observations. This strategy will inevitably lead to different estimates of true scores from each study, with no logical way to combine them. As one example, imagine we did an inter- and intra-rater reliability study with two observers and a 7-point scale. Assume that one observer used the whole scale, but the other used only the points from 3 to 5, and that their individual judgements were almost perfectly reproducible. Both intra-rater studies would result in the same near-zero error variance; however, the subject variance of one study would be about four times as large as the other, leading to very different estimates of 'the' reliability.

Finally, there may be interactions amongst the sources of error variance. We will use the Objective Structured Clinical Examination (OSCE; Harden and Gleeson 1979) as an example. In it, students rotate through a series of 'stations', typically of 5–10 minutes duration each, where they perform a component of a clinical exam-ination such as taking a brief history of abdominal pain from a simulated patient, physically examining a chest, or interpreting a radiograph. Although some stations, such as the radiographic interpretation, may be unobserved and scored later, clinical stations are more typically observed and scored by clinician examiners. If we did an inter-observer reliability study on each station using two independent examiners, we would create a whole set of reliability coefficients, one for each station. We could also do an 'inter-station reliability study', examining the correlation across stations. But to the extent that examiners are chosen with expertise in particular skills, and have different scoring styles, the amount of error variance may differ from station to station, amounting to a subject by examiner by station component of variance, which cannot be captured from the individual studies. What we really need is some way of combining all the sources of variability in a single study, using all the data to estimate the variance between subjects and the various components of error variance.

This broad approach was originally devised by Cronbach and his associates and is known as *generalizability theory* (Cronbach *et al.* 1972). The essence of the theory is the recognition that in any measurement situation there are multiple (in fact, infinite) sources of error variance. An important goal of measurement is to attempt to iden-tify, measure, and thereby find strategies to reduce the influence of these sources on the measurement in question. Although the theory is now over 30 years old, it is only within the last few years that it has become a routine approach to measurement in the health sciences. A few review articles have appeared which elaborate on, or utilize, the concepts of generalizability theory (Boodoo and O'Sullivan 1982; Evans *et al.* 1981; Shavelson *et al.* 1989; van der Vleuten and Swanson 1990).

Imagine that we could identify the most likely sources of error in a measurement of some characteristic of a person. Having made this step (e.g. declaring that the important sources of error in this measurement situation were the observer, the time of day, and the phase of the moon), we have then defined our 'universe' of possible observations to include different observers, morning, noon and night, and four lunar phases. If we then proceeded to average each person's scores over all these pos-sible conditions, this would be an unbiased estimate of that person's score over the universe as we have defined it. Note that there is no pretence that this is a 'true' score, since we may well have guessed wrong about the universe—maybe it's the phases of Mars, not the moon, that really matter—but this is still a best guess at a 'universe' score for our predefined and finite universe of observations.

G studies

Presuming that we have done a reasonable job of identifying the possible sources of error, these would then be incorporated into a research design, called a *generalizability study* or 'G study', where all the sources are contained as repeated measures on each subject. The next step then would be to use the data we have gathered to determine the extent to which each of these variables actually influenced the score. One way of expressing this variability is to use the concepts of analysis of variance, as we did in Chapter 8. Thus, to the extent that the time of day does influence the obtained scores, then the analysis of the data will show that the variance due to time will be large relative to other components. As we have pointed out already, if the sources we have identified are trivial, and we have missed some important sources of error, then there will be a large amount of variance due to *random error* or *residual*. By identifying these sources of error, we can determine the relative importance of each component in adding error to a measurement. In turn, this information can then lead to specific strategies to reduce major components of error and improve measurement, the details of which will be discussed later.

Once we have determined all the sources of variance, we can then construct appropriate coefficients reflecting different decision situations. For example, we can create a coefficient showing the extent to which we can generalize from observations made by one observer on one day in one lunar phase, to another observation made by another observer on the same day in the same phase, the equivalent of the standard inter-rater reliability. In the terminology of generalizability theory, 'observer' is *a facet of generalization*, and since we wish to differentiate among patients, 'patient' is a *facet of differentiation*. Lunar phase and day, since they are fixed, are called *fixed facets*. Another coefficient may be determined by keeping the observer fixed but generalizing across days; here the facet of differentiation is still patients, the facet of generalization is days, and the fixed facets are observer and lunar phase. This is, of course, the equivalent of 'intra-rater' or 'test–retest' reliability.

D studies

Having generated the variance estimates, we can then determine the effect of changing the number of observations. For instance, we can see what will happen to the generalizability coefficient if we add a third observer, or decrease the number of days of observation from four to three. Since these explore the impact of certain decisions, they are called *Decision* or *D studies*. These 'studies' are done using only paper and pencil (or a computer), dividing each term by the new number of observations in each facet. This then permits us to see what we must do to increase the reliability to an acceptable level, or conversely, how much the reliability will decline if we make the real-life situation more feasible by eliminating testings.

Within generalizability theory, the patient or subject no longer has any special status. For example, we may want to know the extent to which the scores can differentiate among sadness states related to different phases of the moon. For this D study, lunar phase is the facet of differentiation, patient is the facet of generalization, and observer and day are fixed facets. (This example is not as bizarre as it may first appear. Much effort has been expended trying to relate psychiatric admissions to the full moon, and even to sun-spot activity.)

It is evident that the conventional approaches to reliability—test–retest, inter-observer, and so on—become simply special cases of a more general formulation which seeks to identify the important sources of variance in a particular measurement situation from the outset, and then attempts to quantify these sources of error.

Example 1—therapists, occasions, and patients

An example may clarify the theory. Imagine a group of respiratory patients enrolled in a rehabilitation program. In order to determine the reliability of measurement of pulmonary function, three physiotherapists make independent assessments on two successive visits five days apart. The design may look like Table 9.1.

It is evident that this design contains elements of both inter-observer and test–retest reliability. To the extent that the scores assigned by various therapists on the same day differ, this will contribute to a reduction in inter-observer reliability. Observations by the *same* observer on the second occasion are a measure of test–retest reliability.

What makes this design approach different from conventional assessment is that both sources of error (therapist and occasion) are incorporated in the *same* design, instead of conducting two separate studies. This tactic has three methodological advantages. First, subject or patient variance is a single estimate using all the data. Second, the estimate of each reliability is derived from multiple observations, since three raters are contributing to the assessment of test–retest reliability, and two occasions are summed together to yield a measure of inter-observer reliability. This effectively increases the sample size and thereby improves precision. Third, combining the two sources of variation into one experiment permits the consideration of

Table 9.1 Assessment of ten patients by three physiotherapists on two days

| Patient | Experimental design | | | | | |
| | Observer 1 | | Observer 2 | | Observer 3 | |
	Day 1	Day 5	Day 1	Day 5	Day 1	Day 5
1						
2						
.						
.						
.						
10						

EXAMPLE 1—THERAPISTS, OCCASIONS, AND PATIENTS | 157

Table 9.2 Analysis of variance table

Source	Sum of squares	d.f.	Mean square (MS)	Expected mean square (EMS)
Patients (p)	3915	9	435	$\sigma^2_{dop} + 2\sigma^2_{op} + 3\sigma^2_{dp} + 6\sigma^2_{p}$
Day (d)	815	1	815	$\sigma^2_{dop} + 3\sigma^2_{dp} + 10\sigma^2_{do} + 30\sigma^2_{d}$
Day × Patients (dp)	585	9	65	$\sigma^2_{dop} + 3\sigma^2_{dp}$
Observer (o)	960	2	480	$\sigma^2_{dop} + 2\sigma^2_{op} + 10\sigma^2_{do} + 20\sigma^2_{o}$
Observer × Patients (op)	540	18	30	$\sigma^2_{dop} + 2\sigma^2_{op}$
Day × Observer (do)	340	2	170	$\sigma^2_{dop} + 10\sigma^2_{do}$
Day × Observer × Patients (dop)	360	18	20	σ^2_{dop}

additional combinations of error variance. For example, it is likely that our real concern is the reliability of an observation made by *any* therapist on *any* occasion, a situation which would suggest the need for a test-retest/inter-observer reliability coefficient. This coefficient can be easily determined from a design such as that in the example, but would not normally be available from applications of classical test theory.

Continuing with the example, we might explore how the various components of variance are derived. For simplicity, we limit ourselves to the two-factor case, including only variation due to multiple observers and repeated occasions of observation. If the data were analyzed using repeated-measures ANOVA, the results would resemble Table 9.2.

Note that this table includes the expected mean squares, expressed as a sum of variance components. The detailed derivation of these expressions can be found in statistics texts (e.g. Glass and Stanley 1970), so we will just give a brief indication of the conceptual basis of the expressions.

The basic notation of the mean square (MS) as a sum of variances was discussed in Chapter 8. Every MS contains both the variance due to the factor of interest and also variance due to all other sources which interact with it; so for example, the MS due to observers contains variance due to observers, and also variance due to the interaction between observers and patients, observers and days, and observers, days, and patients (which is just the residual error term in this example). At first sight, this seems nonsensical, since we have already separately calculated the variance due to all the other interactions. However, the apparent contradiction resides in the basic assumption of statistics, which distinguishes between samples and populations.

Table 9.3 Components of variance

Source	Variance
Patients	60
Day	20
Day × Patients	15
Observer	15
Observer × Patients	5
Day × Observer	15
Day × Observer × Patients	20

The MS terms we have calculated are *estimates* of the population variances, expressed in σ^2 terms. Even if, for example, there really was no difference between observers, or no 'main effect' of observers, we might expect that random fluctuations would result in some difference between the calculated means for each observer, and hence some non-zero value of the MS due to observers. The extent to which this calculated MS differs from the population variance due to observers is imbedded in the magnitude of the interaction terms, and thus these interactions contribute to the expected MS.

Furthermore, each MS is actually summed up over all levels of the factors *not* contained in the expression; the *DP* interaction is summed over the three levels of the observer, and the *O* main effect is summed over the 10 levels of patients and two levels of days. As a result, when these variance components are entered into the expected mean square (EMS) expression, they contain multipliers accounting for the levels of the factors *not* in each term.

Further elaboration of the derivation of these expressions is beyond the scope of this book. Suffice it to say that from these formulae we can derive the resulting variance components. These are shown in Table 9.3.

From this analysis, it is apparent that the main source of variance in the measurements is *P*, which indicates that most of the variability in the measurements is due to systematic differences between patients. This is the expectation, and indicates that we were successful in discriminating among patients. Relatively less variance is due to the main effects of *D* (suggesting systematically higher or lower values on different days) and *O* (reflecting systematic differences between observers). The *DP* interaction shows that some patients did better on day 1 than day 5, while this was reversed for other patients. The *OD* interaction is interpreted in a similar manner. The low variance due to the *OP* interaction is encouraging, reflecting that the observers' ratings are *not* influenced by specific patients. Finally, the residual (*DOP*) interaction is relatively large (20) in comparison to the remaining sources of variance, possibly suggesting that there are other important factors we might have included in the G study.

Applying the approaches of the previous chapter, we could easily conjure up a reliability coefficient consisting of the variance due to patients (60), divided by the sum

EXAMPLE 1—THERAPISTS, OCCASIONS, AND PATIENTS | 159

of all the variance components (150), or 0.4. Unfortunately, this approach simply indicates that the other factors are contributing considerable error variance, but does not indicate where it came from or how one might improve the situation.

Let us examine Table 9.3 in more detail. First, note that the main effects of D and O imply simply that the average score on day 1 differed from the score on day 5, and that there were differences in the average scores of the observers. This may be of no consequence if we simply wish to compare scores on the same day or by the same observer, or alternatively if we are willing to apply a correction factor to eliminate this source of bias in each estimate. Conversely, the interaction terms between P and the other variables represent the extent to which each source directly contributes *random* variation to a score. For example, the OP interaction implies that some patients are rated differently by some observers than by other observers, an effect that we cannot disentangle if we wish to use scores obtained from different observers. However, this interaction term is irrelevant if we wish to look only at the reliability of the ratings by the same observer on successive days. In this case, the DP interaction term expresses the amount of random error in repeated scores by the same observer.

These observations suggest that it may be possible to use the variance components identified in the analysis of variance to construct a series of coefficients, which will depend on the variables that will remain constant (or 'fixed') in a particular measurement situation, and the variables one wishes to make generalizations over.

Continuing with this example, suppose we want to use these data to examine inter-observer reliability. In this case, the fact that the observations were repeated on two occasions is incidental; what we want to focus on is differences between observers. The design looks as if we had done an inter-observer reliability study twice.

In examining inter-observer reliability, then, the change in scores that occurred with the passage of time is incidental, and so the main effect of day would be excluded from the sources of variance in this generalizability coefficient. Second, if the day factor were not explicitly calculated as a variance component, then the interaction between day and patients would end up in the sum of squares due to patients. So if we wish to calculate the coefficient equivalent to an inter-observer reliability, the numerator would contain the main effect of patients, and the interaction between patients and day.

Extrapolating from this example, then, in constructing a generalizability coefficient, the numerator of the coefficient contains the variance due to patients and all interactions between patients and any factors over which one does not wish to generalize (such as day). The denominator contains variance due to patients, interactions between patients and all other factors, and the random error term (in this case, patient $\times$ observer $\times$ day). The generalizability coefficient becomes:

$$\frac{\sigma_P^2 + \sigma_{DP}^2}{\sigma_P^2 + \sigma_{OP}^2 + \sigma_{DP}^2 + \sigma_{DOP}^2} = \frac{60 + 15}{60 + 5 + 15 + 20} = 0.75.$$

In looking at the test–retest reliability, the opposite situation arises. In this circumstance, variance due to systematic differences between observers (i.e. the main effect of O) is irrelevant. Analogously, the *OP* interaction is incorporated into the variance due to patients in the numerator of the coefficient. So, the generalizability coefficient becomes:

$$\frac{\sigma_P^2 + \sigma_{OP}^2}{\sigma_P^2 + \sigma_{OP}^2 + \sigma_{DP}^2 + \sigma_{DOP}^2} = \frac{60 + 5}{60 + 5 + 15 + 20} = 0.65.$$

Finally, one may wish to generalize from a rating by one observer on one day to a rating by a different observer at another time. This coefficient has no classical equivalent, and equals:

$$\frac{\sigma_P^2}{\sigma_P^2 + \sigma_{OP}^2 + \sigma_{DP}^2 + \sigma_{DOP}^2} = \frac{60}{60 + 5 + 15 + 20} = 0.60.$$

As one would expect, this coefficient is lower than either of the preceding ones.

This example provides some insight into the nature of generalizability theory. The approach begins by attempting to define all the significant sources of observational error—observers, days, items, and so forth. These are then incorporated into a factorial experimental design, and components of variance determined. Different coefficients can then be calculated depending on which factors ('facets' in the theory) will remain fixed and which will vary.

The example we used was based on a simple ANOVA design, in which there were two factors, and each factor occurred at all levels of the other factors: a 'crossed' design in the language of analysis of variance. However, the method can be used with more complex designs, including as many as four or five factors, as well as 'nested' designs, where the factor structure is more complex. The general approach remains the same; to begin by isolating the various sources of variance in the scores, and then generating a family of coefficients which depend on the particular factors which are allowed to vary and remain fixed.

D study examples

Having obtained the estimates of variance coefficients, we are now in the position to estimate a wide range of D coefficients to address various possible decision situations. While some of these may be performed by the investigator as part of the original study, the fact that there are estimates of variance components available enables the reader to construct additional G coefficients corresponding to his or her decision situation.

For example, given the clinical situation we began with, where patients are being assessed on multiple occasions over the course of treatment, it might be reasonable to determine whether we get a more reliable estimate of different patients' disease by using multiple therapists rating the patient on a single day, or one therapist rating the patient over several days. We noted in our previous example that the observer was a relatively small source of variance compared to the day of assessment. Therefore, the logically more appropriate strategy would appear to be to take assessments on several days using a single observer. The alternative strategy of gathering observations from multiple observers on a single day would provide relatively little gain.

The effect of these strategies can be quantified. Since the variance of the average of n observations is just the initial variance divided by n, this can be included in the generalizability coefficients. Let us compare the following two strategies:

(a) one observer on three successive days;

vs.

(b) three observers on a single day.

For case (a), the variance due to days × patients and the error variance will be reduced by a factor of 3, so the new coefficient is:

$$G = \frac{60}{60 + 5 + \dfrac{15}{3} + \dfrac{20}{3}} = 0.78.$$

Similarly, the coefficient for the second strategy will have the observer × patients interaction and the error variance divided by 3, to result in:

$$G = \frac{60}{60 + \dfrac{5}{3} + 15 + \dfrac{20}{3}} = 0.72.$$

Therefore the second strategy resulted in a lower coefficient, even though it used the same amount of therapist time.

We have also stated that there can be different facets of differentiation, and patient is only one possibility. In the present example we might, for instance, ascertain whether the instrument can distinguish among therapists, determining those who are systematically lower or higher in their estimates; information which might be useful in deciding whether to initiate a training program for therapists. More interesting, perhaps, is the use of generalizability theory to distinguish between the two occasions of assessment, on the first and fifth day. We might have expected some response to therapy after five days of treatment; the question is whether the measure can detect this effect.

There is a large literature devoted to the measurement of change, and Chapter 11 discusses many of these issues in detail. In the present situation, we simply wish to demonstrate that the measurement of change is a natural aspect of generalizability theory, and the creation of a 'responsiveness to change coefficient' is just one more variation on the central theme. In this case, the facet of differentiation is day (to what extent can we differentiate among different days of treatment?), the facet of generalization is patient (to what extent does the change from day 1 to day 5 generalize across patients?) and observer is the fixed facet.

The appropriate G coefficient now is:

$$G = \frac{\sigma_D^2 + \sigma_{DO}^2}{\sigma_D^2 + \sigma_{DO}^2 + \sigma_{DP}^2 + \sigma_{DOP}^2} = \frac{20 + 15}{20 + 15 + 15 + 20} = 0.50.$$

Thus, the G coefficient related to responsiveness is very similar to the reliability coefficient; in fact, two of the terms in the denominator are identical.

Example 2—items, observers, and stations (the OSCE)

In this example, we will use the OSCE format, which we discussed earlier, to illustrate the idea of 'nested' factors. We presume that each examiner will be rating students at only one station, and second, that the rating form used at each station is specific to the station, although the number of categories is the same for all stations (to ease computation and interpretation). For example, each examiner may complete a global rating on a 7-point scale for each of three different dimensions (e.g. completeness of history taking, communication skills and accuracy of the physical examination). Let us suppose that there are two observers per case, four stations, and 10 students. Thus, in G theory terminology, the universe of observations consists of four facets: the observer, with two levels; the rating, with three levels; the station or case, with four levels; and the student, with 10 levels. To complicate things further, since each observer stays at one station for the exercise, observer is 'nested' within case. Second, since each station examines a different aspect of competence, the four ratings in each station may in turn address different aspects on each station, so rating is also nested within case. The study design is shown in Table 9.4.

Because the observer and the rating are nested within each case, we cannot examine the interaction between these factors and the case. This results in fewer lines in the ANOVA table, and some more complications in the estimated mean squares. For a sample of data we used, the ANOVA table looked like Table 9.5, where (c) means that rating is nested within case.

Now the next step, as usual, is to derive formulae for the expected mean squares. Again, the approach is complicated but is presented in some statistics books. These,

Table 9.4 Design of a typical OSCE with four stations, two observers and three ratings

Student	Station 1		Station 2			Station 4	
	Obs 1	Obs 2	Obs 3	Obs 4	...	Obs 7	Obs 8
1	$R_1 R_2 R_3$	$R_1 R_2 R_3$	$R_1 R_2 R_3$	$R_1 R_2 R_3$	...	$R_1 R_2 R_3$	$R_1 R_2 R_3$
2					...		
3					...		
4					...		
5					...		
.							
.							
10					...		

EXAMPLE 2—ITEMS, OBSERVERS, AND STATIONS (THE OSCE) | 163

Table 9.5 ANOVA table for Example 2

Source	Sum of squares	df	Mean square
Student S	85.23	9	9.47
Observer O: (C)	14.56	4	3.64
Rating R: (C)	11.00	4	1.37
Case C	118.48	3	39.49
S × O(C)	111.76	36	3.10
S × R(C)	70.33	72	0.98
S × C	205.93	27	7.62
O × C	6.93	8	0.87
S × O × R(C) Error	61.73	72	0.86

Table 9.6 Estimated mean squares and variances for Example 2

Source	Expected mean square	Calculated variance
Student S	$\sigma_{Err}^2 + 6\sigma_{SC}^2 + 3\sigma_{SO(C)}^2 + 2\sigma_{SR(C)}^2 + 24\sigma_S^2$	0.077
Observer O: (C)	$\sigma_{Err}^2 + 3\sigma_{SO(C)}^2 + 10\sigma_{SR(C)}^2 + 30\sigma_{O(C)}^2$	0.017
Rating R: (C)	$\sigma_{Err}^2 + 2\sigma_{SO(C)}^2 + 10\sigma_{OR(C)}^2 + 20\sigma_{R(C)}^2$	0.019
Case C	$\sigma_{Err}^2 + 2\sigma_{SR(C)}^2 + 10\sigma_{OR(C)}^2 + 3\sigma_{SO(C)}^2$ $+ 6\sigma_{SC}^2 + 20\sigma_{R(C)}^2 + 30\sigma_{O(C)}^2 + 60\sigma_C^2$	0.516
S × O(C)	$\sigma_{Err}^2 + 3\sigma_{SO(C)}^3$	0.749
S × R(C)	$\sigma_{Err}^2 + 2\sigma_{SR(C)}^2$	0.059
S × C	$\sigma_{Err}^2 + 2\sigma_{SR(C)}^2 + 3\sigma_{SO(C)}^2 + 6\sigma_{SC}^2$	0.734
O × R	$\sigma_{Err}^2 + 10\sigma_{OR(C)}^2$	0.001
S × O × R(C)	σ_{Err}^2	0.857

and the variances calculated from the mean squares using these formulae, are presented in Table 9.6.

Once the variances are computed, we can construct the appropriate G coefficients using the usual strategy. Thus, for differentiating among students, the denominator is always the same:

$$Denominator\ 1 = \sigma_{SR(C)}^2 + \sigma_{SC}^2 + \sigma_{SO(C)}^2 + \sigma_S^2 + \sigma_{SOR(C)}^2 = 2.476.$$

For generalization across ratings (a measure of the average inter-item correlation), case and observer are fixed factors, hence end up in the numerator with the main effect of students, so the coefficient is:

$$G(Ratings) = \frac{\sigma_{SC}^2 + \sigma_{SO(C)}^2 + \sigma_S^2}{Denominator\ 1} = \frac{1.560}{2.476} = 0.63.$$

This in turn may be modified into the equivalent of a Cronbach's alpha by dividing the appropriate error and interaction terms (those involving rating) by the number of ratings, three. So the new denominator is:

$$Denominator\ 2 = \sigma_{SC}^2 + \sigma_{SO(C)}^2 + \sigma_{SR(C)}^2/3 + \sigma_S^2 + \sigma_{SOR(C)}^2/3 = 1.866$$

and the G coefficient is now:

$$G(Ratings) = \frac{\sigma_{SC}^2 + \sigma_{SO(C)}^2 + \sigma_S^2}{Denominator\ 2} = \frac{1.560}{1.866} = 0.836.$$

Similarly, the G coefficient for generalizing across observer, i.e. the inter-rater reliability, keeps rating and case as fixed factors, so the coefficient is:

$$G(Observer) = \frac{\sigma_{SC}^2 + \sigma_{SR(C)}^2 + \sigma_S^2}{Denominator\ 1} = \frac{0.870}{2.476} = 0.351.$$

For generalization across cases, we use the same strategy, keeping observer and rating as fixed factors:

$$G(Cases) = \frac{\sigma_{SO(C)}^2 + \sigma_{SR(C)}^2 + \sigma_S^2}{Denominator\ 1} = \frac{0.885}{2.476} = 0.357.$$

Finally, since OSCEs are frequently used in examination settings, the overall reliability of the test, which amounts to treating observer, rating, and case all as facets of generalization but dividing by the appropriate ns in order to determine the generalizability of the total test score, becomes:

$$G(Test) = \frac{\sigma_S^2}{\frac{\sigma_{SOR(C)}^2}{6} + \frac{\sigma_{SC}^2}{4} + \frac{\sigma_{SO(C)}^2}{2} + \frac{\sigma_{SR(C)}^2}{3} + \sigma_S^2} = \frac{0.077}{0.797} = 0.097.$$

As we can see, from a design such as this, we can estimate all the conventional coefficients, using all the data in turn. The inclusion of appropriate nested factors complicates the ANOVA and the estimation of expected mean squares, but the calculation of variances and G coefficients, while messy, is completely analogous to the previous examples.

Example 3—econometric vs. psychometric perspectives on the utility of health states

We described the standard econometric approaches to measurement in Chapter 4. A series of descriptions of health states are created, then a group of people—patients

EXAMPLE 3—ECONOMETRIC VS. PSYCHOMETRIC PERSPECTIVES | 165

or non-patients—are approached and asked to rate the utility of the state, using standard gambles, time trade-offs, or other methods. The goal of measurement in these circumstances is to obtain a precise estimate of the utility of the various health states, so that resources can be appropriately allocated; in short, to differentiate among health states.

At least, that is the economist's goal. However, the same approach could conceivably be used to find out information about the raters; for example, whether the technique can identify consistent differences among raters, which may be related to other characteristics such as depression, optimism, illness behaviour, and so on. In this case, we are using the method to differentiate among raters. Finally, it has been of continuing interest to determine whether patients and non-patients rate the health states similarly (e.g. Sackett and Torrance 1978).

All of these questions fit naturally into a G theory framework. The design one might use involves three facets: health state (H), patient/non-patient (P), and rater

Table 9.7 Design for an econometric and psychometric G study

State	Patient			Non-patient		
	R_1	R_2	R_3	R_4	R_5	R_6
1						
2						
3						
4						
.	.		.		.	.
.	.		.		.	.
9						
10						

Table 9.8 ANOVA table for Example 3

Source	Sum of squares	df	Mean square	Expected mean square	Variance
Health H	89.08	9	9.89	$\sigma_{Err}^2 + 3\sigma_{HP}^2 + 6\sigma_H^2$	1.39
Patient P non-patient	10.41	1	10.41	$\sigma_{Err}^2 + 3\sigma_{HP}^2 + 10\sigma_{R(P)}^2 + 3\sigma_P^2$	0.31
Rater R(P)	1.73	4	0.43	$\sigma_{Err}^2 + 10\sigma_{R(P)}^2$	0.00
H × P	13.75	9	1.52	$\sigma_{Err}^2 + 3\sigma_{HP}^2$	0.21
H × R(P)	32.26	36	0.89	σ_{Err}^2	0.89

nested within patient (R). Using, for example, 10 health states, and three raters nested within each status (since someone cannot be a patient and a non-patient, at least at the same time), the design may look like Table 9.7.

We have analyzed the design using some artificial data, resulting in the ANOVA table in Table 9.8. The expected mean squares are not too complex, and we have solved these equations for the variance components in the same table. From our above discussion, the next step is to construct three different coefficients related to the three different perspectives. In this case, all the denominators may differ slightly as well as the numerators.

Perspective 1: econometric

- Question: to what extent can we differentiate among health states, using ratings from patients and non-patients?
- Facet of differentiation: health.
- Facet of generalization: patient, rater.
- Coefficient:

$$G = \frac{\sigma_H^2}{\sigma_{H \times P}^2 + \sigma_H^2 + \sigma_{Err}^2} = \frac{1.39}{0.21 + 1.39 + 0.89} = 0.558.$$

Perspective 2: psychometric

- Question: to what extent can we differentiate among individuals, regardless of patient status, using ratings of different health states?
- Facet of differentiation: rater.
- Facet of generalization: patient, health.
- Coefficient:

$$G = \frac{\sigma_{R(P)}^2}{\sigma_{R(P)}^2 + \sigma_{Err}^2} = \frac{0.00}{0.00 + 0.89} = 0.000.$$

Perspective 3: experimental

- Question: to what extent can we differentiate between non-patients and patients using ratings of health states?
- Facet of differentiation: patient/non-patient.
- Facet of generalization: health, rater.
- Coefficient:

$$G = \frac{\sigma_P^2}{\sigma_{H \times P}^2 + \sigma_{R(P)}^2 + \sigma_P^2 + \sigma_{Err}^2} = \frac{0.31}{0.21 + 0.00 + 0.31 + 0.89} = 0.220.$$

It is clear that the success of this instrument is directly related to its intended use. It is reasonably good at differentiating among health states (particularly since we might use the G coefficient corresponding to the mean of all six ratings, which works out to 0.88); it is of very limited utility in differentiating between patients and non-patients; and it is completely useless in discriminating amongst individual raters.

General rules for generalizability

In contrast to Classical Test Theory (CTT), it is not possible to present a standard litany of G theory designs. Of course, some G theory designs are precisely the same as the analogous CTT design. For example, we can create a one-factor repeated measures G study with Rater as a facet of generalization; this is just an inter-rater reliability study. Or if Time is the facet of generalization, then we are looking at test–retest reliability. But the unique aspects of G theories are two-fold: first, we can consider *all* relevant sources of error variance simultaneously in a single design; and second, we can create families of G coefficients, some with no classical equivalent, based on different measurement situations.

As a consequence, it makes no sense to provide formulae for possible designs, since the possibilities are limitless. But what we can do is to provide a set of rules of thumb to derive G coefficients from variance components. (We will not provide the methods to compute variance components from Mean Squares; these are covered in some statistics books and are often an option in statistical packages like SPSS.)

1. First, it is necessary to decide on the facet of differentiation (usually, but not always, Subject), which we will call D; the facet(s) of generalization, called $G_1, G_2 \ldots G_j$; and the fixed facet(s), $F_1, F_2, \ldots F_k$.

2. The relevant coefficient will involve the following variance components:

   (a) the variance due to the main effect of D;
   (b) the main effect of all random factors in the facets of generalization, $G_1 \ldots G_j$;
   (c) all two-way and higher interactions between D and $G_1, G_2 \ldots G_j$;
   (d) all two-way and higher interactions between D and $F_1, F_2 \ldots F_k$;
   (e) all three-way and higher interactions between D and $F_1, F_2 \ldots F_k$ and $G_1, G_2 \ldots G_j$; and
   (f) the error term, which is the highest interaction term involving D, all F_js, and all G_ks.

The G coefficient corresponding to the generalizability *of a single observation* is then calculated as:

1. The numerator consists of the main effect of the facet of differentiation and all interactions with the fixed facets, i.e:

$$\text{Numerator} = (a) + (d).$$

2. The denominator consists of the numerator, plus all the interactions with all the facets of generalization including interactions with fixed facets, plus the main effects of all *random* facets of generalization, plus the error term, i.e:

$$\text{Denominator} = (a) + (d) + (b) + (c) + (e) + (f).$$

3. So the relevant G coefficient is:

$$G = \frac{(a) + (d)}{(a) + (d) + (b) + (c) + (f)}.$$

If we now want to compute a coefficient corresponding to multiple observations on particular factors, every time that factor appears in a main effect or interaction (whether in the numerator or denominator), we divide the relevant variance component by the number of levels.

We will work through an example, which is, if anything, more complex than any we have seen so far.

Imagine a study with an 8-item scale (I), involving three raters (R), on two occasions (O). The study is done with 20 subjects (S). Rater and Occasion are random facets; Item is a fixed facet. Assume throughout that the facet of differentiation is Subject. Further, let us assume we did the study and ran a three-factor repeated measures ANOVA with Item, Rater, and Occasion as the repeated measures, so there are $8 \times 3 \times 2 = 48$ observations on each subject (and all raters rated all subjects on both occasions with all items; a completely crossed design). Finally, assume we applied the formulae correctly using the methods we have outlined already, to convert Mean Squares to variances. The list of all main effects and interactions, with associated variances, would look like Table 9.9.

Table 9.9 Effects and variances for a Subject × Rater × Time G study

Effect	Variance
Main effects:	
Subject (S)	250
Rater (R)	100
Item (I)	300
Occasion (O)	50
Two-way interactions:	
S × R	40
S × I	90
S × O	30
Three-way interactions:	
S × O × R	30
S × O × I	20
S × R × I	15
Error:	
S × R × O × I	125

Now, for test–retest reliability, I and R are fixed facets, and O is a facet of generalization. If we only want relative standards, we need not worry about any main effect of O. So the numerator and denominator are:

$$\text{Numerator} = S + S \times I + S \times R + S \times R \times I = 250 + 90 + 40 + 15 = 395$$

and

$$\text{Denominator} = S + S \times I + S \times R + S \times R \times I + S \times O + S \times O \times R + S \times O \times I + \text{Error} = 250 + 90 + 40 + 15 + 30 + 30 + 20 + 125 = 600.$$

$$G = \frac{S + S \times I + S \times R + S \times I \times R}{S + S \times I + S \times R + S \times I \times R + S \times O + S \times O \times R + S \times O \times I + \text{Error}}$$
$$= \frac{395}{600} = 0.66.$$

Now, for inter-rater reliability, I and O are fixed facets, and R is a facet of generalization. So the numerator is:

$$\text{Numerator} = S + S \times I + S \times O + S \times I \times O = 250 + 90 + 30 + 20 = 390.$$

The denominator is as before, and the G coefficient is:

$$G = \frac{S + S \times I + S \times O + S \times I \times O}{S + S \times I + S \times R + S \times I \times R + S \times O + S \times O \times R + S \times O \times I + \text{Error}}$$
$$= \frac{395}{600} = 0.65.$$

If we consider multiple observations, then we divide the relevant variance components by the number of levels of the factor. For example, if we were to compute the reliability of the average score over all eight items, the equivalent of the internal consistency, then we divide any variance component containing Item by eight. So, with Item as the facet of generalization, and Rater and Occasion both fixed facets, the G coefficient would be:

$$G = \frac{S + S \times R + S \times O + S \times O \times R}{S + \dfrac{S \times I}{8} + S \times R + \dfrac{S \times R \times I}{8} + S \times O + S \times O \times R + \dfrac{S \times O \times I}{8} + \dfrac{\text{Error}}{8}}$$
$$= \frac{250 + 40 + 30 + 30}{250 + \dfrac{90}{8} + 40 + \dfrac{15}{8} + 30 + 30 + \dfrac{20}{8} + \dfrac{125}{8}} = \frac{350}{381.25} = 0.92.$$

Of course, some of the previous considerations related to classical reliability, as covered in Chapter 8, still apply. For example, if we wish to consider Rater as a random factor (or alternatively, if we wish to consider absolute rather than relative scoring), then the main effect of Rater would be one of the error terms in the denominator. In this case, the G coefficient would look like:

$$G = \frac{S + S \times I + S \times R + S \times I \times R}{S + R + S \times I + S \times R + S \times I \times R + S \times O + S \times O \times R + S \times O \times I + \text{Error}}$$
$$= \frac{395}{700} = 0.56.$$

Nested designs

Occasionally we run across 'nested' designs, extensions of the reliability study of residents rating supervisors in Chapter 8. As one example of these designs, we could consider an extension of the design we just worked through, except in this case, each subject is rated by different raters. Under these circumstances, some of the interactions—those containing both Subject and Rater—drop out, so there are no $S \times R$, $S \times R \times O$, or $S \times R \times I$ terms. The reason for the absence of these terms follows from the definition of the $S \times R$ term, which measures the extent to which different subjects are rated differently by different raters. However, since each rater rates only one subject, we cannot estimate this.

Under these circumstances, the best approach is to use a good statistical package that will handle nested designs to do the ANOVA, and then proceed as we did above to create G coefficients. Of course, if there is no term for a particular interaction, this amounts to adding a '0' to the sum.

Error estimates for G coefficients

In the previous chapter, we found how difficult it is to obtain exact estimates of the standard error of a simple intraclass correlation. Not surprisingly, exact estimating procedures for complex G coefficients do not exist. Approximate errors can be computed as sums and differences of squared Mean Squares, using formulae far too complicated to be derived in a general measurement book. Some advanced G theory packages like GENOVA (Brennan 2001) compute these estimates, and likely this is really the only practical way to get estimates of errors.

Summary

Although generalizability theory is at first difficult to comprehend, the value of the method lies in the re-interpretation of the nature of measurement afforded by the theory. Instead of conceptualizing a measurement as a sum of a 'true' score and an 'error' score, generalizability theory forces a critical examination of the *sources* of measurement error. In addition, the effect of particular strategies to reduce error, based on multiple observations, can be directly estimated. As a result, the theory represents a powerful tool in advancing the methods of measurement.

References

Boodoo, G. M. and O'Sullivan, P. (1982). Obtaining generalizability coefficients for clinical evaluations. *Evaluation and the Health Professions*, 5, 345–58.

Brennan, R. L. (2001). *Generalizability theory*. Springer-Verlag, New York.

Chambers, L. W., Haight, M., Norman, G. R., and MacDonald, L. (1987). Effect of mode of administration on a health status measure's responsiveness to change. *Medical Care*, 25, 470–80.

Cronbach, L. J., Gleser, G. C., Nanda, H., and Rajaratnam, N. (1972). *The dependability of behavioral measurements: Theory of generalizability for scores and profiles*. Wiley, New York.

Evans, W. J., Cayten, C. G., and Green, P. A. (1981). Determining the generalizability of rating scales in clinical settings. *Medical Care*, **19**, 1211–19.

Glass, G. V. and Stanley, J. C. (1970). *Statistical methods in education and psychology*. Prentice-Hall, Englewood Cliffs, NJ.

Harden, R. M. and Gleeson, F. A. (1979). Assessment of clinical experience using an objective structured clinical examination (OSCE). *Medical Education*, **13**, 41–54.

Sackett, D. L. and Torrance, G. W. (1978). The utility of different health states as perceived by the general public. *Journal of Chronic Diseases*, **31**, 697–704.

Shavelson, R. J., Webb, N. M., and Rowley, G. L. (1989). Generalizability theory. *American Psychologist*, **44**, 922–32.

van der Vleuten, C. P. M. and Swanson D. B. (1990). Assessment of clinical skills with standardized patients: The state of the art. *Teaching and Learning in Medicine*, **2**, 58–76.

Chapter 10

Validity

In the previous chapters, we examined various aspects of reliability; that is, how reproducible the results of a scale are under different conditions. This is a necessary step in establishing the usefulness of a measure, but it is not sufficient. The next step is to determine if the scale is measuring what we think it is; that is, the scale's *validity*. To illustrate the difference, imagine that we are trying to develop a new index to measure the degree of headache pain. We find that patients get the same score when they are tested on two different occasions, that different interviewers get similar results when assessing the same patient, and so on; in other words, the index is reliable. However, we still have no proof that differences in the total score reflect the degree of headache pain: the scale may be measuring pain from other sources; or it may be tapping factors entirely unrelated to pain, such as depression or the tendency to complain of bodily ailments. In this chapter, we will examine how to determine if we can draw valid conclusions from the scale.

Why assess validity?

The question that immediately arises is why we have to establish validity in the first place. After all, the health care fields are replete with measures that have never been 'validated' through any laborious testing process. Despite this, no one questions the usefulness of taking a patient's temperature to detect the presence of fever, or of keeping track of the height and weight of an infant to check growth, or getting TSH levels on people with suspected thyroid problems. Why, then, are there a multitude of articles addressing the problems of trying to test for validity? There are two answers to this question: the nature of *what* is being measured; and the *relationship* of that variable to its purported cause.

Many variables measured in the health sciences are physical quantities, such as height, serum cholesterol level, or bicarbonate. As such, they are readily observable, either directly or with the correct instruments. Irrespective of who manufactured the thermometer, different nurses will get the same reading, within the limits of reliability discussed in Chapters 8 and 9. Moreover, there is little question that what is being measured is temperature; no one would state that the height of the mercury in the tube is really due to something else, like blood pressure or pH level.

The situation is different when we turn to variables like 'range of motion', 'quality of life', or 'responsibility as a physician'. As we discuss later in this chapter, the measurements of these factors are dependent upon their definitions, which may vary from one person to another, and the way they are measured. For example, some theorists hold that 'social support' can be assessed by counting the number of people a person has contact with during a fixed period of time. Other theories state that the person's perceptions of who is available in times of need are more important; while yet another school of thought is that the reciprocity of the helping relationship is crucial. Since social support is not something which can be observed and measured directly, various questionnaires have been developed to assess it, each reflecting a different underlying theory. Needless to say, each instrument yields a somewhat different result, raising the question of which, if any, gives the 'correct' answer.

The second reason why validity testing is required in some areas but not others depends on the relationship between the observation and what it reflects. Based on years of observation or our knowledge of how the body works, the validity of a test may be self-evident. For instance, since the kidneys regulate the level of creatinine in the body, it makes sense to use serum creatinine to determine the presence of renal disease. On the other hand, we do not know ahead of time whether a physiotherapist's evaluations of patients' level of functioning bear any relationship to their actual performance once they are discharged from hospital. Similarly, we may hypothesize that students who have spent time doing volunteer work for service agencies will make better physicians or nurses. However, since our knowledge of the determinants of human behaviour is far from perfect, this prediction will have to be validated against actual performance.

Reliability and validity

We discussed in previous chapters that reliability places an upper limit on validity, so that the higher the reliability, the higher the maximum possible validity (more formally, the maximum validity of a test is the square root of the reliability coefficient). We can also see how the different types of error—random and systematic (bias)—affect both. The traditional way of expressing the variance of observed scores is:

$$\sigma^2_{Observed} = \sigma^2_{True} + \sigma^2_{Error}$$

That is, as we explained in Chapter 8, the total, or observed, variance of scores is composed of the variance of the true scores (which we never see) plus error variance, which can increase or decrease the true variance. Judd *et al.* (1991) expanded this to read:

$$\sigma^2_{Observed} = \sigma^2_{CI} + \sigma^2_{SE} + \sigma^2_{RE}$$

where *CI* indicates the Construct of Interest, *SE* the Systematic Error, *RE* the Random Error; and

$$\sigma^2_{CI} + \sigma^2_{SE} = \sigma^2_{True}.$$

Using this formulation:

$$Reliability = \frac{\sigma^2_{CI} + \sigma^2_{SE}}{\sigma^2_{Observed}}$$

and

$$Validity = \frac{\sigma^2_{CI}}{\sigma^2_{Observed}}.$$

From this, we can see that random error affects both reliability and validity (since the larger the random error is, the smaller the ratio between the numerators and denominators), whereas systematic error affects only the validity of a scale.

The 'types' of validity

One of the most difficult aspects of validity testing is the terminology. Until the 1970s, almost all textbooks adopted a 'trinitarian' point of view (Landy 1986), dividing this topic into the 'three Cs' of *content* validity, *criterion* validity, and *construct* validity (terms we will discuss later). These were seen as three relatively separate attributes of a measure, which had to be independently established. More recently, though, two seemingly different trends have emerged. First, a proliferation of new 'types' of validity were proposed. For example, construct validity was differentiated into various classes such as trait validity, discriminant validity, convergent validity, and so forth (see, for example, Messick 1980). At the same time, a second trend led to a reconceptualization of the process of validity testing itself and what could actually be concluded from a demonstration of validity in one form or another.

Previously, testing for validity was seen as demonstrating the psychometric properties of a *scale*. Led by Cronbach (1971), though, the focus changed to emphasize the characteristics of the *people* who are assessed. As Landy (1986) puts it, 'Validation processes are not so much directed toward the integrity of tests as they are directed toward the inferences that can be made about the attributes of the people who have produced those test scores' (p. 1186). In other words, validating a scale is really a process whereby we determine the degree of confidence we can place on inferences we make about people based on their scores from that scale.

Seen from this perspective, the two trends are actually just different aspects of the same thing. Validation is a process *of hypothesis testing*: 'Someone who scores high on this measure will also do well in situation A, perform poorly on test B, and will differ from those who score low on the scale on traits C and D'. So, rather than being constrained by the trinitarian Cs mentioned above, scale constructors are limited only by their imagination in devising experiments to test their hypotheses. In the past, students (and their teachers) have spent much time arguing whether a specific study demonstrated, for example, criterion or construct validity. Now, the important questions are, 'Does the hypothesis of this validation study make sense in light of what the scale is designed to measure', and 'Do the results of this study allow us to draw the inferences that we wish to make?'.

Unfortunately, this creates difficulties for writers of textbooks. From the new perspective, a chapter on validity would focus primarily on the logic and methodology of hypothesis testing. The student, though, will continue to encounter terms like 'construct validity' and 'criterion validity' in his or her readings for some time to come. We have chosen here to take the middle ground; to organize the chapter around the traditional headings, but at the same time to emphasize that rather than being disparate attributes, the various 'types' of validity are all addressing the same issue of the degree of confidence we can place in the inferences we draw from scores on scales.

Content validity

We mentioned content validity previously within the context of issues surrounding item construction (Chapter 3). Here, let us briefly touch on it again from our new vantage point. When we conclude that a student has 'passed' a test in, say, respirology, or that an arthritic patient has a grip strength of only 10 kg, we are making the assumption that the measures comprise representative samples of the disorders, behaviours, attitudes, or knowledge that we want to assess. That is, we do not too much care if the student knows the specific bits of information tapped by the examination, or how much the patient can squeeze a dynamometer. Going back to what validity testing is all about, our aim is *inferential*; a person who does well on the exam can be expected to know more about lungs than a student who does poorly, and a patient who has a weaker grip has more severe arthritis than someone who can exert more pressure.

A measure that includes a more representative sample of the target behaviour lends itself to more accurate inferences; that is, inferences which hold true under a wider range of circumstances. If there are important aspects of the outcome that are missed by the scales, then we are likely to make some inferences which will prove to be wrong; our *inferences* (not the instruments) are invalid. For example, if there was nothing on the respirology examination regarding oxygen exchange, then it is quite possible that a high scorer on the test may *not* know more about this topic than a student with a lower score. Similarly, grip strength has relatively poor content validity; as such, it does not allow us to make accurate inferences about other attributes of the rheumatoid patient, such as erythrocyte sedimentation rate, joint count, or morning stiffness, except insofar as these indices are correlated with grip strength.

Thus, the higher the content validity of a measure, the broader are the inferences that we can validly draw about the person under a variety of conditions and in different situations.

We discussed in previous chapters that reliability places an upper limit on validity, so that the higher the reliability, the higher the maximum possible validity. There is one notable exception to this general rule: the relationship between internal consistency (an index of reliability) and content validity. If we are tapping a behaviour, disorder, or trait that is relatively heterogeneous, like rheumatoid arthritis, then it is quite conceivable that the scale will have low internal consistency; not all patients with a high joint count have a high sedimentation rates or morning stiffness. We could increase the internal consistency of the index by eliminating items which are not highly correlated with each other or the total score. If we did this, though, we would end up with an index tapping only one aspect of arthritis—stiffness, for example—and which therefore has very low content validity. Under such circumstances, it is better to sacrifice internal consistency for content validity. The ultimate aim of the scale is inferential, which depends more on content validity than internal consistency.

Criterion validity

The traditional definition of criterion validity is the correlation of a scale with some other measure of the trait or disorder under study, ideally, a 'gold standard' which has been used and accepted in the field. Criterion validity is usually divided into two types: *concurrent* validity and *predictive* validity. With concurrent validity, we correlate the new scale with the criterion measure, both of which are given at the same time. For example, we could administer a new scale for depression and the *Beck Depression Inventory* (an accepted measure of depression) during the same interview, or within a short time of each other. In predictive validity, the criterion will not be available until some time in the future. The major areas where this latter form of criterion validity is used are in college admission tests, where the ultimate outcome is the person's performance on graduation four years hence; or diagnostic tests, where we must await the outcome of an autopsy or the further progression of the disease to confirm or disconfirm our predictions.

A major question is why, if a good criterion measure already exists, are we going through the often laborious process of developing a new instrument? Leaving aside the unworthy (if prevalent) reasons of trying to cash in on a lucrative market, or having an instrument with one's name as part of the title, there are a number of valid reasons. The existing test can be expensive, invasive, dangerous, or time-consuming; or the outcome may not be known until it is too late. The first four reasons are the usual rationales for scales which require concurrent validation, and the last reason for those which need predictive validity. On the basis of these reasons for developing new tests, Messick (1980) has proposed using the terms *diagnostic utility* or *substitutability* for concurrent validity, and *predictive utility* for predictive validity; while they are not yet widely used, these are far more descriptive terms for the rationales underlying criterion validity testing.

As an example of the use of concurrent validity, let us look at the usual standard test for tuberculosis, the chest X-ray. While it is still used as the definitive criterion, it suffers from a number of drawbacks which make it a less than ideal test, especially for routine screening. It is somewhat invasive—exposing the patient to low levels of ionizing radiation, and expensive—requiring a costly machine, film, a trained technician, and a radiologist to interpret the results. For these reasons, it would be desirable to develop a cheaper and less risky test for screening purposes. This new tool would then be compared, in a concurrent validation study, to the chest X-ray.

Within the realm of predictive validity, we would like to know *before* students are admitted to graduate or professional school whether or not they will graduate four years later, rather than having to incur the expense of the training and possibly denying

Table 10.1 Fourfold table to evaluate criterion validity for scales with dichotomous outcomes

		X-ray results	
		TB	No TB
Mantoux	TB	A	B
test	No TB	C	D

admission to someone who will do well. So, administering our scale prior to admission, we would determine how well it predicts graduate status or performance on a licensing examination.

Let us go through the usual procedures for establishing these two forms of validity and their rationales. As we have mentioned, the most commonly used design for concurrent validity is to administer the new scale and the standard at the same time. Staying with the example of a new test for TB, we would give both the Mantoux test (assuming it is the one being validated) and the X-ray to a large group of people. Since the outcome is dichotomous (the person either has or does not have abnormalities on the X-ray consistent with TB), we would draw up a four-fold table, as in Table 10.1.

We could analyze the results using either the indices of sensitivity and specificity, or some measure of correlation which can be derived from a 2 × 2 table, such as the phi coefficient (φ). This coefficient is related to χ^2 by the formula:

$$\phi = \frac{\sqrt{\chi^2}}{N},$$

or can be calculated from Table 10.1 using the equation:

$$\phi = \frac{|BC - AD|}{\sqrt{[(A + B)(C + D)(A + C)(B + D)]}}.$$

If our measures were continuous, as would be found if we were validating a new measure of depression against the *Beck Depression Inventory* or *CES-D* (another accepted index of depression), we would use a Pearson correlation coefficient. In either case, we would be looking for a strong association between our new measure and the already existing one. This would indicate that a person who has a high score or comes out 'diseased' on the new test would be expected to have a high score (or have been labeled as diseased) on the more established instrument.

In assessing predictive validity, the person is given the new measure at Time 1, and then the standard some time later, at Time 2. Again, we would use a four-fold table to evaluate a scale with a dichotomous outcome, and a correlational measure if the outcome were continuous. However, there is one additional point which appears obvious, but is often overlooked; *no decision can be made based on the new instrument*. For example, if we were trying to establish the validity of an autobiographical letter as a criterion for admission to medical or nursing school, we would have all applicants write these missives. Then, no matter how good we felt this measure was, we would immediately put the evaluations of the letters in a safe place, without looking at them, and base our decisions on other criteria. Only after the students had or had not graduated would we take out the scores, and compare them with actual performance.

What would happen if we violated this proscription and used the letters to help us decide who should be admitted? We would be able to determine what proportion of students who wrote excellent letters graduated four years later (cell A in Table 10.1) and what proportion failed (cell B). However, we would *not* be able to state what proportion of those who wrote 'poor' letters would have gone on to pass with flying colors (cell C), nor how good letters are in detecting people who will fail (cell D): they would never be given the chance. In this case, the sample has been *truncated* on the basis of our new test and, as we will describe later in more detail, the correlation between our new test and the standard will be reduced, perhaps significantly.

A somewhat different situation can also occur with diagnostic tests. If the final diagnosis (the gold standard) were predicated in part on the results of our new instrument, then we have artificially built in a high correlation between the two; we are correlating the new measure with an outcome based on it. For example, in the process of validating two-dimensional echo cardiography for diagnosing mitral valve prolapse (MVP), we would use the clinician's judgement of the presence or absence of MVP as the criterion. However, the clinician may know the results of the echo tests, and temper his diagnosis in light of them. This differs from our previous example in that we have not truncated our sample; rather, we are indirectly using the results of our new scale in both the predictor and the outcome. The technical term for this is *criterion contamination*.

In summary, then, criterion validity assesses how a person who scores at a certain level on our new scale does on some criterion measure. The usual experimental design is a correlational one; both measures are taken on a series of individuals. In the case of concurrent validity, the two results are gathered close together in time. In predictive validity, the results from the criterion measure are usually not known for some time, which can be between a few days to a few years later.

Construct validity
What is construct validity?

Attributes such as height or weight are readily observable, or can be 'operationally defined'; that is, defined by the way they are measured. Systolic blood pressure, for example, is the amount of pressure, measured in millimeters of mercury, at the moment of ventricular systole. Once we move away from the realm of physical attributes into more 'psychological' ones like anxiety, intelligence, or pain, however, we begin dealing with more abstract variables, ones that cannot be directly observed. We cannot 'see' anxiety; all we can observe are behaviours which, according to our theory of anxiety, are the results of it. We would attribute the sweaty palms, tachycardia, pacing back and forth, and difficulty in concentrating experienced by a student just prior to writing an exam, to his or her anxiety. Similarly, we may have two patients who, to all intents and purposes, have the same degree of angina. One patient has quit his job and spends most of the day sitting in a chair; the other continues working and is determined to 'fight it'. We may explain these differences in terms of such attitudes as 'motivation', 'illness behaviour', or the 'sick role model'. Again, these factors are not seen directly, only their hypothesized manifestations in terms of the patients' observable behaviours.

These proposed underlying factors are referred to as *hypothetical constructs*, or, more simply, as *constructs*. A construct can be thought of as a 'mini-theory' to explain the relationships among various behaviours or attitudes. Many constructs arose from larger theories or clinical observations, before there were any ways of objectively measuring their effects. This would include terms like 'anxiety' or 'repression', derived from psychoanalytic theory; or 'sick role behaviour', which was based mainly on socio-logical theorizing. Other concepts, like the difference between 'fluid' and 'crystal-lized' intelligence (Cattell 1963), were proposed to explain observed correlations among variables which were already measured with a high degree of reliability.

It is fair to say that most psychological instruments and many measures of health are designed to tap some aspect of a hypothetical construct. There are two reasons for wanting to develop such an instrument: the construct is a new one, and no scale exists that measures it; or we are dissatisfied with the existing tools, and feel that they omit some key aspect of the construct. Note that we are doing more than replacing one tool with a shorter, cheaper, or less invasive one, which is the rationale for cri-terion validity. Rather, we are using the underlying theory to help us develop a new or better instrument, where 'better' means able to explain a broader range of find-ings, explain them in a more parsimonious manner, or make more accurate predic-tions about a person's behaviour.

Establishing construct validity

As an example, consider the quest to develop a short checklist or scale to identify patients with irritable bowel syndrome (IBS). First, though, we should address the issue of why we consider IBS to be a construct rather than a disease like ulcers or amoebic dysentery. The central issue is that we cannot (at least not yet) definitively prove that a person has IBS; it is diagnosed by excluding other possible causes of the patient's symptoms. There is no X-ray or laboratory test to which we can point and say, 'Yes, that person has IBS'. Moreover, there is no known pathogen that produces the constellation of symptoms. We tie them together conceptually by postulating an underlying disorder, which cannot be measured directly, in much the same way that we say a large vocabulary, a breadth of knowledge, and skill at problem-solving are all outward manifestations of a postulated but unseen concept we label 'intelligence'. Many of what physicians call 'syndromes' would be called 'hypothetical constructs' by psychologists and test developers. Indeed, even some 'diseases' like schizophrenia, Alzheimer's, or systemic lupus erythematosus, are closer to constructs than actual entities, since their diagnosis is based on constellations of symptoms, and there are no unequivocal diagnostic tests that can be used with living patients. This is more than just semantics, though. It implies that tests for diagnosing or measuring syndromes should be constructed in an analogous manner to those for more 'psychological' attributes.

The first indices developed for assessing IBS consisted, in the main, of two parts: exclusion of other diseases, and the presence of some physical signs and symptoms like pain in the lower left quadrant and diarrhoea without pain. These scales proved to be inadequate, as many patients 'diagnosed' by them were later discovered to have stomach cancer or other diseases, and patients who were missed were, a few years later, indistinguishable from IBS patients. Thus, new scales were developed which added other—primarily demographic and personality—factors, predicated on a broader view (a revised construct) of IBS, as a disorder marked by specific demography and a unique psychological configuration, in addition to the physical symptoms. The problem the test developers now faced was how to demonstrate that the new index was better than the older ones.

To address this problem, let us go back to what we mean by a 'valid' scale: it is one that allows us to make accurate inferences about a person. These inferences are derived from the construct, and are of the form; 'Based on my theory of construct X, people who score high on a test of X differ from people who score low on it in terms of attributes A, B, and C', where A, B, and C can be other instruments, behaviours, diagnoses, and so on. In this particular case, we would say, 'Based on my concept of IBS, high scorers on the index should:

(1) have symptoms that will not clear with conventional therapy; and
(2) have a lower prevalence of organic bowel disease on autopsy'.

Since we are testing constructs, this form of testing is called *construct validation.* Methodologically, it differs from the types of validity testing we discussed previously in a number of important ways. First, content and criterion validity can often be established with one or two studies. However, we are often able to make many different predictions based on our theory or construct. For example, if we were validating a new scale of anxiety, just a few of the many hypotheses we can derive would be, 'Anxious people would have more rapid heart rates during an exam than low anxious ones'; 'Anxious people should do better on simple tasks than non-anxious subjects, but poorer than them on complex tasks'; or 'If I artificially induce anxiety with some experimental manoeuvre, then the subjects should score higher on my test'.

Thus, there is no one single experiment which can unequivocally 'prove' a construct. Construct validation is an on-going process, of learning more about the construct, making new predictions, and then testing them. Albert Einstein once said that there have been hundreds of experiments supporting his theory of relativity, but it would take only one non-confirmatory study to disprove it. So it is with construct validation; each supportive study serves only to strengthen what Cronbach and Meehl (1955) call the 'nomological network' of the interlocking predictions of a theory, but a single, well-designed experiment with negative findings can call into question the entire construct.

A second major difference between construct validity and the other types is that, with the former, we are assessing both the theory and the measure at the same time. Returning to our example of a better index for IBS, one prediction was that patients who have a high score would not respond to conventional therapy. Assume that we gave the index to a sample of patients presenting at a gastrointestinal (GI) clinic, and gave them all regular treatment. (Remember, we cannot base any decisions on the results of a scale we are validating; this would lead to criterion contamination.) If it turned out that our prediction were confirmed, then it would lend credence to both our concept of IBS and the index we developed to measure it. However, if high-scoring subjects responded to treatment in about the same proportion as low scorers, then the problem could be that:

- our instrument is good, but the theory is wrong;
- the theory is fine, but our index cannot discriminate between IBS patients and those with other GI problems; or
- both the theory is wrong and our scale is useless.

Moreover, we would have no way of knowing which of these situations exists until we do more studies.

A further complication enters the picture when we use an experimental study to validate the scale. Using the example of a new measure of anxiety, one prediction was that if we artificially induce anxiety, as in threatening the subject with an electric shock if he or she performs poorly on some task, then we should see an increase in scores on the index. If the scores do not go up, then the problem could be in either of the areas already mentioned—the theory and the measure—plus one other; both the theory and the scale are fine, but the experiment did not induce anxiety, as we had hoped it would. Again, any combination of these problems could be working: the measure is valid and the experiment worked, but the theory is wrong; the theory is right and the experiment went the way we planned, but the index is not measuring anxiety; and so forth.

Putting this all together, Cronbach and Meehl's (1955) seminal article on construct validity said that it involves three mandatory steps:

(1) explicitly spelling out a set of theoretical concepts and how they are related to each other;

(2) developing scales to measure these hypothetical constructs; and

(3) actually testing the relationships among the constructs and their observable manifestations.

That is, unless there is an articulated theory, there is no construct validity (Clark and Watson 1995). But Clark and Watson go on to say (p. 310):

> This emphasis on theory is not meant to be intimidating. That is, we do not mean to imply that one must have a fully articulated set of interrelated theoretical concepts before embarking on scale development. Our point, rather, is that thinking about these

theoretical issues prior to the actual process of scale construction increases the likelihood that the resulting scale will make a substantial contribution to the...literature.

They recommend writing out a brief, formal description of the construct, how it will manifest itself objectively, and how it is related to other constructs and behaviours.

We said that construct validity differs from content and criterion validity methodologically. At the risk of being repetitive, we should emphasize that construct validation does not *conceptually* differ from the other types. To quote Guion (1977), '*All* validity is at its base some form of construct validity.... It is the basic meaning of validity' (p. 410).

It should not be surprising that given the greater complexity and breadth of questions asked with construct validity as compared with the other types of validity, there are many more ways of establishing it. In the next section, we will discuss only a few of these methods: extreme groups, convergent and discriminant validity, and the multitrait—multimethod matrix. Many other experimental and quasi-experimental approaches exist; the interested reader should consult some of the references listed in Appendix A.

Extreme groups

Perhaps the easiest experiment to conceive of in assessing the validity of a scale is to give it to two groups: one of which has the trait or behaviour, and the other, which does not. The former group should score significantly higher (or lower, depending on how the items are scored) on the new instrument. This is sometimes called construct validation by *extreme groups* (also referred to as *discriminative validity*, which is not to be confused with *discriminant validity*, discussed in the next section). We can use the attempt to develop a better scale for IBS as an example. Using their best tools, experienced clinicians would divide a group of patients presenting to a GI clinic into two subgroups: those whom they feel have IBS and those who have some other bowel disorder. To make the process of scale development easier, all patients with equivocal diagnoses would be eliminated in this type of study.

Although this type of design appears quite straightforward, it has buried within it two methodological problems. The first difficulty with the method is that if we are trying to develop a new or better tool, how can we select the extreme groups? To be able to do so would imply that there is already an instrument in existence which meets our needs. There is no ready solution to this problem. In practice, the groups are selected using the best *available* tool, even if it is the relatively crude criterion of 'expert judgement', or a scale that almost captures what our new scale is designed to tap. We can then use what Cronbach and Meehl (1955) call 'bootstrapping'. If the new scale allows us to make more accurate predictions, or explain more findings, or achieve better inter-observer agreement, then it can replace the original criterion. In turn, then, it can be used as the gold standard against which a newer or revised version can be validated; hence 'pulling ourselves up by the bootstraps'.

The second methodological problem is one that occurs with diagnostic tests, and which is often overlooked in the pressure to publish; the extreme group design may be a necessary step, but it is by no means sufficient. That is, it is minimally necessary for our new scale to be able to differentiate between those people who obviously have the disorder or trait in question and those who do not; if the scale cannot do this, it is probably useless in all other regards. However, the question must be asked, 'Is this the way the instrument will be used in practice?'. If we are trying to develop a new diagnostic tool, the answer most often is 'no'. We likely would not need a new test to separate out the obvious cases from the obvious non-cases. Especially in a tertiary care setting, the people who are sent are in the middle range; they *may* have the disorder, but then again there are some doubts. If it is with this group that the instrument will be used, then the ultimate test of its usefulness is in making these much finer discriminations.

For example, many instruments have been designed to detect the presence of organic brain syndrome (OBS). As a first step, we would try out such a tool on one group of patients with confirmed brain damage and on another where there is no evidence of any pathology. These two groups should be clearly distinguishable on the new test. However, such patients are rarely referred for neuropsychological assessment, since their diagnoses (or lack thereof) are readily apparent based on other criteria. The next step, then, would be to try this instrument on the types of patients who *would* be sent for assessment, where the differential diagnosis is between OBS and depression, a difficult discrimination to make. These groups would be formed based on the best guess of a psychiatrist, perhaps augmented by some other tests of OBS, ones we are trying to replace.

Convergent and discriminant validity

Assessing the validity by using extreme groups is closely related to *convergent validity*, seeing how closely the new scale is related to other variables and other measures of the same construct to which it should be related. For example, if our theory states that anxious people are supposed to be more aware of autonomic nervous system (ANS) activity than non-anxious people, then scores on the new index of anxiety should correlate with scores on a measure of autonomic awareness. Again, if the scores do *not* correlate, then the problem could be our new scale, the measure of autonomic sensitivity, or our theory. On the other hand, we do not want the scales to be too highly correlated: this would indicate that they are measuring the same thing, that the new one is nothing more than a different measure of autonomic awareness. How high is 'too high'? As usual, it all depends. If ANS sensitivity is, by our theory, a major component of anxiety, then the correlation should be relatively robust; if it is only one of many components of anxiety, then the correlation should be lower.

The other aspect of convergent validity is that the new index of anxiety should correlate with other measures of this construct. Again, while the correlation should be high, it should not be overly high if we believe that our new anxiety scale covers components of this trait not tapped by the existing ones.

Ideally, the new instrument should be tested against existing ones that are maximally different (Campbell and Fiske 1959). Although it is difficult to define what 'maximally different' means (Foster and Cone 1995), it would imply that a self-report scale should be evaluated against one completed by an observer or a performance task, for example, rather than a different self-report measure. The rationale is that scores on a scale are determined not only by the attribute being measured, but also by aspects of the measuring process itself. In the next section, on the multitrait–multimethod matrix, we show how correlations between instruments due to similarity of the assessment method can be disentangled from similarity due to tapping the same attribute.

Not only should our construct correlate with related variables, it should *not* correlate with dissimilar, unrelated ones; what we refer to as *discriminant validity* (which is also sometimes referred to as *divergent validity*). If our theory states that anxiety is independent of intelligence, then we should not find a strong correlation between the two. Finding one may indicate, for example, that the wording of our instrument is so difficult that intelligence is playing a role in simply understanding the items. Of course, the other reasons may also apply; our scale, the intelligence test, or the construct may be faulty. One measure commonly used in discriminant validity testing is social desirability bias, for reasons we discussed in Chapter 6 on biases in responding.

The multitrait–multimethod matrix

A powerful technique for looking at convergent and discriminant validity simultaneously is called the *multitrait–multimethod* matrix, or MTMM (Campbell and Fiske 1959). Two or more different, usually unrelated, traits are each measured by two or more methods at the same time. The two traits, for instance, can be 'self-directed learning' and 'knowledge' (assuming that they are relatively unrelated), each assessed by a rater and a written exam. This leads to a matrix of 10 correlations, as shown with fictitious data in Table 10.2.

The numbers in parentheses (0.53, 0.79, etc.) along the main diagonal are the reliabilities of the four instruments. The two italicized figures, *0.42* and *0.49*, are the 'homotrait–heteromethod' correlations: the same trait (e.g. knowledge) measured in different ways. Those in curly brackets {0.18} and {0.23} are 'heterotrait–homomethod'

Table 10.2 A fictitious multitrait–multimethod matrix

| | | Self-directed learning | | Knowledge | |
		Rater	Exam	Rater	Exam
Self-directed learning	Rater	(0.53)			
	Exam	*0.42*	(0.79)		
Knowledge	Rater	{0.18}	[0.17]	(0.58)	
	Exam	[0.15]	{0.23}	*0.49*	(0.88)

correlations: different traits assessed by the same method. Finally, the heterotrait–heteromethod correlations are in square brackets [0.17] and [0.15]: different traits measured with different methods.

Ideally, the highest correlations should be the reliabilities of the individual measures; an examination of 'knowledge' given on two occasions should yield higher correlations than examinations of different traits or two different ways of tapping knowledge. Similarly, the lowest correlations should be the heterotrait–heteromethod ones; different traits measured by different methods should not be related.

Convergent validity is reflected in the homotrait–heteromethod correlations; different measures of the same trait should correlate with each other. In this example, the results of the written exam should correlate with scores given by the rater for 'knowledge', and similarly for the two assessments of 'self-directed learning'. Conversely, discriminant validity is shown by low correlations when the same method (e.g. the written exam) is applied to different traits—the heterotrait–homomethod coefficients. If they are as high or higher than the homotrait–heteromethod correlations, this would show that the *method* of measurement was more important than *what* was being measured. This is obviously an undesirable property, since the manner of assessing various attributes should be secondary to the relationship that should exist between various ways of tapping into the same trait.

It is often difficult to do studies appropriate for the MTMM approach because of the time required on the subjects' part, as well the problem of finding different methods of assessing the same trait. When these studies can be done, though, they can address a number of validity issues simultaneously.

Summary

Unlike criterion validity, then, there is no one experimental design or statistic which is common to construct validational studies. If one of the hypotheses is that our new measure of a construct is related to other indices of that construct or that the construct should be associated with other constructs, then the study is usually correlational in nature; our new scale and another one (of the same or a related construct) are given to the subjects. If one hypothesis is that some naturally occurring group has 'more' of the construct than another group, then we can simply give our new instrument to both groups, and look for differences between the two means. Still another hypothesis may be that if we give some experimental or therapeutic intervention, it will affect the construct and the measure of it; transcutaneous stimulation should reduce pain, while intense radiant heat should increase it. In this instance, our study could be a before/after trial or, more powerfully, a true experiment whereby one group receives the intervention and the other does not. If our construct is correct, and the manoeuver worked, and our scale is valid, then we should see differences between the groups.

In summary, it is obviously necessary to conduct validational studies for each new instrument we develop. However, when the scale is one measuring a hypothetical construct, the task is an on-going one. New hypotheses derived from the construct require new studies. Similarly, if we want to use the measure with groups it was not initially validated on, we must first demonstrate that the inferences we make for them are as valid as for the original population. Finally, modifications of existing scales often require new validity studies. For example, if we wanted to use the D scale of the MMPI as an index of depression, we cannot assume that it is as valid when used in isolation as when the items are imbedded amongst 500 other, unrelated ones. It is possible that the mere fact of presenting them together gives the patient a different orientation and viewpoint.

Responsiveness and sensitivity to change

Over the past 10 or so years, two new terms have crept into the psychometric lexicon: *responsiveness* and *sensitivity to change*. While these define useful concepts in evaluating scales, their introduction has also led to two sources of confusion: whether these are synonyms or refer to different attributes of an instrument; and if they refer to a third attribute of a scale (that is, separate from reliability and validity) or are a component of one or both of them.

Although many authors use the terms interchangeably, Liang (2000) draws a useful distinction between them. He defines sensitivity to change as 'the ability of an instrument to measure change in a state regardless of whether it is relevant or meaningful to the decision maker' (p. 85); and responsiveness as 'the ability of an instrument to measure a meaningful or clinically important change in a clinical state' (p. 85). This, needless to say, leaves open the question of what is meant by a 'clinically important change'. We will discuss this point, as well as the overall issue of how to measure change at all, in the next chapter.

Accompanying the introduction of these terms has been a tendency for articles to state that their aim is to examine the 'reliability, validity, and sensitivity to change' (or 'responsiveness') of a given instrument. The implication of this statement is that it is not sufficient to establish reliability and validity, and that sensitivity and responsiveness are different from them. The short response is that this implication is wrong. As a number of theorists have said, responsiveness and sensitivity are part and parcel of validity (e.g. Hays and Hadorn 1992; Patrick and Chiang 2000), and not separate attributes. In the next chapter, on measuring change, we discuss the mathematical relationship of responsiveness and sensitivity to reliability. On a conceptual level, they are an aspect of validity, most akin to criterion validity—does the change detected by the new measure correlate with change as measured by some other instrument?

Validity and 'types of indices'

Some authors have proposed that there are different kinds of scales or indices, which vary according to their potential application. For example, Kirshner and Guyatt (1985) state that indices can be *discriminative* (i.e. used to distinguish between individuals or groups when there is no gold standard), *predictive* (used to classify individuals into predefined groups according to an existing gold standard), or *evaluative* (for tracking people or groups over time). Moreover, they state that the purpose of the scale dictates how the items are scaled, which procedures are used to select the items, how reliability and validity are assessed, and how 'responsiveness' is measured. We believe that these are false distinctions that do not reflect the reality of how tests are used in the real world; and more importantly, reflects a misunderstanding of validity testing.

While a scale may have been developed for one purpose, in actual practice, it is often used in a variety of different ways. Using their own example of the MMPI, Kirshner and Guyatt state that this is a 'discriminative' tool, 'developed in order to distinguish those with emotional and psychological disorders from the general population' (p. 27). This is undoubtably true, but it has also been used to diagnose people (what they call the 'predictive' use of a test; e.g. Scheibe *et al.* 2001), as well as a measure of improvement in therapy (e.g. Munley 2002). Similarly, they cite the Denver Developmental Screening Test as a 'predictive' tool 'designed to identify children who are likely to have learning problems in the future' (p. 28). Again, though, its use has not been restricted to this, but has also been used as a discriminative tool (Cadman *et al.* 1988) and to measure change (Mandich *et al.* 1994).

The bottom line is that scales are used in many ways. Whether or not they can be depends on one, and only one, issue—has it been validated for that purpose? If larger decreases on the Depression scale on the MMPI are seen in a group that receives cognitive behaviour therapy as compared to a control group, for example, then it can be used to measure changes over time, irrespective of the fact that the scale was initially developed to identify patients with depression. It is worth repeating the statement by Nunnally (1970): 'Strictly speaking, one validates not a measurement instrument but rather some use to which the instrument is put' (p. 133).

Biases in validity assessment
Restriction in range

We mentioned in Chapter 8 that an unacceptable way of seeming to increase the reliability of a measure is to give it to a more heterogeneous group than the one it is designed for. In this section, we return to this point from a different perspective; how the range of scores affects the validity of the scale. There are actually three ways this can occur:

- the predictor variable (usually our new measure) is restricted;
- the criterion is restricted; and
- a third variable, correlated with both the predictor and criterion variables, is used to select the group which will be given the predictor and criterion variables.

As an example, assume that we have read about a new assay for serum monoamine oxidase (MAO), which is highly correlated with scores on a depression inventory. In the original (fictitious) article, a correlation of 0.80 was found in a large community-based sample. Such an assay would be extremely useful in a hospital setting, where

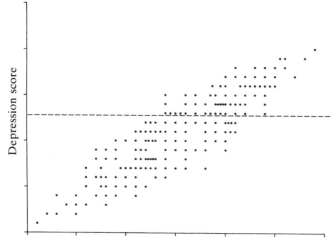

Fig. 10.1 Scatterplot showing the relationship between two variables.

difficulty with the English language and the various biases (e.g. faking good or bad) are often problems with self-administered scales. We replicate the study on our in-patient psychiatry ward, but find a disappointingly low correlation of only 0.37. Should we be surprised?

Based on our discussion of restriction of range, the answer is 'no'. We can illustrate this effect pictorially by drawing a scatter diagram of the two variables in the original study as in Fig. 10.1.

As a brief reminder, a scatterplot is made by placing a dot at the intersection of a person's scores on the two variables. Alternatively, an ellipse can be drawn so that it includes (usually) 95 per cent of the people. The more elliptical the swarm of points or the ellipse, the stronger the correlation; the more circular the ellipse, the lower the association, with the extreme being a circle reflecting a total lack of any relationship. This scatterplot is fairly thin, as would be expected with a correlation of 0.80.

In our study, all of the subjects were hospitalized depressives, so their scores on the depression inventory are expected to be higher than those in a community sample, falling above the line in Fig. 10.1. As can be seen, the portion of the ellipse falling above the line is more circular than the whole scatterplot, indicating that for this more restricted sample, the correlation between the two variables is considerably lower.

Using some equations developed by Thorndike (1949), we can predict how much the validity coefficient will be affected by selecting more restricted groups based on the criterion (X), the predictor (Y), or some other variable (Z). The first situation would apply if patients were hospitalized only if their scores on the depression inventory exceeded a certain level. This would be the case if high scores on the scale were one of the criteria for admission, and would be analogous to validating a new

TB test only on patients who have lesions on an X-ray. In this case, the validity of the predictor would be:

$$r' = \frac{r(s'_X/s_X)}{\sqrt{[1-r^2 + r^2(s'^2_X/s_X^2)]}}$$

where r' is the restricted validity coefficient, r is the validity coefficient in the unrestricted sample, s' is the SD of the criterion for the restricted sample, and s_X is the SD of the criterion for the unrestricted sample.

If the standard deviation in the unrestricted sample was 10, and it was reduced to 3 in the restricted sample, we would get:

$$\frac{0.80 \times (3/10)}{\sqrt{[1 - 0.64 + 0.64 \times (9/100)]}} = 0.37.$$

By the same token, we can work backwards by transforming this formula. If we did a study on a sample that was in some way constrained on the criterion variable, we could figure out what the validity coefficient would be if the full range of the variable were available. In this case, the formula would be:

$$r' = \frac{r'(s_X/s'_X)}{\sqrt{[1-r'^2 + r'^2(s_X^2/s'^2_X)]}}$$

where the terms have the same meaning as above.

The second case occurs when the group is selected on the basis of the *predictor* variable (Y); using the same example, only patients with increased MAO levels are included. This is the situation that obtains with criterion contamination; students are selected based on their scores on the admission test, which is actually being evaluated to see if it is a valid predictor. The formulae are the same, except that s'_Y is substituted for s'_X, and s_Y for s_X.

The last case is where the subjects are selected on the basis of some other variable (Z), which is correlated with both X and Y. Using our original example, this is the most realistic condition, since patients are admitted because of the severity of their symptomatology, which is related to both MAO level and scores on the depression inventory. The question can again be asked in two ways:

(1) if we know the results from an (unrestricted) community-based study, what would the correlation be in our (more restricted) hospital environment; or

(2) if we correlated X and Y in our restricted sample, what would the correlation be in an unrestricted one?

Since an additional variable is involved (Z, the severity of depression), more information needs to be known:

(1) the correlation of X and Y in the unrestricted sample;

(2) the correlations of X with Z and Y with Z in this sample; and

(3) the standard deviation of Z in the restricted and unrestricted samples.

As these data are rarely known, the equation is mainly of academic interest. For those who are interested, a thorough treatment of this topic can be found in Ghiselli (1964).

Unreliability of the criterion

One pervasive problem in validation occurs when we correlate our new scale with a gold standard. Quite frequently, though, the criterion is not as good as this term suggests, since it is unreliable in its own right. Thus, the validity coefficient may be attenuated since, even if the predictor (Y) were excellent, it is predicting to an unreliable criterion (X). We can estimate what the validity coefficient would be if the criterion were perfectly reliable by using the formula:

$$r'_{XY'} = \frac{r_{XY}}{\sqrt{(r_{XX})}}$$

where r_{XY}' is the estimated correlation with a perfectly reliable criterion, r_{XY} is the actual correlation between tests X and Y, and r_{XX} is the reliability coefficient of the criterion (test X).

If we assume that the criterion is perfectly reliable, and we want to see how much the correlation *could* improve if the new test were perfectly reliable, we would simply substitute r_{YY} for r_{XX} under the radical:

$$r'_{XY'} = \frac{r_{XY}}{\sqrt{(r_{YY})}}.$$

A more general (and realistic) case assumes that both scales are unreliable, and we want to see what the correlation would be if both were perfectly reliable. The equation now reads:

$$r'_{XY'} = \frac{r_{XY}}{\sqrt{(r_{XX}\, r_{YY})}}.$$

Another way this equation can be used is to compare two or more studies that are examining the same construct, but using different tests whose reliabilities vary (Schmidt and Hunter 1999). Let us assume that Study A finds a correlation of 0.42 between a quality of life (QOL) scale and an index of activities of daily living (ADL). Study B, using a different set of scales to measure the same constructs, finds a correlation of 0.22. Why is r nearly twice as high in the first study? Assuming that both studies were sufficiently large enough to rule out sampling error, then a possible answer is the differing reliabilities of the measures. If the QOL scale in Study A had a reliability of 0.90, and the ADL scale a reliability of 0.80, then the disattenuated correlation between them is:

$$r'_{XY'} = \frac{0.42}{\sqrt{(0.90)(0.80)}} = 0.49.$$

If Study B used shorter scales with lower reliabilities (e.g. 0.50 for QOL and 0.40 for ADL), then its disattenuated correlation is:

$$r'_{XY'} = \frac{0.22}{\sqrt{(0.50)(0.40)}} = 0.49.$$

Thus, while the studies report different correlations between the *measures*, the correlations between the *constructs* are the same (Schmidt and Hunter 1999).

The most general (and realistic) case is that perfect reliability never exists, in either the new instrument or in the criterion. However, it may be possible to improve the reliability of one or both, and we would want to know what the correlation between the two indices would be, given these improved (albeit not perfect) reliabilities. In this case, we would use the equation:

$$r'_{XY'} = \frac{r_{XY}\sqrt{(r'_{XX'}\, r'_{YY'})}}{\sqrt{(r_{XX}\, r_{YY})}}$$

where r_{XX}' and r_{YY}' are the changed reliabilities for the two variables (somewhere between their actual reliabilities and 1.0).

These equations have two possible uses. First, they tell us how much the validity would increase if we were able to increase the reliabilities of the instruments. If the increase is only marginal, then the investment of time and perhaps money needed to improve the psychometric properties may not be worth it; whereas a large potential increase may signal that it could be worthwhile making the investment. The second useful function is in the area of theory development. If our theory tells us that variable *A* should correlate strongly with variable *B*, then correcting for unreliability of the measures gives us an indication of the true validity of the instrument, and hence of our construct. A low, uncorrected validity estimate may incorrectly lead us to discard the theory, when in fact it may be correct, and the problem is with the scales.

Whether or not to use any of these formulae depends on the question being asked. If the issue is whether the test, as it currently exists, can predict some other measure as it currently exists, then neither should be corrected for unreliability. Any correction would overestimate how the test performs in the real world, which consists of measures that have some degree of measurement error. Quoting Guion (1965) in this regard, 'The effect of a possible correction for attenuation should never be a consideration when one is deciding how to evaluate a measure as it exists' (p. 32). On the other hand, if we are interested in the degree of improvement that is possible with the new test in predicting an existing criterion, then we should correct only for the predictor variable. However, this corrected coefficient should not be reported as if it were the actual correlation between the two measures, and we cannot perform any tests of significance on it (Magnusson 1967). Finally, if the issue is one of testing a construct—that is, seeing if the construct being measured is related to some other construct—as opposed to establishing the validity of the test itself, then correcting both the predictor and the criterion may make sense (Schmidt and Hunter 1996, 1999).

The final issue is which reliability coefficient to use in the equation—internal consistency, test–retest, or inter-rater. Muchinsky (1996) correctly states that one should 'use the type of reliability estimate that treats as error those factors that one decides should be treated as error' (p. 87). That is, if you feel that the test can be improved by increasing the coverage of the construct (or the criterion is constrained by limited sampling from the domain), then it makes most sense to use Cronbach's α as the estimate of reliability. Conversely, if you feel that error is introduced by unreliability of the raters, then the estimate of inter-rater reliability is the correct one to use, and so on. However, quoting Muchinsky (1996) again, 'There is no acceptable psychometric basis for creating validity coefficients that are the product of correcting for multiple types of unreliability' (p. 87).

Changes in the sample

Life would be simple if we could establish the validity of a measure once by conducting a series of studies, and then assume that we could use that instrument under a range of circumstances and with a variety of people. Unfortunately, this is not the case. Estimates of validity, like those of reliability, are dependent upon the nature of the people being measured and, to a greater or lesser degree, the circumstances under which they are being assessed. A tool that can accurately measure the activities of daily living among cancer patients may be quite useless when used in respirology; and one that has proven valid in distinguishing OBS from depressed patients may not discriminate between OBS patients and schizophrenics. Every time a scale is used in a new context, or with a different group of people, it is necessary to re-establish its psychometric properties.

Summary

Validity is a process of determining what, if anything, we are measuring with our scale; that is, can we make valid statements about a person based on his or her score on the index. *Concurrent* validity is most often used when we are trying to replace one tool with a simpler, cheaper, or less invasive one. We generally use another form of criterion validation, called *predictive* validity, in developing instruments that allow us to get answers earlier than current instruments allow. *Construct validity* refers to a wide range of approaches which are used when what we are trying to measure is a 'hypothetical construct', like anxiety or some syndromes, rather than something which can be readily observed.

References

Cadman, D., Walter, S. D., Chambers, L. W., Ferguson, R., Szatmari, P., Johnson, N., and McNamee, J. (1988). Predicting problems in school performance from preschool health, developmental and behavioural assessments. *CMAJ*, **139**, 31–6.

Campbell, D. T. and Fiske, D. W. (1959). Convergent and discriminant validation by the multitrait-multimethod matrix. *Psychological Bulletin*, **56**, 81–105.

Cattell, R. B. (1963). Theory of fluid and crystallized intelligence: Critical experiment. *British Journal of Educational Psychology*, **54**, 1–22.

Clark, L. A. and Watson, D. (1995). Constructing validity: Basic issues in objective scale development. *Psychological Assessment*, **7**, 309–19.

Cronbach, L. J. (1971). Test validation. In *Educational measurement* (ed. R. L. Thorndike) pp. 221–37. American Council on Education, Washington DC.

Cronbach, L. J. and Meehl, P. E. (1955). Construct validity in psychological tests. *Psychological Bulletin*, **52**, 281–302.

Foster, S. L. and Cone, J. D. (1995). Validity issues in clinical assessment. *Psychological Assessment*, 7, 248–60.

Ghiselli, E. E. (1964). *Theory of psychological measurement.* McGraw-Hill, New York.

Guion, R. M. (1965). *Personnel testing.* McGraw-Hill, New York.

Guion, R. M. (1977). Content validity: Three years of talk—what's the action? *Public Personnel Management*, 6, 407–14.

Hays, R. D. and Hadorn, D. (1992). Responsiveness to change: An aspect of validity, not a separate dimension. *Quality of Life Research*, 1, 73–5.

Kirshner, B. and Guyatt, G. (1985). A methodological framework for assessing health indices. *Journal of Chronic Disease*, 38, 27–36.

Landy, F. J. (1986). Stamp collecting versus science. *American Psychologist*, 41, 1183–92.

Liang, M. H. (2000). Longitudinal construct validity: Establishment of clinical meaning in patient evaluation instruments. *Medical Care*, 38 (Supplement II), S84–S90.

Magnusson, D. (1967). *Test theory.* Addison-Wesley, Reading MA.

Mandich, M., Simons, C. J. R., Ritchie, S., Schmidt, D., and Mullett, M. (1994). Motor development, infantile reactions and postural responses of pre-term, at-risk infants. *Developmental Medicine & Child Neurology*, 36, 397–405.

Messick, S. (1980). Test validity and the ethics of assessment. *American Psychologist*, 35, 1012–27.

Muchinsky, P. M. (1996). The correction for attenuation. *Educational and Psychological Measurement*, 56, 78–90.

Munley, P. H. (2002). Comparability of MMPI-2 scales and profiles over time. *Journal of Personality Assessment*, 78, 145–60.

Nunnally, J. C. (1970). *Introduction to psychological measurement.* McGraw-Hill, NY.

Patrick, D. L. and Chiang, Y.-P. (2000). Measurement of health outcomes in treatment effectiveness evaluations: Conceptual and methodological challenges. *Medical Care*, 38 (Supplement II), S14–S25.

Scheibe, S., Bagby, R. M., Miller, L. S., and Dorian, B. J. (2001). Assessing posttraumatic stress disorder with the MMPI-2 in a sample of workplace accident victims. *Psychological Assessment*, 13, 369–74.

Schmidt, F. L. and Hunter, J. E. (1996). Measurement error in psychological research: Lessons from 26 research scenarios. *Psychological Methods*, 1, 199–223.

Schmidt, F. L. and Hunter, J. E. (1999). Theory testing and measurement error. *Intelligence*, 27, 183–98.

Thorndike, R. L. (1949). *Personnel selection: Test and measurement techniques.* Wiley, New York.

Chapter 11

Measuring change

Introduction

The measurement of change has been a topic of considerable confusion in the medical literature. As clinicians and researchers, we view that the ultimate goal of most treatment—medical, surgical, psychosocial, or educational—is to induce change in the patient's or student's status. It would appear to follow that the measurement of change in patients' health state or in a student's level of understanding is an appropriate goal of research. A number of recent articles (Guyatt *et al.* 1987; MacKenzie *et al.* 1986) have advocated this position, both on the grounds that the measurement of change in patient's condition is the goal of clinical care and should be addressed by research methods, and on the methodological basis that instruments which are responsive to changes in health status are more sensitive measures of the effects of clinical interventions than those which simply assess health status after an intervention.

However, this opinion is by no means unanimous. Several authors in education and psychology have taken stands against the use of difference scores (Burckhardt *et al.* 1982; Cronbach and Furby 1970). In this chapter, we explore the issues surrounding the use of change scores and show that these divergent positions are based on different views of the goals of measurement, and different assumptions regarding the methodological advantages and disadvantages of change measures.

The goal of measurement of change

In order to understand the source of the controversy in the literature, it is necessary to recognize that the measurement of change can be directed at different goals. These have been described by Linn and Slinde (1977).

1. *To measure differences between individuals in the amount of change.* Although apparently similar to the notion of reliability, the intent is to distinguish between those individuals who *change a lot* and those who *change little*. For example, if we wanted to identify individuals who were responsive to therapy (e.g. in a secondary analysis of a trial of therapy for arthritis), we would proceed by a comparison of individual differences in change scores. Much of the literature in psychology addressing the measurement of change accepts this as the basic goal of change measurement.

2. *To identify correlates of change.* This goal really represents an elaboration of the first. If we were successful at identifying responsive subgroups in a trial of therapy, a logical second step is to attempt to identify those factors which are associated or

correlated with good response. The issues of measurement also follow from the earlier concerns: if we cannot differentiate between those who change a great deal and those who change little, the resulting restriction in range will attenuate any attempt to find correlates.

3. *To infer treatment effects from group differences.* This goal is probably the primary goal of most clinical trials. By randomly assigning individuals to treatment and control groups, measuring the health state before and after treatment, and then comparing the average change in health state in the groups, we can determine a treatment effect—individuals in a treatment group will change, on the average, more than those in a control group.

The first and last goals work against one another. To the extent that there are individual differences in response to treatment, this is an indication that the treatment had different effects on different people, and it will be more difficult to detect an overall treatment effect. However, if there are individual differences in response to treatment, then we will be able to identify responsive subgroups and possible prognostic factors; if there are no individual differences, we will be unsuccessful in this search.

Note however, that there is no conflict in the goal of discrimination between individuals, as expressed in the reliability coefficient, and the goal of evaluation of change within individuals. It is certainly possible that there may be large and stable differences between individuals on some measure, yet all may change equally in response to treatment. If we consider the everyday example of dieting, overweight people may range from 60 kg to 150 kg; yet a conservative and successful diet would have all losing from 1 kg to 2 kg per week. As long as there was reasonable consistency in the amount of weight loss experienced by different individuals in the plan, it would not be difficult to demonstrate the efficacy of a treatment program which showed losses of this order, despite the large differences in individual weights. So the presence of large differences among individuals does not, of itself, preclude the demonstration of small treatment effects. Differences in *change* of different individuals *does* reduce the chance of demonstrating overall treatment effects.

Why not measure change directly?

The remainder of this chapter will address different ways to combine measures taken at various times (usually two) to best measure the amount of change in individuals or groups. This seems, on the surface, to be a complicated way to go about things. Why not simply ask people how much they have changed, which appears a much more straightforward method? Clinicians do it all the time; for example, the following seem likely ways to ask the question:

Since I put you on the new drug at your last visit, have you got better or worse? How much?

Since your illness began a few months ago, have you been getting better or worse? How much?

Thinking back to when you first noticed this symptom, how much worse has it got?

Although this is a time-honoured approach, there is a very good reason to avoid asking about change directly: people simply do not remember how they were at the beginning. We have already noted in Chapter 6 that retrospective judgements of change are vulnerable to potential bias. The two biases that are most evident are:

1. *Implicit theory of change.* It is very difficult for people to remember their past state unless there is a salient event associated with it. Ross (1989) showed that, when asked how much they felt 'last September', people commonly begin with their present state ('How do I feel today?'), then invoke an implicit theory of change ('How do I think the drug worked?'), and then work backwards to an estimate of what their prior state must have been. As a consequence, the correlation between measures of change and the present state is high, but between the change measure and the prior state is low (Guyatt *et al.* 2002). So a retrospective assessment of an initial state is not to be trusted.

2. *Response shift.* Conversely, the initial assessment may be wrong. If you are asked to assess your 'self-actualization skills', you may make an initial estimate, but with little knowledge, it may be little more than a wild guess. After a course in 'self-actualization training' (whatever that is) you may be better able to assess your initial, uninformed state. This phenomenon is called 'response shift' (Schwarz and Sprangers 1999). Again, the consequence is that the initial assessment is not to be trusted.

As we discussed earlier, the two theories lead to opposite predictions, and there are many circumstances in assessing health status where the same phenomenon can be interpreted in diametrically opposite ways (Norman 2003). One thing, however, is clear: both theories are based on documented bias, and both lead to some suspicion about the veracity of direct change measures.

Measures of association—reliability and sensitivity to change

The different goals of measurement are reflected in different coefficients, analogous to the reliability coefficient, which express the ability of an instrument to detect change within subjects or the effects of treatment. In order to clarify these distinctions, let us consider a group of six individuals who have entered into a diet plan and are weighed before treatment and again after 2 weeks of dieting. The data might look like Table 11.1.

As we discussed before, the goal of discriminating among subjects has been incorporated in the notion of *reliability*, which we discussed at length in Chapter 8, and is defined as:

$$\text{Reliability } (R) = \frac{\sigma^2_{\text{pat}}}{\sigma^2_{\text{pat}} + \sigma^2_{\text{err}}}.$$

In the present example, the reliability focuses on the difference between patients' average weights, and σ^2_{pat} would be determined from a sum of squares calculated as:

$$\text{SS}_{\text{pat}} = (147 - 127)^2 + (116 - 127)^2 + \ldots + (114 - 127)^2.$$

Table 11.1 Weight (in kg) of six patients in a diet clinic

Patient	Before	After two weeks	Average	Change
1	150	144	147	−6
2	120	112	116	−8
3	110	108	109	−2
4	140	142	141	+2
5	138	132	135	−6
6	116	112	114	−4
Mean	129	125	127	−4.0

By analogy, we can also develop a measure to describe the reproducibility of the change score, i.e. an index of the ability of the measure to discriminate between those subjects who change a great deal and those who change little.

Reliability of the change score

The assessment of the ability of an instrument to detect individual differences in change scores is appropriately labeled as the *reliability of the change score* (Lord and Novick 1968). By analogy to the reliability coefficient, this can be expressed as:

$$\text{Reliability}\,(D) = \frac{\sigma_D^2}{\sigma_D^2 + \sigma_{\text{err}(D)}^2}.$$

where $\sigma^2{}_D$ expresses the systematic difference between subjects in their change score, and $\sigma^2{}_{\text{err}}(D)$ is the error associated with this estimate. In our example, $\sigma^2{}_D$ would be derived from a sum of squares calculated as:

$$\text{SS}_D = (-6 - (-4))^2 + (-8 - (-4))^2 + \ldots + (-4 -)-4))^2.$$

The reliability of the change score can be shown to be related to the variance of pre-test (x) and post-test (y) scores, their reliability (R) and the correlation between pre-test and post-test (r), in the following manner:

$$\text{Reliability}\,(D) = \frac{\sigma_x^2 R_{xx} + \sigma_y^2 R_{yy} - 2\sigma_x\sigma_y r_{xy}}{\sigma_x^2 + \sigma_y^2 - 2\sigma_x\sigma_y r_{xy}}$$

where r_{xy} is the correlation between the pre-test and post-test. If the pre-test and post-test have the same variances, this expression reduces to:

$$\text{Reliability} = \frac{R_{xx} + R_{yy} - 2r_{xy}}{2.0 - 2r_{xy}}$$

where R_{xx} and R_{yy} are the reliabilities of the initial and final measurements. In our previous example, the measured reliability was 0.95. If we assume that this reliability coefficient applies equally to both pre-test and post-test, and we further assume a correlation of, say 0.80 between the two measures, then the reliability of the difference score becomes:

$$\text{Reliability}\,(D) = \frac{0.95 + 0.95 - 2 \times 0.80}{2.0 - 2 \times 0.80} = 0.30/0.40 = 0.75.$$

In the limiting case, it can be demonstrated that, under the circumstances where there is a perfect correlation between the pre-test and post-test scores, the reliability of the difference score is zero. Although this appears strange, it actually follows from the basic notion of discriminating between those who change a great deal and those who change little. If an experimental intervention resulted in a uniform response to treatment, all patients would improve an equal amount. As a result, the variance of the change score will be zero, since every patient's post-test score would be equal to his or her pre-test score, except for a constant; no patients would have changed more or less than any other, and the reliability of the difference score would be zero.

Since a perfectly uniform response to treatment would represent an ideal state of affairs for the use of change scores to measure treatment effects, yet would yield a reliability coefficient for change scores of zero, it should not be used as an index appropriate for assessing the ability of an instrument to measure treatment effects, and some other approach must be used.

Different indices of sensitivity to change

In assessing change, it is reasonable to presume that some measures, for whatever reason, may be more sensitive to changes resulting from treatments than others. If so, it is useful to have standard indices, perhaps analogous to the reliability coefficient, to compare one instrument to another.

Although it is possible to create an index of sensitivity to change resulting from treatment effects, which is a direct analogy of the reliability coefficient and has the form of an intraclass correlation, this is rarely used in the literature. Instead, there have been a number of indices proposed, most of which are variants on an effect size (average change divided by the standard deviation; Cohen 1988).

First, a word about terminology. As we mentioned in the previous chapter, Liang (2000) differentiates between *sensitivity to change*, which taps an instrument's ability to measure any degree of change; and *responsiveness*, which assesses its ability to measure clinically important change. In this section, we will follow Liang, and discuss the issue of clinical importance at the end. Further, a number of authors (e.g. Kirshner and Guyatt 1985), primarily in the area of health-related quality of life, have proposed that sensitivity or responsiveness should be considered a third essential measurement property of an instrument, equal with reliability and validity. Not everyone agrees. As we discussed earlier, we and others (e.g. Hays and Hadorn

1992; Patrick and Chiang 2000) view it as just one form of construct validity, assessing the hypothesis that the instrument is capable of detecting clinically meaningful change.

Regardless of its status, the starting point for examining sensitivity to change is a comparison of the mean score (or mean change score) of a group of patients who were given a successful therapy and the mean of a second group who were not. These means, or mean changes, are then used to compute a difference between treatment and control groups. This difference is then compared to some estimate of variability to create a dimensionless ratio.

Regrettably, while there is not universal consensus on the importance of responsiveness as a separate test attribute, there is even less agreement as to how to measure it. As we indicated, most, but not all measures, are variants on an effect size (ES), but here the similarity ends. Different measures of variability are used, and some numerical multipliers are also used. Below is a brief catalogue of current favourites.

Cohen's effect size

The grandfather of all of these measures is Cohen's effect size (Cohen 1988), which is simply the ratio of the mean difference to the standard deviation (SD) of baseline scores. Since it is a fairly general construct, initially proposed simply as a basis for sample size calculations, it can be applied to the change observed in a single group from pre-test to post test, or the difference between the post-test score of a treatment or control group or, for that matter, the difference between change scores of a treatment and control group. In any case, the denominator would be the SD at baseline of the control group (in which case it is also referred to as *Glass's* Δ; Glass 1976), or the pooled SD at baseline of the treatment and control groups, which is referred to as *Cohen's d* (Rosenthal 1994). The advantage of *d* that it uses all of the data, and so is a more stable estimate of the SD.

Guyatt's responsiveness

Guyatt's measure (Guyatt *et al.* 1987) is specific to a pre-test/post-test, two-group design, and is a variant of the ES. In this case, it is the ratio of the mean change *in the treatment group* to the standard deviation of the change scores *in the control group*. It is not at all clear, since there is a control group, why this index would not use a numerator based on the difference between mean change in the treatment group and mean change in the control group.

The standardized response mean

McHorney and Tarlov (1995) have suggested a different effect size, called the standardized response mean, or SRM, which is the ratio of the mean change (in a single group) to the standard deviation of the change scores. This has more of the form of a statistical test of a difference, and is simply the paired *t*-test multiplied by $\sqrt{n}$, where *n* is the sample size.

From our previous discussion, we can actually show a relationship between the SRM and the ES. The standard deviation of the difference score is just $\sqrt{2} \times$ SEM (standard error of measurement), and the SEM, in turn, is equal to:

$$\text{SEM} = \text{SD}_{Baseline} \times \sqrt{1 - R}$$

so the SRM is just $\sqrt{2}\,(1-R)$ times the ES.

These indices do not exhaust the possibilities, but are clearly the most common. As we have seen, all are, at their core, variants on the ES, differing only in whether you use the SD of baseline scores or the SD of difference scores, and whether there is a numerical multiplier. But the differences among them are more ecclesiastical than substantive.

Conceptual problems with sensitivity to change

Aside from the theoretical problems with sensitivity to change and the potpourri of coefficients, discussed above, there are two real problems with trying to calculate it as a property of the instrument.

The first is that, just as reliability is a property of an instrument *as applied to a particular population* and is sensitive to the variance of the sample, sensitivity to change to a treatment is a characteristic of both the treatment and the inherent sensitivity and measurement error of the instrument. Simply put, all instruments are more responsive to large treatment effects than to small ones. But the situation is more tenuous with sensitivity to change than with reliability. It is not all that difficult to select a sample which can be assumed to have, on average, characteristics (mean, standard deviation) of the population to which you ultimately want to apply the measure. But it is a lot more difficult to contemplate selecting a treatment which is representative of the treatments you want to apply the instrument to. That is, presumably you want to show that the sensitivity to change is adequate for the kind of treatments you want to measure. But how can you determine *a priori* how big those treatment effects are likely to be? And how do you select a single treatment which is right in the middle of them? It clearly matters. Any instrument will be much more sensitive to large treatments than small ones, so it is hard to disentangle characteristics of the instrument from characteristics of the treatment.

One solution is to apply multiple instruments—the new one, and existing validated measures—to the same group of patients who are undergoing a standard and effective treatment, and then look at the relative sensitivity to change of the various measures. But herein lies the second problem: it is very difficult to get funding to examine a group of patients who are given a known efficacious therapy. National agencies might fund it; drug companies will not.

A second solution that has seen widespread application (regrettably) is to simply follow a group of patients for some period of time, and administer the instrument at beginning and end. You then ask them individually whether they got better, stayed the same, or got worse. Finally, you compute the average change on the instrument for those who got better. However appealing the strategy, since it circumvents problems with choosing a representative therapy, it is fatally flawed (Norman *et al.* 1997).

The problem is that, in any cohort of subjects followed over time, some people will get better and some worse, just by chance. Indeed, the variability in response of individuals is just what makes it difficult to detect treatment effects, and will eventually end up in the denominator of any statistical test of treatment; but it is this same variability which is being used for the measure of responsiveness. As a consequence, you can end up with nonsensical results, such as a high responsiveness in a situation where the average treatment effect is exactly zero.

Difficulties with change scores in experimental designs
Potential loss of precision

Although it would appear that it is always desirable to measure change, since it removes the effect of variance between patients, this is actually not the case. The calculation of a difference score is based on the difference between two quantities, the pre-test and post-test, and both are measured with some error, σ^2_{err}. If this quantity is sufficiently large relative to the variance between patients, the net result might be to introduce more, rather than less, error into the estimate of treatment effect.

The conditions under which it makes sense to measures change within patients as a measure of treatment effect can be expressed in terms of a generalizability coefficient. The use of change scores to estimate treatment main effects is only appropriate when the variance between subjects exceeds the error variance within subjects. This is equivalent to the following expression:

$$\frac{\sigma^2_{sub}}{\sigma^2_{sub} + \sigma^2_{err}} \geqslant 0.5$$

Thus, one should only use change scores when the reliability of the measure exceeds 0.5. Reliability is not irrelevant or inversely related to sensitivity—*reliability is a necessary pre-condition for the appropriate application of change scores.* This analysis does not, of course, imply that measures which are reliable are, of necessity, useful for the assessment of change. Even if an instrument is reliable, it remains to be shown that differences in response to treatment can be detected before the instrument can be used for the assessment of change.

Biased measurement of treatment effects

The simple subtraction of post-treatment from pre-treatment scores to create a difference score as a measure of the overall effect of treatment assumes that the effect of treatment will be the same, except for random error, for all patients. This assumption can be shown to be false in many, if not most circumstances. One reason is that one major cause of an individual having an extreme score on pre-test is simply an accumulation of random processes; i.e. the very good scores are to some extent due to good luck, and the very bad scores are due to bad luck. To the extent that chance is operative (and any reliability coefficient less than 1 is an indication of the presence of random variation), then the very good are likely to get worse, and the very bad get better, on retest. This effect is known as 'regression to the mean'. In effect, the best line fitting post-test to pre-treatment data in the absence of treatment effects has a slope less than 1 and an intercept greater than 0.The use of change scores assumes a best-fit line with a slope of 1 and intercept of 0. The consequence of regression to the mean is that the use of change or difference scores overestimates the effect of pre-test differences on post-test scores.

The solution to this problem for assessing individual change recommended by Cronbach and Furby (1970) is the use of *residualized gain scores*. Instead of subtracting pre-test from post-test, we first fit the line relating the pre-test and post-test scores using regression analysis. We then estimate the post-test score of each patient from the regression equation. The residualized gain score is the difference between the actual post-test score and the score that was predicted from the regression equation. In other words, the residualized gain score removes from consideration that portion of the gain score which was linearly predictable from the pre-test score. What remains is an indication of those individuals who changed more or less than was expected.

This operation is really designed to identify individual differences in change in an unbiased manner. Cronbach and Furby (1970) among others have commented on the use of change scores to estimate overall treatment effects, and conclude that analysis of covariance methods should be employed when the reliability is sufficiently large, and simple post-test scores otherwise.

The reason for the use of ANCOVA is again related to the phenomenon of regression to the mean. As we discussed, the change score assumes that the line relating pre-test to post-test has a slope of 1 and intercept 0, which is not the optimal line when error of measurement is present. The result is that the denominator of the statistical test of treatment effects includes variance due to lack of fit, resulting in a conservative test. Since ANCOVA fits an optimum line to the data, in general, this will result in a smaller error term and a more sensitive test of treatment effects.

Change scores and quasi-experimental designs

So far, we have addressed the use of change scores in the context of randomized trials, where the primary goal is to increase the sensitivity of statistical tests by reducing the magnitude of the error term. There is another potential application of these methods in situations such as cohort analytical studies, where there are likely to be initial differences between treatment and control groups. In this situation, the change score has an apparent advantage, in that the subtraction of the initial score for each subject will have the effect of eliminating the initial differences between groups.

However, when the change score is used in a situation where there are differences between the two groups on the pre-test measure, as might result if subjects were not allocated at random to the two conditions, additional complications arise. These are directly related to the effect of regression to the mean, discussed in the section on residualized gain scores. In the absence of treatment effects, individuals measured with some random error will not stay the same on retest. Those who were very good will worsen, on average, and those who were very bad will improve.

Unfortunately this effect also applies to group means, which are simply the average of individual scores. In the absence of any treatment effect, the differences between groups will be reduced at the second testing, confounding any interpretation of differences between groups observed following treatment. One way around this problem is again the use of *analysis of covariance*, however this method is a refinement to the use of change scores, not a fundamentally different approach.

There are other fundamental reasons to view any attempt at post-hoc adjustment for differences between groups on pre-test, whether by difference scores, repeated measures ANOVA or ANCOVA, with considerable suspicion. Implicit in these analytical methods is a specific model of the change process which cannot be assumed to have general applicability. This is illustrated in Fig. 11.1.

Any of the analytical methods assume that, in the absence of any treatment effect, the experimental and control group will grow at the same rate, so that the difference in means at the beginning would equal the difference in means at the end, and any additional difference between the two groups (shown as the difference between the post-test mean of the treated group and the dotted line) is evidence of a treatment effect.

Unfortunately, there are any number of plausible alternative models, which will fit the data equally well. For example, in a rehabilitation setting or in an educational program for mentally handicapped children, individuals who are less impaired, thus score higher initially, may have the greatest capacity for change or improvement over time. Under these circumstances, referred to in the literature as a 'fan-spread' model, the observed data would be obtained in the absence of any treatment effect, and ANCOVA or analysis of difference scores would wrongly conclude a benefit from treatment.

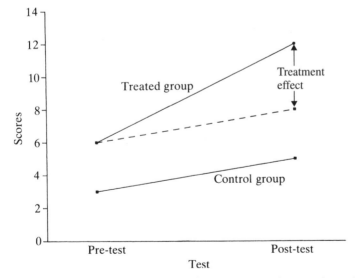

Fig. 11.1 Relation between pre-test and post-test scores in a quasi-experimental design.

Conversely, a situation may arise where a 'ceiling effect' occurs; that is, individuals with high scores initially may already be at the limit of their potential, thus would be expected to improve relatively less with treatment than those with initially lower scores. In this circumstance, the post-test scores in the absence of an effect of treatment would converge, and the analysis would underestimate the treatment effect.

It is evident that any analysis based on just one or two means for each group will not permit a choice among these models of growth, and additional points on the individual growth curve would be required (Rogosa *et al.* 1982). Of course, if such situations were rare, one could argue for the adequacy of change score approaches; however it is likely that situations of non-constant growth are the rule, not the exception, in health research. As Lord (1967) put it, 'There simply is no logical or statistical procedure that can be counted on to make proper allowances for uncontrolled pre-existing differences between groups'.

Measuring change using multiple observations: growth curves

In the last section, we alluded to the problems associated with inferring change from two observations. In part, these problems result from the very simple model of change which is implied by a simple pre-test/post-test approach. Change looks like a quantum process: first you are in one state, then you are in another state. Individual change obviously does not occur this way. It is a continuous process, whether we are speaking of physical change (e.g. growth or recovery from trauma), intellectual change (learning or development), or emotional change. Moreover, it is probably non-linear. Some individuals may make an initially rapid recovery from an illness and then improve slowly; some may improve gradually at first and then more rapidly; and of course some may deteriorate or fluctuate around a stable state of partial recovery.

It is evident that any reasonable attempt to characterize these individual *growth curves* will require multiple points of observation, so that a statistical curve can be fitted. While this sounds laborious, in many circumstances multiple observations are available, and only await an appropriate method for analysis. For example, many treatment programs extend across multiple visits, and frequently the clinician makes systematic observations in order to assess response to therapy and possibly adjust treatment. If multiple observations are available, it makes little sense to base an assessment of treatment effect only on assessments at the beginning and end of treatment, which would throw away a great deal of data. Even if the change is uniform and linear, so that there is no apparent advantage of assessment methods based on individual growth, the use of multiple observations amounts to an increase in sample size, with a corresponding reduction of within-subject error and an increase in statistical power.

There is a growing consensus on approaches to the appropriate analysis of data of this form, although the theory underlying such methods has a brief history, dating back only about two decades (Bryk and Raudenbush 1987; Francis *et al.* 1991; Rogosa *et al.* 1982). The basic idea common to all methods is to develop an analytical model of the relationship between individual growth and time, then estimate the parameters of the model using a variant of regression analysis. In its simplest form, it involves no more than using standard options within some computerized ANOVA packages to break down the variance into linear and higher order terms. That is, instead of simply estimating the means of all patients at each time point, we first fit a straight line to the means over time, then a quadratic (time^2) term, then a cubic (time^3) term, and so on. If there were repeated observations for a total of k time points, then the data would be fitted with a $(k-1)$ degree polynomial. Thus, in the simplest case where there are only two time points, the best we can do is fit a $(k-1) = 1$ degree polynomial; i.e. a straight line. As it turns out, a straight line goes rather well through two points.

More complex analysis involves the idea that each person should be fitted separately, since growths are individual (Rogosa *et al.* 1982). Then each parameter of the overall growth curve (the factor, or *beta weight*, multiplying each term) becomes a random variable with its own mean and standard deviation, rather than a point estimate.

To make things more concrete, imagine a series of patients with acute knee injuries enrolled in a physiotherapy program for treatment. Suppose the therapist aims for biweekly treatments over a total period of three weeks. Table 11.2 shows data for eight such patients.

It is always useful to graph the data prior to analysis, and we have done this in Fig. 11.2, which shows the individual data as curves, as well as the means at each time. Examining first the progression of the means, it is evident that they fall on a nearly straight line as a function of time, with a small amount of curvature. This fact suggests that the data could be modeled quite successfully with a linear function, which has only two parameters, the slope and the intercept, and possibly a small quadratic (time^2) term.

Table 11.2 Range of motion (in degrees) of knee joints for eight patients enroled in a treatment program at baseline and over five follow-up visits

Patient	Baseline	Follow-up visit				
		1	2	3	4	5
1	22	23	25	36	42	44
2	30	35	44	51	56	60
3	44	48	50	55	63	66
4	28	32	35	39	42	44
5	40	45	50	57	61	64
6	32	33	35	38	38	37
7	22	27	30	37	42	43
8	40	45	46	55	56	58
Mean	32.25	36.00	39.75	46.00	50.00	52.00

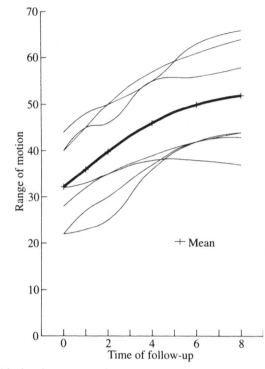

Fig. 11.2 Individual and mean growth curves.

We do not usually approach the analysis this way, however. With analysis of variance (ANOVA) or analysis of covariance (ANCOVA), we simply look for differences among means; the data at each time could be interchanged and the results would be the same; the analysis is completely indifferent to the actual functional relationship between time and the dependent variable. In fact, it does not account for the difference in timing of the follow-up visits, since time is treated as simply a categorical variable. What we really want is an analysis which separately tests the degree of linear change, and any other components. We can show this contrast between the two methods by doing the regular ANCOVA and also conducting a second analysis, called an 'orthogonal decomposition', where the linear, quadratic, and higher order polynomials are modelled. The results are shown in Table 11.3.

The orthogonal analysis confirms our observations from the graph. The linear relationship with time is highly significant ($F = 52.63$, $p = 0.0002$); the quadratic term is also highly significant ($F = 39.42$, $p = 0.0004$); and no other terms are significant. Note that the sums of squares are additive, so that the conventional result can be obtained by simply adding up all the trend sums of squares to get the overall effect of time; and all the patient × time sums of squares to get the overall patient × time term. This results in a significant overall effect of time; the F value is slightly lower,

Table 11.3 Analysis of covariance of range of motion data, with orthogonal decomposition

Source	Sum of squares	df	Mean square	F	Tail prob
Orthogonal decomposition					
Baseline	2509.26981	1	2509.26981	23.40	0.0029
Patients	643.50519	6	107.25086		
Linear trend	1430.17820	1	1430.17820	52.63	0.0002
Patient $\times$ time^1	190.23034	7	27.17576		
Quadratic trend	65.53945	1	65.53945	39.42	0.0004
Patients $\times$ time^2	11.63924	7	1.66275		
Cubic trend	0.37651	1	0.37651	0.19	0.6759
Patient $\times$ time^3	13.85499	7	1.97928		
Quadratic trend	0.80584	1	0.80584	0.50	0.5041
Patient $\times$ time^4	11.37543	7	1.62506		
Conventional analysis					
Time	1496.90000	4	374.22500	46.14	<0.0001
Patient $\times$ time	227.10000	28	8.11071		

but it is more significant (because the degrees of freedom in the numerator is 4 instead of 1).

Why are the results not all that different between the two analyses? In this case, because the individual growth curves are quite different. There is a large patient $\times$ time interaction, showing that individual patients are changing at quite different rates. This can be tested manually by taking the ratio of the patient $\times$ time interaction (27.17) to the appropriate error term ($[11.64 + 13.85 + 11.38]/21 = 1.75$) resulting in an overall test of the difference in patients in linear trend of $(27.17/1.75) = 15.5$, which is highly significant. As a result, the gain in statistical power is only marginal.

In general, if all the error variance results from systematic differences in the slopes of individual growth curves (i.e. all subjects are changing at different rates), then the overall ANOVA will be more powerful than the trend analysis. Conversely, if all subjects are changing linearly at the same rate, the trend analysis is more powerful.

Modeling individual growth

While the methods outlined above are a more satisfactory strategy for modeling change when multiple observations are available than the use of standard ANOVA methods, they do have a severe restriction. Ordinary analysis software for repeated measures ANOVA, with or without trend analysis, requires a complete data set; all subjects must be measured at the same times and all subjects must have data at each time point. Any missing data will result in the complete loss of the case. This is an obvious constraint when applied to the real world of scattered follow-up visits or repeated assessments. In addition, it appears conceptually unnecessary. We have reconceptualized the problem as one of modeling individual change, using whatever data are available on each subject, then aggregating these data (i.e. the growth parameters) over all subjects. Under this model, it is unnecessarily restrictive to constrain time of assessment to a few standard points.

The solution to the problem is to analyze the data as two regression problems. The first step is to conduct individual regression analyses for each subject, estimating the linear, quadratic, and other higher-order growth parameters. The second step is to then aggregate the parameters across all subjects, essentially treating the growth parameters as random, normally distributed variables. If the goal is to predict individual growth, the parameters are estimated using a second regression equation, where the dependent variable is the growth parameter, and the various predictors (e.g. initial severity, age, fitness) are independent variables. The method is called *hierarchical regression modeling* (Bryk and Raudenbush 1987). Over the past few years, a number of software packages, including SPSS, SAS, and others, have implemented routines that are capable of modeling individual growth parameters as random variables. The method uses maximum likelihood estimation procedures, and as a result does not create the usual ANOVA table; instead, the parameters with their standard errors are estimated directly, similar to a regression analysis. A typical computer output, using the same data set, is shown in Table 11.4.

The p-values suggest that the results are similar to those observed previously. This can be confirmed by squaring the Z-scores, which are interpretable as F values. Thus, this analysis results in an F-test for the baseline measurement of 3.86 (1.967^2) vs. 23.40 previously; a linear term of 98.2 (9.911^2) vs. the 52.6 observed previously; and an F-test for the quadratic term of 41.33 vs. 39.42 previously, so we have gained some statistical power using this approach. In general, when the data are complete the results will be similar; however, this method accommodates incomplete data sets.

Table 11.4 Analysis of individual growth curves using maximum likelihood procedures

Parameter	Estimate	Asymptotic SE	Z-Score	Two-sided p-value
1 Baseline	70.9203	36.0466	1.967	0.050
2 Linear	4.63821	0.4680	9.911	0.000
3 Quadratic	−0.25805	0.0401	−6.429	0.000

How much change is enough?

In this and previous chapters, we have discussed how to measure change and how to set cut-points that differentiate between groups. Astute readers may have noticed that nowhere did we discuss the issue of how much change is 'enough', or whether the groups were 'really' different despite statistically significant differences in scores. In part, this reflects the fact that this is still an open and contentious issue, about which there is little consensus.

In Chapter 7, we discussed one approach to the issue, called the Minimally Important Difference (MID; Jaeschke *et al.* 1991), and the problems that exist in trying to establish it. In fact, Norman *et al.* (2003) showed, in a review of 56 MIDs computed in 29 studies, that the mean MID was almost exactly equal to Cohen's 'moderate' effect size of 0.5; and further, that this was equivalent to the detection threshold of humans in a variety of discrimination tasks. In short, it may well be that an ES of 0.5 is a reasonable first approximation to a threshold of important change. Although circumstances will undoubtedly emerge that differ from this approximation, there is remarkable consistency in the empirical estimates of minimal change across a large variety of scaling methods, clinical conditions, and methodologies to estimate minimal change.

In contrast to determining important change for *groups*, techniques have been developed, primarily in the psychotherapy research literature, to evaluate change in *individuals*. Jacobson *et al.* (1984) outlined three criteria:

(1) the patient's score should initially be within the range found for dysfunctional groups;

(2) the score at the end of treatment should fall within the 'normal' range; and

(3) the amount of change is more than would be expected by measurement error.

The first two criteria seemingly raise the issue of cut-points again, albeit in a somewhat different context. One solution, proposed by Kendall *et al.* (1999), is to use data from already existing large 'normative' groups, obviating the circularity of defining change based on the study that is trying to induce it. A different solution, using Bayesian statistics to account for differences in the prevalences of the functional and dysfunctional groups, is to establish a cut-point (again from pre-existing data or from the study itself). If the variances of the two groups are similar, Hsu (1996) proposes the formula to derive the cut-point (c) as:

$$c = \frac{s^2 \times 2.3026 \times \log_e BR_F/BR_D}{\overline{X}_D - \overline{X}_F} + \frac{\overline{X}_D + \overline{X}_F}{2}$$

where the subscript F refers to the Functional group and the subscript D to the Dysfunctional group; the BRs are the base rates; and s is the pooled standard deviation. (The article also gives the far more complicated formula for the case of unequal variances.)

The third criterion has led to the development of the *reliable change index* (Jacobson and Truax 1991), to take into account the measurement error of the instrument. This was modified by Christensen and Mendoza (1986) to use both the pre- and post-test distributions of scores; and by Hageman and Arrindell (1993) to account for regression to the mean. The RC_{ID} is defined as:

$$RC_{ID} = \frac{(x_{Post} - x_{Pre})r_{DD} + (\overline{X}_{Post} - \overline{X}_{Pre})(1 - r_{DD})}{\sqrt{SEM^2_{Pre} + SEM^2_{Post}}}$$

where the x_s are the pre- and post-intervention scores for the individual, and *SEM* the standard errors of measurement. The reliability of the difference scores, r_{DD}, is:

$$r_{DD} = \frac{s^2_{Pre}r_{xx_{Pre}} + s^2_{Post}r_{xx_{Post}} - 2s_{Pre}s_{Post2}r_{Pre - Post}}{s^2_{Pre} + s^2_{Post} - 2s_{Pre}s_{Post2}r_{Pre - Post}}$$

where r_{XX} is the reliability of the test. A reliable change has occurred if RC_{ID} is greater than 1.96.

Although this approach was developed to determine if an individual subject has changed, it is possible to calculate the score for each person in various groups, and use χ^2 type statistics to see if more people in the experimental group improved compared to the comparison group.

Summary

This chapter has attempted to resolve some controversies surrounding the measurement of change. There are two distinct purposes for measuring change: examining overall effects of treatments; and distinguishing individual differences in treatment response. Focusing on the former, we demonstrated that reliability and sensitivity to change are different but related concepts. We determined the conditions under which the measurement of change will result in increased and decreased statistical power. We also reviewed the literature on the use of change scores to correct for baseline differences and concluded that this purpose can rarely be justified.

As an extension of the methods to measure change, we have considered in detail the use of growth curves in the circumstances where there are more than two observations per subject. The method is conceptually more satisfactory than the classical approach of considering only a beginning and an end point. In addition, growth curve analyses appropriately use all the data available from individual subjects, even when they are measured at different times after the initial assessment.

References

Bryk, A. S. and Raudenbush, S. W. (1987). Application of hierarchical linear models to assessing change. *Psychological Bulletin*, 101, 147–58.

Burckhardt, C. S., Goodwin, L. D., and Prescott, P. A. (1982). The measurement of change in nursing schools: Statistical considerations. *Nursing Research*, 31, 53–5.

Christensen, L. and Mendoza, J. L. (1986). A method of assessing change in a single subject: An alteration of the RC index. *Behavior Therapy*, 17, 305–8.

Cohen, J. (1988). *Statistical power analysis for the behavioral sciences* (2nd edn). Lawrence Erlbaum, Hillsdale, NJ.

Cronbach, L. J. and Furby, L. (1970). How should we measure 'change'—or should we? *Psychological Bulletin*, 74, 68–80.

Francis, D. J., Fletcher, J. M., Stuebing, K. K., Davidson, K. C., and Thompson, N. M. (1991). Analysis of change: Modeling individual growth. *Journal of Consulting and Clinical Psychology*, 59, 27–37.

Glass, G. V. (1976). Primary, secondary, and meta-analyses of research. *Educational Researcher*, 5, 3–8.

Guyatt, G. H., Norman, G. R., and Juniper, E. F. (2000). A critical look at transition ratings. *Journal of Clinical Epidemiology*, 55, 900–8.

Guyatt, G. H., Kirshner, B., and Jaeschke, R. (1992). Measuring health status: What are the necessary measurement properties? *Journal of Clinical Epidemiology*, 45, 1341–5.

Guyatt, G., Walter, S. D., and Norman, G. R. (1987). Measuring change over time: Assessing the usefulness of evaluative instruments. *Journal of Chronic Diseases*, 40, 171–8.

Hageman, W. J. J. M. and Arrindell, W. A. (1993). A further refinement of the Reliable Change (RC) index by improving the pre-post *d*ifference score: Introducing the RC_{ID}. *Behaviour Research and Therapy*, 31, 693–700.

Hays, R. D. and Hadorn, D. (1992). Responsiveness to change: An aspect of validity, not a separate dimension. *Quality of Life Research*, 1, 73–5.

Hsu, L. M. (1996). On the identification of clinically significant client changes: Reinterpretation of Jacobson's cut scores. *Journal of Psychopathology and Behavioral Assessment*, 18, 371–85.

Jacobson, N. S. and Truax, P. (1991). Clinical significance: A statistical approach to defining meaningful change in psychotherapy research. *Journal of Consulting and Clinical Psychology*, 59, 12–9.

Jacobson, N. S., Follette, W. C., and Revenstorf, D. (1984). Psychotherapy outcome research: Methods for reporting variability and evaluating clinical significance. *Behavior Therapy*, 15, 336–52.

Jaeschke, R., Singer, J., and Guyatt, G. H. (1989). Measurement of health status. Ascertaining the minimally important difference. *Controlled Clinical Trials*, 10, 407–15.

Kendall, P. C., Marrs-Garcia, A., Nath, S. R., and Sheldrick, R. C. (1999). Normative comparisons for the evaluation of clinical change. *Journal of Consulting and Clinical Psychology*, 67, 285–99.

Kirshner, B. and Guyatt, G. (1985). A methodological framework for assessing health indices. *Journal of Chronic Disease*, 38, 27–36.

Liang, M. H. (2000). Longitudinal construct validity: Establishment of clinical meaning in patient evaluation instruments. *Medical Care*, 38 (Supplement II), S84–S90.

Linn, P. L. and Slinde, J. A. (1977). Determination of the significance of change between pre- and post testing periods. *Reviews of Educational Research*, 47, 121–50.

Linton, S. J. and Melin, L. (1982). The accuracy of remembering chronic pain. *Pain*, 13, 281–5.

Lord, F. M. (1967). A paradox in the interpretation of group comparisons. *Psychological Bulletin*, 68, 304–5.

Lord, F. M. and Novick, M. N. (1968). *Statistical theories of mental test development*. Addison-Wesley, Reading, MA.

MacKenzie, C. R., Charlson, M. E., DiGioia, D., and Kelley, K. (1986). Can the Sickness Impact Profile measure change: An example of scale assessment. *Journal of Chronic Diseases*, 39, 429–38.

McHorney, C. A and Tarlov, A. (1995). Individual-patient monitoring in clinical practice: Are available health status measures adequate? *Quality of Life Research*, 4, 293–307.

Norman, G. R. (1987). Issues in the use of change scores in randomized trials. *Journal of Clinical Epidemiology*, **42**, 1097–105.

Norman, G. R. (2003). Hi! How are you? Response shift, implicit theories and differing epistemologies. *Quality of Life Research*, **12**, 239–49.

Norman, G. R., Regehr, G., and Stratford, P. S (1997). Bias in the retrospective calculation of responsiveness to change: The lesson of Cronbach. *Journal of Clinical Epidemiology*, **8**, 869–79.

Norman, G. R., Sloan, J. A., and Wyrwich, K. W. (2003). Interpretation of changes in health-related quality of life: The remarkable universality of half a standard deviation. *Medical Care*, **41**, 582–92.

Patrick, D. L. and Chiang, Y.-P. (2000). Measurement of health outcomes in treatment effectiveness evaluations: Conceptual and methodological challenges. *Medical Care*, **38** (Supplement II), S14–S25.

Rogosa, D., Brandt, D., and Zimowski, M. (1982). A growth curve approach to the measurement of change. *Psychological Bulletin*, **92**, 726–48.

Rosenthal, R. (1994). Parametric measures of effect size. In *The handbook of research synthesis* (ed. H. Cooper and L. V. Hedges), pp. 231–44. Russell Sage Foundation, New York.

Ross, M. (1989). Relation of implicit theories to the construction of personal histories. *Psychological Review*, **96**, 341–57.

Schwartz, C. E. and Sprangers, M. A. G. (1999). Methodological approaches for assessing response shift in longitudinal health related quality of life research. *Social Science and Medicine*, **48**, 1531–48.

Spiro, S. E., Shalev, A., Solomon, Z., and Kotler, M. (1989). Self-reported change versus changed self-report: Contradictory findings of an evaluation of a treatment program for war veterans suffering from post traumatic stress disorder. *Evaluation Review*, **15**, 533–49.

Chapter 12

Item response theory

Classical test theory (CTT) has been the underpinning for most test construction and theory for nearly a century. One reason for its popularity is that the assumptions that CTT makes about the items and the test are relatively 'weak' ones (e.g. that the error is independent of the true score), meaning that the theory is appropriate in most situations (Hambleton and Swaminathan 1985). However, there are a number of limitations to CTT (Shea *et al.* 1988). The primary one, as we have pointed out in the chapters on reliability and validity, is that the item and scale statistics apply only to the specific group of subjects who took the test. That means that if the scale is to be administered to people who are different in some way, such as being members of a minority group or patients rather than students, then it is necessary to re-establish its psychometric properties and perhaps develop new norms (e.g. Scott and Pampa 2000). Similarly, we would have to go through the same renorming process if any of the items were altered, or if items were deleted in order to develop a shorter version of the scale (e.g. Streiner and Miller 1986). This is related to a second problem, in that it is impossible to separate out the properties of a test from the attributes of the people taking it (Hambleton *et al.* 1991). That is, there is a *circular dependency*, in that the scores on an instrument depend on how much of the trait the people in the sample have; while 'how much they have' depends on the norms of the scale. Thus, the instrument's characteristics change as we test different groups, and the groups' characteristics change as we use different tests.

A third problem is the assumption that each item contributes equally to the final score. That is, unless we attach different weights to each item (and we saw in Chapter 7 why that does not change much in CTT), they are all simply summed up, irrespective of how much each item correlates with the underlying construct. Related to this, the fourth problem, is that if a person answers 50 per cent of the items in a positive direction, all we can say in CTT is that his or her probability of responding positively to any given item is 50 per cent, because of the assumption that all of the items have equal variances. It is impossible to predict, though, how a person will respond on any given item if the items differ in their propensity to tap the attribute being measured. Fifth, it is also assumed that each item is measured on the same interval scale. This assumption often fails on two grounds: items are most often ordinal rather than interval, and the 'psychological distance' between response options differs from one item to the next (Bond and Fox 2001). Sixth, it is extremely difficult to compare a person's score on two or more different tests. The usual approach is to convert the totals to T or z scores, as we mentioned in Chapter 7, or to use equipercentile equating. However, this assumes that all of the tests are normally distributed, which is, as Micceri (1989) said, as improbable as unicorns. Finally, there is the problem in the assumption of homoscedasticity; that the error of measurement is the same at the ends of the scale as it is in the middle. Indeed, we know this assumption is false, but ignore it because it is usually too difficult to calculate the actual standard error of measurement at each point along the scale.

In the 1960s, two quite independent groups were modifying CTT in an attempt to overcome these limitations. In North America, Allan Birnbaum (1968) included four previously unpublished papers in what is arguably one of the most seminal books in psychometric theory (Lord and Novick 1968), outlining a new approach to test development; while in Denmark, Georg Rasch (1960) was developing a new mathematical way of separately estimating parameters about the test items and the people taking the test at the same time. These two areas have come together in what is now called *item response theory* or IRT. (For a more thorough description of the history of the technique, see Embretson and Reise 2000.) IRT does not refer to a specific technique, but rather to a framework which encompasses a group of models, some of which we will discuss in this chapter. CTT focuses primarily on test-level information, whereas IRT focuses on item-level information (Fan 1998).

Unlike the 'soft' assumptions of CTT, IRT is based on two 'hard' assumptions: that the scale is unidimensional (i.e. the items tap only one trait or ability); and that the probability of answering any item in the positive direction (i.e. reflecting more of the trait) is unrelated to the probability of answering any other item positively for people with the same amount of the trait (a property called *local independence*). If these two assumptions are met, then two postulates follow. First, the performance of a subject on the test can be predicted by a set of factors, which are variously called 'traits,' 'abilities', or 'latent traits' (and the amount of which is referred to in IRT by the Greek letter θ, *theta*). The second postulate is that the relationship between a person's performance on any item and the underlying trait can be described by an *item characteristic curve* or *item response function*.

Item characteristic curves

Figure. 12.1 depicts hypothetical curves showing a group's response to two questions, A and B, on a test of some trait, denoted by θ. These are called *item characteristic curves* (ICCs) or *item response functions* (IRFs). As is usually done when drawing these curves, θ has been standardized to have a mean of 0 and a standard deviation of 1. Theoretically, θ can extend from $-\infty$ to $+\infty$, but we know from the normal curve that over 99.73 per cent of the cases fall between $\theta = \pm 3$, and over 99.99 per cent between ± 4, so the x-axis is usually drawn between ± 3 or 4. There are a few important characteristics of the curves that are worth noting. First, they are both S-shaped (the technical name for the shape is an 'ogive'). While other shapes of the ICC are possible, the ogive is the most widely used one in test construction. Second, they are *monotonic*; the probability of answering in a positive direction consistently increases

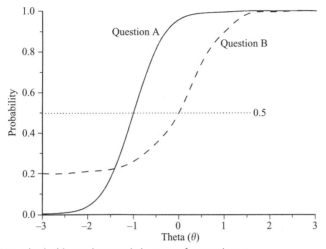

Fig. 12.1 Hypothetical item characteristic curves for two items.

as the score on the trait (θ) increases. However, they differ from each other along three dimensions: the steepness of their slopes; their location along the trait continuum; and where they flatten out on the bottom. We shall return to the significance of these differences later in the chapter.

To show some of the attributes of the curves, we have drawn a horizontal line where the probability is 0.5: it intersects the ICC for Question A at a value of the trait (θ) of −1.0, and Question B at a value of 0.0. What this means is that, for a group of people whose value of the trait is −1.0, 50 per cent will answer positively to Question A and 50 per cent will answer negatively; and similarly, 50 per cent of people whose θ level is 0.0 will respond each way to Question B. (Later, we will discuss models where there are more than two possible responses for each item.)

What can we tell from these two curves? First, Question A is a better discriminator of the trait than Question B. The reason is that the proportion of people responding in the positive direction changes relatively rapidly on Question A as θ increases. The slope for Question B is flatter, indicating that it does not discriminate as well. For example, as we move from $\theta = -2.0$ to $\theta = +1.0$, the proportion of people answering positively to Question A increases from 4 per cent to nearly 100 per cent; while for Question B, a comparable change in the trait is associated with an increase only from 21 per cent to 90 per cent. When the curve has the maximum steepness, it takes the form of a 'step function': no people below the critical point respond positively, and everyone above it responds in the positive direction. The items would then form a perfect Guttman-type of scale (see Chapter 4). Thus, one way of thinking about item-characteristic curves is that they are 'imperfect' Guttman scales, where the probability of responding increases gradually with more of the trait, rather than jumping suddenly from a probability of 0 to 100 per cent.

A second observation is that Question B is 'harder' than Question A throughout most of the range of the trait (for values of θ greater than -1.5). That is, the average person needs more of the trait in order to respond in the positive direction. This can also be seen by the fact that the 50 per cent point is further along the trait continuum for Question B than it is for Question A. Finally, the lower asymptote for Question A is 0.0, while it is 0.2 for Question B. When none of the trait is present, nobody responds positively to A, but 20 per cent do to B; later, we will discuss possible reasons for this.

The one-parameter model

The simplest IRT model is the *one-parameter model*. According to this model, the only factor differentiating the ICCs of the various items is the item difficulty (also called the *threshold parameter*), denoted b_i. That is, it assumes that all of the items have equal discriminating ability (designated as a) and reflecting the fact that the slopes of the curves are parallel, but are placed at various points along the trait continuum, as in Fig. 12.2.

Formally, the proportion of people who have θ amount of the trait who answer item i correctly is defined by the *item response function*:

$$P_i(\theta) = \frac{e^{a(\theta - b_i)}}{1 + e^{a(\theta - b_i)}}$$

Since the form of the equation is called 'logistic', this model and the ones we will discuss in the next section are referred to as *logistic models*. (There are other models, such as those based on a cumulative normal, or *normal ogive*, distribution, but they

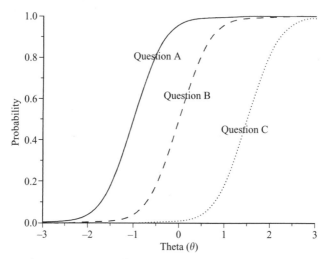

Fig. 12.2 Item characteristic curves for three items with equal discrimination but different levels of difficulty.

are not as widely used, because they yield comparable results but are computationally more difficult. For more information about the differences, see Embretson and Reise (2000). Because this equation has only one parameter that varies among items (*b*, reflecting item difficulty), it is referred to as the one-parameter logistic model, or 1PLM. When the response option is dichotomous (e.g. True/False, Yes/No), it is also commonly called the *Rasch model*, although Rasch later developed more complicated models (Rasch 1960; Wright 1977). One of the key features of IRT is that *b*, which reflects the property of an item, is expressed on the same scale as θ, which reflects a property of the individual. That is, for all people for whom $\theta = b$ (i.e. their level of the trait is equal to the item's difficulty), 50 per cent will endorse the item. If $\theta < b$, then fewer than 50 per cent will endorse it; and conversely, if $\theta > b$, then a majority will. Because, by definition, half the people have negative values of θ and half have positive ones, this means that Question A in Fig. 12.2 is an easy one that a majority of people will endorse, and Question C a difficult one that most people will not. Note that *b* in the IRT models is related to *p* (the proportion correct score) in CTT, but inversely—the harder the item (i.e. the higher the value of *b*), the lower the value of *p*. An important implication of this equation, and one area where IRT differs significantly from CTT, is that a person's true position along the latent trait continuum does not depend upon the specific set of items that comprise the scale (Reise 2003).

The two- and three-parameter models

The *two-parameter model* (2PLM) allows the ICCs to differ from each other on the basis of both difficulty and discriminating ability; that is, instead of *a* being a constant, there is a different a_i for each item. Consequently, the ICCs are different with respect to their position along the trait line and the slope of the curve, as seen in Fig. 12.3.

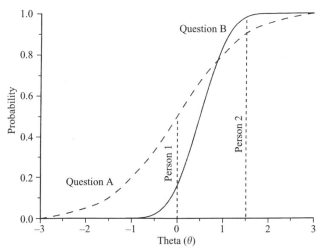

Fig. 12.3 Item characteristic curves for two items differing in both discrimination and difficulty.

The equation for this takes the form:

$$P_i(\theta) = \frac{e^{\,a_i(\theta - b_i)}}{1 + e^{\,a_i(\theta - b_i)}}$$

which differs from the previous equation in that a is now a variable, rather than a constant. The discrimination parameter, a_i, is equivalent to the item-total correlation in CTT, which is usually expressed as a Pearson correlation or point-biserial correlation (Fan 1998).

There is one unfortunate consequence of the two-parameter model. Note than in Fig. 12.3, Question A is easier than Question B. As would be expected, Person 1 has a higher probability of answering Question A than Question B. However, because the ICCs may cross at some point, we have the paradoxical situation where Person 2 has a higher probability of responding positively to the harder question than the easier one. This does not happen in all cases, but should be guarded against in selecting items.

Both the one- and two-parameter models assume that at the lowest level of the trait, the probability of responding positively is zero; that is, the left tail of all of the curves is asymptotic to the x-axis. This may be a valid assumption with attitudinal or personality questionnaires, if all of the people are paying attention to the questions at all times and there are no errors in responding. However, it is likely that people will guess on items to which they do not know the answer on multiple-choice achievement tests; and that, on personality tests, some people with very small amounts of the trait may endorse an item because of lapses in attention, bias, or some other factors. The *three-parameter model* (3PLM) takes this into account, and allows the lower end of the curve to asymptote at some probability level greater than zero. This 'pseudo-guessing parameter' is designated as c_i, and the resulting equation is given as:

$$P_i(\theta) = c_i + (1 - c_i)\frac{e^{\,a_i(\theta - b_i)}}{1 + e^{\,a_i(\theta - b_i)}}$$

In Fig. 12.1, Question A has a value of c_i of 0.0 (i.e. the probability of responding positively at the lowest level of the trait is zero), while Question B has a value of 0.2 for c_i. In this last equation, if c_i is 0, then the equation is identical to the one for the 2PLM; and when c_i is 0 and a_i is 1, then it is the same as the 1PLM.

Polytomous models

Up to this point, we have discussed IRT models for scales that have a dichotomous response option: Yes/No, True/False, and so forth. Most instruments, though, consist of items that allow a range of responses, by using Likert scales, VASs, adjectival scales, and the like. It is widely accepted that the response options rarely have interval-level properties, in that the psychological distance between adjacent points is not constant from one end of the response continuum to the other. However, with CTT, we often close our eyes to this fact, and assume that the actual ordinal data are 'close enough' to interval level for us to ignore the distinction, or that by summing over a number of items, at least the total score will be more or less normally distributed.

Using IRT, we do not have to play 'make believe'. There are many different models for evaluating polytomous response options. When the answers can be considered to be ordered categories, which is most often the case with Likert, adjectival, and VAS scales, the most commonly used model is the *graded-response model* (GRM), which is a generalization of the two-parameter logistic model (2PLM) we discussed earlier (for a discussion of this and five other models see: Embretson and Reise 2000). Let us assume that each item is answered on a five-point Likert scale: Strongly Agree (SA), Agree (A), Neutral (N), Disagree (D), and Strongly Disagree (SD). Conceptually, the GRM would treat each item as if it were a scale with five items. In this case, the two parameters are the slope, or discrimination index, for each response option (a_i); and the between-category threshold parameter (b_i), which is equivalent to the difficulty parameter. Because there are five response options, then there will be four thresholds: between SA and A, between A and N, between N and D, and between D and SD. These threshold curves can be plotted, as in Fig. 12.4, where we have kept the discrimination index constant for the sake of simplicity. It is obvious that there is a larger threshold between Agree and Neutral (the gap labeled A–N) than between Neutral and Disagree (N–D) and between Disagree and Strongly Disagree (D–SD), and that the latter two thresholds are about the same, reflecting the ordinal nature of the answers; that is, it takes more of the trait to move from Agree to Neutral than it does to move from Neutral to Disagree or from Disagree to Strongly Disagree. The probabilities of giving each response can also be examined, as in Fig. 12.5, where they are plotted for differing levels of θ. The peaks of the curves fall in the middle of the gaps between the thresholds. At any point along the *x*-axis, the sum of the probabilities is 1.0, since there is a 100 per cent probability that one of the options will be chosen.

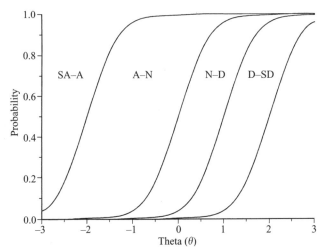

Fig. 12.4 Thresholds for a five-item Likert scale.

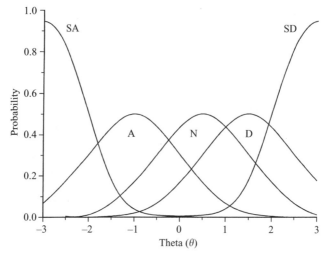

Fig. 12.5 Response curves for the five items in Fig. 12.4.

Item fit

The purpose of IRT is to find a small set of items (usually much smaller than with scales derived using CTT, for reasons we will explain a bit later) that span the range of the construct. Because the item difficulty parameter, b, is standardized on a logit scale to have a mean of 0 and a standard deviation (SD) of 1, an ideal situation is to have a set of items where the bs range from about −3 to +3 (i.e. 3 SDs above and below the mean). If the bs cluster toward the lower end of this logit scale, with few items near +3, it indicates that the items were too 'easy', with many items measuring small amounts of the trait, and few that are endorsed only by people who have much of it. For example, if we were developing a pain scale, this situation would arise if there were many items about common aches and pains that are experienced by a large number of people, but few items that tap extreme levels of pain, such as endured by patients with bone cancer. Conversely, few items near the −3 end of the scale would reflect the opposite situation—not very many items relating to mild pain, and many at the extreme end. The third situation is where all of the items cluster near the middle, indicating that the scale is restricted at both ends.

Because the logit scale is an interval one, items can be selected from the pool that are relatively evenly spaced along the continuum. How many items to choose depends on how precisely you want to measure the construct. Few, more broadly spaced items would be chosen for a brief screening test, for example; while many, closely spaced ones would be used to make fine distinctions among people, or to measure small amounts of change. The right side of Fig. 12.6 shows the plot of a 10-item scale (for now, we will ignore the left side, where the subjects are plotted). A few points stand out from this. First, the test contains more easy items than hard ones, since seven of the items have logit scores below 0. One consequence is that we jump from a score

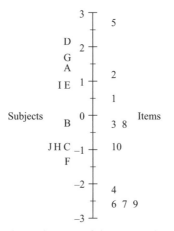

Fig. 12.6 Plot of item difficulty to the right of the axis, and person location to the left.

of just over 1 (item 2) to a score just below 3. This tells us that we may want to write some moderately difficult items in order to discriminate among people within this range. Similarly, it would be helpful to add some moderately easy items, to plug the gap between items 4 and 10. Second, there are a number of items with the same difficulty scores: 3 and 8, and the triplet of 6, 7, and 9. We can eliminate either 3 or 8, and any two of the triplet, and the scale would still have the same discriminating ability.

If a 2PLM was used, then selecting between two items that have similar values of *b* would depend on the discrimination index for each item, *a*. Items with higher values have steeper item characteristic curves than those with lower values, and thus discriminate better between people whose values of the trait, θ, are similar, but not identical.

We mentioned that one of the strong assumptions of IRT is that the scale is unidimensional. This is usually determined by first factor analysing the data; if the scale taps only one attribute, then there should be few significant factors, and the first one should be considerably higher than the others. Even after this has been done, some items may remain that do not fit the assumption of unidimensionality. There are a number of statistics, which vary from one computer program to the next, that indicate the degree to which each item deviates from it. The most common one is a measure of the *residual* of each item, which is evaluated with a likelihood-ratio goodness-of-fit chi-square statistic (χ^2_{GoF}). This assesses the discrepancy between the expected and actual response patterns across respondents, based on their performance on the test as a whole (Fan 1998). Items that meet the assumption of unidimensionality have a low residual value (below 1.96), and a non-significant χ^2_{GoF}, which is conceptually similar to the item having a high item-total correlation. However, χ^2_{GoF} is very sensitive to the sample size, so that if *N* is large, even slight deviations from unidimensionality may be statistically significant; and conversely, when it is small, large deviations may not be significant.

Person fit

We mentioned previously that both items and people are scored along the same logit scale, which usually ranges from -3 to $+3$. Consequently, we can determine the degree to which people may be outliers, using a similar type of statistic as was used to see which items fail the criterion of unidimensionality. We can also plot people along the same continuum, which is shown in the left side of Fig. 12.6. In this example, the subjects tend to cluster at the high end of the scale, reflecting the fact that most of them endorsed most of the items. Thus, this group either had a significant degree of pain or, consistent with our evaluation of the items, there are not enough more difficult ones.

The standard error of measurement

In CTT, there is one standard error of measurement (SEM) for the test, defined as:

$$SEM = \sigma\sqrt{1 - r_{xx}}$$

where r_{xx} is the estimated reliability of the scale and σ^2 its estimated variance. As we mentioned in the introduction to this chapter, this is an unrealistic simplification, because the error is actually smaller in the middle of the scale, and larger at the extremes where there are usually far fewer items and people. Further, the SEM varies from one population to another, because each has a different reliability and variance.

In IRT, the SEM varies as a function of θ, but is constant across populations. If θ is estimated by the simple sum of the items, as in the Rasch model, then the squared SEM for any score y, conditional on the value of θ, is:

$$\sigma^2(y/\theta) = \sqrt{\sum_{g=1}^{n} p_g(\theta)q_g(\theta)}$$

where p_g is the probability of responding positively to item g, and $q_g = 1 - p_g$ (Lord 1980). In general, the graph of the SEM is a U-shaped function, smallest when θ is zero (and roughly equal to the SEM estimated from CTT), and increasing as we move toward the extremes (Embretson 1996).

Sample size

Although we have been discussing both the 'simple' Rasch model and the more complex 2- and 3PLMs in the same chapter, they differ greatly with respect to sample-size requirements. For the Rasch model, Linacre (1994) and Wright and Tennant (1996) state that, to be 95 per cent confident that no item calibration score (b) is more than ± 1 logit from its stable value, 30 subjects are required; and about 100 subjects are needed for $\pm\frac{1}{2}$ logit. However, as the number of parameters increases, and when we move from dichotomous to polytomous items, the sample size requirements increase rapidly. Embretson and Reise (2000) state that 'some of the category threshold parameters were not well estimated in the GRM with 350 examinees' (p. 123); and Reise and Yu (1990) recommend 500 responders for the GRM with a 25-item test; longer questionnaires may require even larger sample sizes. As with CTT, all we have are recommendations based on experience and simulations. Our (tentative) suggestions at this point are:

(1) for a 1PLM with a dichotomous response option, the minimum requirement is 30 subjects;

(2) the more parameters that are estimated, the larger the sample size that is needed;

(3) with the GRM and the 2- and 3PLMs, aim for a minimum of 500 people; and

(4) the finer the discriminations among people you want to make, the more subjects are needed to derive the scale.

Advantages

IRT has many advantages over CTT, which are both theoretical and practical. On the theoretical side, the primary one is that there is no need to play 'let's pretend' that what is really an ordinal scale can be treated as if it were interval; the scale that emerges from an IRT analysis truly has interval-level properties. Consequently, moving from a score of $+2$ to $+1$ logits on a pain scale would represent the same distance as changing from 0 to -1. Because many of the mathematical models of change described in Chapter 11 assume that the scale is interval (i.e. difference scores are constant across the range of possible answers), the results are more likely to be valid. It should be noted, though, that some authors, such as Bond and Fox (2001), maintain that interval level scales arise only from the one-parameter Rasch model, and that adding the other two parameters eliminates this property.

A second theoretical advantage is that IRT provides a more precise estimate of measurement error. In CTT, as we discussed, there is one value for the reliability and the SEM, which then pertains to all respondents, irrespective of where they fall on the scale. IRT is more realistic, in that these values vary, depending on what the respondent's score is. Because most people fall in the middle range, scores with intermediate values of θ are estimated more accurately than those at the two extremes.

On the practical side, a major advantage is that IRT allows *test-free measurement*; that is, people can be compared on a trait or attribute even if they took completely different items! Assume that we have developed a test of physical mobility using IRT, and have derived a 30-item scale that spans the range from complete immobility at the low end, to unrestricted, pain-free movement at the top. These items can be thought of as comprising a Guttman-ordered scale; responding positively to the eighth item, for example, means that the person must have responded positively to the previous seven. Conversely, if a person answers in the negative direction to item 15, then he or she would not answer positively to any item above number 15. Knowing this, we do not need to give all the items to all people; only those items that straddle the point where the person switches from answering in one direction to answering in the other. That point places the person at a specific point on the mobility continuum; and that point can be compared directly to one from another person, who was given a different subset of items. In actuality, because the slopes of the item characteristic curves are never perfectly vertical, a number of items spanning the critical point must be used.

This form of administration has received its widest application in achievement testing. Many tests developed over the past three decades, such as the revised version of the *Wide Range Achievement Test* (Wilkinson 1993), the *Keymath Diagnostic Arithmetic Test* (Connolly *et al.* 1976), and the *Woodcock Reading Mastery Tests* (Woodcock 1987) have used it, so that people at different levels can be given different items, yet be placed on the same scale at the end. This means that people with less of the trait (e.g. spelling ability) are not frustrated by being given a large number of items that are beyond their ability; nor are people with more of the trait bored by having to spell very easy words like 'cat' or 'run'. In addition to reducing frustration, it also lessens testing time, since candidates do not spend large amounts of time on items that are trivial or beyond their capacity. This 'adaptive' or 'tailored' testing is not dependent on IRT (e.g. the Wechsler intelligence tests were not developed using IRT, but use a degree of adaptive testing), but it is greatly facilitated by it.

One concern that may be raised is that a shortened subtest would have a much larger standard error of measurement (SEM) and lower reliability than the whole test, and this would be true in CTT. However, in IRT, the SEM is dependent solely on the probability of endorsing an item at a given value of θ, so that short tests can be as reliable, or even more reliable, than long ones (Embretson 1996; Embretson and Reise 2000). Another reason is that, in CTT, the assumption is that all items come from a common pool, so that the Spearman–Brown prophecy formula, discussed in Chapter 5, applies—increasing the number of items increases the test's reliability. However, in adaptive testing, the items that are presented are tailored to the person's ability level, and those that are too extreme for that person are not given (Embretson 1996).

A second practical advantage of IRT is that, in CTT, it is usually undesirable to have items with different response options in the same scale (e.g. mixing True/False items with 5- and 7-level Likert scales) because this leads to the items contributing differentially to the total score, simply because of the answering scheme. This is not a problem using IRT, since the weight assigned to each item is a function of its difficulty level, not the raw answer. This gives the test designer much greater flexibility in phrasing the questions, rather than the usual Procrustean solution of forcing all items into the same format.

Disadvantages

Given the many practical and theoretical advantages of IRT, the question can be raised why it is used so widely in aptitude and achievement testing, but is rarely used for measuring attitudes, traits, quality of life, and other areas tapped by this book. In fact, Reise (2003) found that over 57 per cent of articles in two leading journals that focus on innovations in psychometrics (the *Journal of Educational Measurement* and *Applied Psychological Measurement*) involved IRT, but fewer than 4 per cent of articles in two equally prestigious scale-oriented journals (the *Journal of Personality Assessment* and *Psychological Assessment*) did.

One reason is that, with the large sample sizes generally found in developing educational tests, the differences between scales constructed with IRT and CTT are trivial. Fan (1998), for example, found that the correlations between the parameters a, b, and θ derived from IRT, and the equivalent values of r_{pb}, p, and the T score derived from CTT were in the high 0.80s and 0.90s. Further, as mentioned previously, none of the versions of the widely used intelligence tests developed by Wechsler were developed using IRT, yet no one within the psychometric community challenges their validity, and the IQ scale that results from them is most often considered an interval one.

Second, one purported advantage of IRT is its *invariance* property; that is, that item characteristics are independent of the sample from which they were derived. This has been shown on a theoretical level (e.g. Hambleton and Swaminathan 1985), but Fan (1998) states that 'the superiority of IRT over CTT in this regard has been taken for granted by the measurement community, and no empirical scrutiny has been deemed necessary' (p. 361). In fact, a number of studies have found relatively large differences from one population or test condition to another, suggesting that invariance does not hold (e.g. Cook *et al.* 1988; Miller and Linn 1988).

A third reason that IRT is not as widely used is its 'hard' assumption of unidimensionality. One implication of this is that IRT cannot be used to construct indices, where the items are causal rather than effect indicators (this was discussed in Chapter 5: When homogeneity does not matter). Thus, it would be wrong to use IRT to construct indices of quality of life, symptom checklists, and other tools where the items themselves define the construct, rather than being manifestations of an underlying latent trait. A second implication is that IRT cannot be used when the underlying construct is itself multifaceted and complex, as are many in the health field. For example, Koksal and Power (1990) postulate that anxiety consists of four components—affective, behavioural, cognitive, and somatic—which Antony (2001) states can operate independently from one another. Although IRT can be used to create four subscales, it cannot be used in this case to make a 'global' anxiety scale.

Fourth, adaptive testing makes sense when, as with aptitude, achievement, and admissions tests, there is a very large pool of items, and it is impractical to administer them all to each person. However, most scales used in personality and health-related areas are relatively short, consisting of 20 or 30 items at most, so that there is little advantage is using adaptive or tailored tests. Finally, as Reise (2003) points out, testing in these fields has not come under the close public and legal scrutiny about fairness and validity that exists (at least in the US) in the realms of achievement and aptitude testing, so there is less pressure to develop scales that meet the more stringent psychometric demands of IRT.

Computer programs

When this chapter was first written, there were relatively few computer programs that could handle IRT models. Now, there is a proliferation of them, especially for the 1PLM. Perhaps the most popular are RUMM for the polytomous Rasch model (Sheridan *et al.* 1996); BILOG (Mislevy and Bock 1990), which can handle up to a three-parameter model for dichotomous data; an extension of it, called PARSCALE

(Muraki and Bock 1993) for polytomous items; and MULTILOG (Thissen 1991), for up to three parameters and dichotomous or polytomous data. Guides to these and other of the more popular programs can be found in Embretson and Reise (2000) and Bond and Fox (2001).

References

Birnbaum, A. (1968). Some latent trait models and their use in inferring an examinee's ability. In *Statistical theories of mental test scores* (ed. F. M. Lord and M. R. Novick), pp. 397–479. Addison-Wesley, Reading, MA.

Bond, T. G. and Fox, C. M. (2001). *Applying the Rasch model: Fundamental measurement in the human sciences.* Lawrence Erlbaum Associates, Mahwah, NJ.

Choppin, B. H. (1976). Recent developments in item banking. In *Advances in psychological and educational measurement* (ed. D. N. M. De Gruitjer and L. J. van der Kamp), pp. 233–45. Wiley, New York.

Connolly, A. J., Nachtman, W., and Pritchett, E. M. (1976). *Keymath Diagnostic Arithmetic Test.* American Guidance Service, Circle Pines, MN.

Cook, L. L., Eignor, D. R., and Taft, H. L. (1988). A comparative study of the effects of recency of instruction on the stability of IRT and conventional item parameter estimates. *Journal of Educational Measurement*, 25, 31–45.

Embretson, S. E. (1996). The new rules of measurement. *Psychological Assessment*, 8, 341–9.

Embretson, S. E. and Reise, S. P. (2000). *Item response theory for psychologists.* Lawrence Erlbaum Associates, Mahwah, NJ.

Fan, X. (1998). Item response theory and classical test theory: An empirical comparison of their item/person statistics. *Educational and Psychological Measurement*, 58, 357–81.

Hambleton, R. K. and Swaminathan, H. (1985). *Item response theory: Principles and applications.* Kluwer Nijhoff, Boston.

Hambleton, R. K., Swaminathan, H., and Rogers, H. J. (1991). *Fundamentals of item response theory.* Sage, Newbury Park, NJ.

Koksal, F. and Power, K. G. (1990). Four systems anxiety questionnaire (FSAQ): A self-report measure of somatic, cognitive, behavioral, and feeling components. *Journal of Personality Assessment*, 54, 534–45.

Lang, P. J. (1971). The application of psychophysiological methods. In *Handbook of psychotherapy and behavior change* (ed. S. Garfield and A. Bergin), pp. 75–125. Wiley, New York.

Linacre, J. M. (1994). Sample size and item calibration stability. *Rasch Measurement Transactions*, 7, 328. Available at: http://www. rasch.org/rmt/rmt74m.htm.

Lord, F. M. (1980). *Application of item response theory to practical testing problems.* Erlbaum, Hillsdale, NJ.

Lord, F. M. and Novick, M. N. (1968). *Statistical theories of mental test development.* Addison–Wesley, Reading, MA.

Micceri, T. (1989). The unicorn, the normal curve, and other improbable creatures. *Psychological Bulletin*, 105, 156–66.

Miller, M. D. and Linn, R. L. (1988). Invariance of item characteristic functions with variations in instructional coverage. *Journal of Educational Measurement*, 25, 205–19.

Mislevy, R. J. and Bock, R. D. (1990). *BILOG 3: Item analysis and test scoring with binary logistic models.* Scientific Software, Mooresville, IN.

Muraki, E. and Bock, R. D. (1993). *PARSCALE: IRT based test scoring and item analysis for graded open-ended exercises and performance tasks.* Scientific Software Int., Chicago.

Rasch, G. (1960). *Probabilistic models for some intelligence and attainment tests.* Nielson and Lydiche, Copenhagen.

Reise, S. P. (in press). A discussion of modern versus traditional psychometrics as applied to personality assessment scales. *Journal of Personality Assessment.*

Reise, S. P. and Yu, J. (1990). Parameter recovery in the graded response model using MULTILOG. *Journal of Educational Measurement,* 27, 133–44.

Scott, R. L. and Pampa, W. M. (2000). The MMPI-2 in Peru: A normative study. *Journal of Personality Assessment,* 74, 95–105.

Shea, J. A., Norcini, J. J., and Webster, G. D. (1988). An application of item response theory to certifying examinations in internal medicine. *Evaluation and the Health Professions,* 11, 283–305.

Sheridan, B., Andrich, D., and Luo, G. (1996). *Welcome to RUMM: a Windows-based item analysis program employing Rasch unidimensional measurement models. User's guide.* RUMM Laboratory, Perth, Australia.

Streiner, D. L. and Miller, H. R. (1986). Can a good short form of the MMPI ever be developed? *Journal of Clinical Psychology,* 42, 109–13.

Thissen, D. (1991). *MULTILOG user's guide: Multiple category item analysis and test scoring using item response theory.* Scientific Software Int., Chicago.

Wilkinson, G. S. (1993). *Wide Range Achievement Test 3 manual.* Jastak Associates, Wilmington, DE.

Woodcock, R. W. (1987). *Woodcock Reading Mastery Tests—Revised.* American Guidance Service, Circle Pines, MN.

Wright, B. D. (1977). Solving measurement problems with the Rasch model. *Journal of Educational Measurement,* 14, 97–116.

Wright, B. D. and Tennant, A. (1996). Sample size again. *Rasch Measurement Transactions,* 9, 468. Available at: http://www. rasch.org/rmt/rmt94m. htm.

Chapter 13

Methods of administration

Having developed the questionnaire, the next problem is how to administer it. This is an issue which not only affects costs and response rates but, as we shall see, may influence which questions can be asked and in what format. The three methods commonly used to administer questionnaires are: face-to-face interviews, over the telephone, and by mail.

As the cost of microcomputers has come down, scales can now be 'administered' by a computer, with the respondent sitting in front of a screen. At the present time, this is possible primarily within clinical contexts where the subject is already near the researcher's office, or as part of smaller studies. However, as 'lap top' computers become more powerful, computer presentation will become more prevalent. Each of these methods has its own distinct advantages and disadvantages, which will be discussed in this chapter.

Face-to-face interviews

As the name implies, this method involves a trained interviewer administering the scale or questionnaire on a one-to-one basis, either in an office or, more usually, in the subject's home. The latter setting serves to put the respondents at ease, since they are in familiar surroundings, and may also increase compliance, because the subjects do not have to travel. However, home interviewing involves greater cost to the investigator and the possibility of interruptions, for instance, by telephones or family members.

Advantages

The advantages of face-to-face interviewing begin even before the first question is asked—the interviewer is sure who is responding. This is not the case with telephone or mail administration, since anyone in the household can answer or provide a second opinion for the respondent. In addition, having to respond verbally to another person reduces the number of items omitted by the respondent; it is more difficult to refuse to answer than simply to omit an item on a form (Quine 1985). The interviewer can also determine if the subject is having any difficulty understanding the items, whether due to a poor grasp of the language, limited intelligence, problems in concentration, or boredom. Further, since many immigrants and people with limited education understand the spoken language better than they can read it, and read it better than they can write it, fewer people will be eliminated because of these problems. This method of administration also allows the interviewer to rephrase the question in terms the person may better understand, or to probe for a more complete response. The converse of this, though, is that without sufficient training, the interviewer may distort the meaning of questions.

Another advantage is the flexibility afforded in presenting the items, since questions in an interview can range from 'closed' to 'open'. Closed questions, which require only a number as a response, such as the person's age, number of children, or years of residence, can be read to the subject. If it is necessary for the respondent to choose among three or more alternatives, or to give a Likert-type response, a card with the possible answers could (and most likely *should*) be given to the person so that memory will not be a factor. Open questions can be used to gather additional information, since respondents will generally give longer answers to open-ended questions verbally rather than in writing. This can sometimes be a disadvantage with verbose respondents.

Complicated questionnaires may contain items that are not appropriate for all respondents: men should not be asked how many pregnancies they have had; native-born people when they immigrated; or people who have never been hospitalized when they were last discharged. These questions are avoided with what are called 'skip patterns': instructions or arrows indicating to the person that he or she should omit a section by skipping to a later portion of the questionnaire. Unless they are very carefully constructed and worded, skip patterns can be confusing to some respondents—and therefore likely to induce errors—if they have to follow these themselves. In contrast, interviewers, because of their training and experience in giving the questionnaire many times, can wend their way through these skip patterns much more readily, and are less likely to make mistakes. Moreover, with the advent of 'laptop' computers, the order of questions and the skip patterns can be programmed to be presented to the interviewer, so that the potential for asking the wrong questions or omitting items is minimized.

Disadvantages

Naturally, there is a cost associated with all of these advantages, in terms of both time and money. Face-to-face interviews are significantly more expensive to administer than any other method. Interviewers must be trained, so that they ask the same questions in the same way, and handle unusual circumstances similarly. In many studies, random interviews are tape-recorded, to ensure that the interviewers' styles have not changed over time; that they have not become lazy or slipshod, or do not sound bored. This entails further expense, for the tape-recorder itself, and for the supervisor's time to review the session and go over it with the interviewer.

If the interview is relatively short, the interviewer can arrive unannounced. This, though, takes the chance that the respondent is at home and is willing to be disturbed. The longer the session, the greater the danger that it will be seen as an imposition. For these reasons, especially when an hour or more of the person's time is needed, it is best to announce the visit beforehand, checking the respondent's willingness to participate and arranging a convenient time to come. This requirement imposes the added costs of telephoning, often repeatedly, until an answer is obtained. Further, since many people work during the day, and only evening interviews are convenient, the number of possible interviews that can be done in one day may be limited.

Another potential cost arises if, for instance, English is not the native language for a sizable proportion of the respondents. Not only must the scales and questions be translated into one or more foreign languages (as would be the case, regardless of the format), but bilingual interviewers must be found. This may not be unduly difficult if there are only a few major linguistic cultures (e.g. English and French in Quebec, Spanish in the southwestern United States, Flemish and French in Belgium), but can be more of a problem in cities which attract many immigrants from different countries. There are more languages to take into account and, if immigration has been recent, there may be few people sufficiently bilingual who can be trained as interviewers.

Finally, attributes of the interviewer may affect the responses given. This can be caused by two factors: biases of the interviewer, and his or her social or ethnic characteristics (Weiss 1975). It has been known for a long time that interviewers can subtly communicate what answers they want to hear, often without being aware that they are doing so (e.g. Rice 1929). This is the easier of the two factors to deal with, since it can be overcome with adequate training (Hyman *et al.* 1954). The more difficult problem is that differences between the interviewer and respondent, especially race, also have an effect (Pettigrew 1964; Saltier 1970). During a gubernatorial campaign in the United States, for example, white telephone interviewers found that 43.8 per cent of those polled preferred the black Democratic candidate, while black interviewers found that his level of support was 52.2 per cent, a difference of 8.4 per cent (Finkel *et al.* 1991). The interaction between the perceived race of the interviewer and the background characteristics of the interviewees was even more striking: among Republicans, there was only a 0.5 per cent difference, while Democrats' reported level of support increased 24.2 per cent with Black interviewers. Among those who reported themselves to be 'apolitical', support increased from 16.7 per cent to 63.6 per cent, although the sample size for this group was small. The reasons usually given for this phenomenon include social desirability, deferring to the perceived preferences of the interviewer because of 'interpersonal deference', or 'courtesy to a polite stranger' (Finkel *et al.* 1991). As is obvious from the results of this and other studies (e.g. Meislin 1987), the race of the interviewer can be detected relatively accurately over the telephone, although it is not known whether the subjects respond to the interviewers' accent, speech patterns, inflections, or other verbal cues.

The effect of sex differences is less clear. Female interviewers usually have fewer refusers and higher completion rates than males (Backstrom and Hursh-Cesar 1981; Hornik 1982), which in part may explain why the majority of interviewers are women (Colombotos *et al.* 1968). The responses women elicit may be different from those given to male interviewers, especially when sexual material is being discussed (Hyman *et al.* 1954), but also when the topic of the interview is politics (Hutchinson and Wegge 1991). Pollner (1998) found that both men and women reported more symptoms of depression, substance abuse, and conduct disorder to female interviewers than to

males, and suggested that 'female interviewers may create conditions more con-
ducive to disclosure and be perceived as more sympathetic than male interviewers'
(p. 369). Furthermore, the differences in response rates seem to occur more with
male interviewees than with females.

Age differences between the interviewer and interviewee have not been extensively
studied. The general conclusion, though, is that to the degree that it is possible, the
two should be as similar as possible, since perceived similarity generally leads to
improved communication (Hutchinson and Wegge 1991; Rogers and Bhowmik 1970).

Telephone questionnaires

An alternative to meeting with the subjects in person is to interview them over the telephone. A major advantage is the savings incurred in terms of time and therefore
money; in one Canadian study, a home interview cost $16.10, a telephone interview
only $7.10 (Siemiatycki 1979). In the past, researchers have avoided this interviewing
method because a significant proportion of homes did not have telephones. Moreover,
this proportion was not evenly distributed, but was higher in the lower socio-
economic classes. Thus, any survey using the telephone directory as a sampling frame
systematically under-represented poorer people. Indeed, the famous prediction in
1936 by the *Literary Digest* that Alf Landon would beat Roosevelt decisively was based
on a telephone survey. Unfortunately for the pollsters, more Roosevelt voters than
Landon voters did not have phones, leading to a biased sample.

The situation has changed considerably since then, but not always in directions
that make it easier for the researcher. On the positive side, most households in North
America and the UK now have telephones. In the US, the proportion has grown
from 80.3 per cent in 1963 to 94.8 per cent in 1994 (Keeter 1995); with comparable
figures for the UK (Nicolaas and Lynn 2002). Not having a telephone is more prevalent among the lower social classes (Beerten and Martin 1999). Smith (1990)
describes those with no telephones as 'outsiders'; they are 'outside the economic
mainstream, from regional and racial subcultures, with weak attachment to society
and its processes and institutions' (p. 385). However, the converse is that a larger
number of people have unlisted numbers; close to 20 per cent in the US in 1975
(Glasser and Metzger 1975), and nearly one-third in the UK by 1998 (Beerten and
Martin 1999). As opposed to not having a telephone, not listing a number is, because
of the additional expense, more of an urban, middle-class phenomenon.
Surprisingly, the rate of unlisted numbers among the highest income group is about
the same as among the lowest (roughly 16 per cent); middle-income people have the
highest unlisted rate (Glasser and Metzger 1975).

Over the past decade, a new technological 'advance' has come between the telephone interviewer and the potential respondent: the answering machine. Whereas
previously this was limited to a device that the person had to buy and install, it is
now a service offered by many telephone companies for a monthly fee, making it
more attractive to potential users. As is the case with unlisted numbers, the distribution of answering machines is uneven, with those using answering machines to

screen calls being mainly younger, urban dwelling, and having higher incomes than the general population (Oldendick and Link 1994).

Random digit dialling

A technique has been developed to get around this problem of unlisted numbers, called *random digit dialling*. A computer-driven device dials telephone numbers at random, using either all seven digits of the number, or the last four once the three-digit exchange has been chosen by the researcher. This latter refinement was added because some exchanges consist primarily of businesses, whereas others are located in mainly residential neighbourhoods; in some areas, 80 per cent of numbers are not assigned to households (Glasser and Metzger 1972). Pre-selecting the exchange has resulted in an increase in the proportion of households reached with this technique, although it is may still not exceed 50 per cent (Waksberg 1978). One disadvantage of sampling by telephone number rather than by address or name is that homes with more than one telephone have multiple chances of being selected, a bias favoring more affluent households. Another disadvantage is that, since the selected numbers tend to be physically near one another, households tend to be more homogeneous than with a purely random sample. To overcome this 'design effect' due to cluster randomization, larger sample sizes are needed (Waksberg 1978).

Advantages

Many of the advantages of face-to-face interviewing also pertain to telephone surveys. These include:

(1) a reduction in the number of omitted items;

(2) skip patterns are followed by the trained interviewer rather than the respondent;

(3) open-ended questions can be asked;

(4) a broad, representative sample can be obtained;

(5) the interviewer can be prompted by a computer (a technique often referred to as CATI, or Computer Assisted Telephone Interviewing); and

(6) the interviewer can determine if the person is having problems understanding the language in general or a specific question in particular.

Another advantage of telephone interviewing is that, even when the person is not willing to participate, he or she may give some basic demographic information, such as age, marital status, or education. This allows the researcher to determine if there is any systematic bias among those who decline to participate in the study.

Moreover, there are at least three areas in which the telephone may be superior to face-to-face interviews. First, any bias which may be caused by the appearance of the interviewer, due to factors such as skin colour or physical deformity, is eliminated. However, one interviewer characteristic that cannot be masked by a telephone is gender. There is some evidence that male interviewers elicit more feminist responses from women and more conservative answers from men than do female interviewers; and more optimistic reports from both sexes regarding the economic outlook (Groves and Fultz 1985). These authors also report higher refusal rates for male interviewers, which is consistent with other studies.

A second advantage is that nationwide surveys can be conducted out of one office, which lowers administrative costs and facilitates supervision of the interviewers to ensure uniformity of style. Last, there is some evidence that people may report more health-related events in a telephone interview than in a face-to-face one (Thornberry 1987), although it is not clear that the higher figure is necessarily more accurate.

Disadvantages

A potential problem with telephone interviewing is that another person in the household may be prompting the respondent. However, this risk is fairly small, since the person on the phone would have to repeat each question aloud. A more difficult issue is that there is no assurance who the person is at the other end of the line. If the sampling scheme calls for interviewing the husband, for instance, the masculine voice can be that of the chosen respondent's son or father. This may be a problem if the designated person is an immigrant unsure of his or her grasp of the language and asks a more fluent member of the household to substitute.

Another difficulty with telephone interviews, as with face-to-face ones, is that unless a specific respondent is chosen beforehand, the sample may be biased by *when* the call is made. During the day, there is a higher probability that housewives, shift-workers, the ill, or the unemployed will be reached. Evening calls may similarly bias the sample by excluding shift-workers. Traugott (1987) found that people reached during the day did not differ significantly from those who could be contacted only in the evening with respect to age, race, or sex; but that the latter group were more likely to be college graduates, since they tended to be employed and not work shifts.

A major problem with telephone interviewing, as opposed to face-to-face interviewing, is the difficulty with questions that require the person to choose among various options. With the interviewer present, he or she can hand the respondent a card listing the response alternatives; an option not available over the telephone. A few suggestions have been offered to overcome this problem. The easiest to implement is to have the respondent write the alternatives on a piece of paper, and then to refer to them when answering. This is feasible when one response set is used with a number of items, such as a Likert scale, which will be referred to in responding to a set of questions. However, if each item requires a different list, the method can become quite tedious and demanding, and the respondent may either hang up or not write the alternatives down, relying on his or her (fallible) memory. In the latter situation, a 'primacy effect' is likely to occur, with subjects tending to endorse categories that are read toward the beginning rather than toward the end of the list (Locander and Burton 1976; Monsees and Massey 1979).

A second method is to divide the question into parts, with each section probing for a more refined answer. For example, the person can be asked if he or she agrees or disagrees with the statement. Then the next question would tap the strength of the endorsement: mild or strong. It also helps if the response format is given to the person as an introduction to the question; for example, 'In the following question, there will be four possible answers: strongly agree, mildly agree, mildly disagree, and strongly disagree. The question is...'.

A third method involves a pre-interview mailing to the subjects. This can consist of the entire questionnaire itself, or a card with the response alternatives. With the former, the interviewer then reads each question, with the respondent following in his or her version. The telephone call allows for probing and recording answers to open-ended questions. If a card with the alternatives is mailed, it is often combined with features like emergency telephone numbers or other items which encourage the person to keep it near the telephone, readily available when the call comes (Aneshensel *et al.* 1982).

These various techniques make it more feasible to ask complicated questions over the telephone. However, the major consideration with this form of interviewing remains to reduce complexity as much as possible. If detailed explanations are necessary, as may be the case if the person's attitudes toward public policy issues are being evaluated, face-to-face or mailed questionnaires may be preferable.

Whatever technique is used, it is highly likely that repeated calls may be necessary to reach a desired household: people may be working, out for the evening, in hospital, or on vacation. It has been recommended that three to six attempts may be required; after this, the law of diminishing returns begins to play an increasingly large role. Moreover, the call should not be made at times such that the respondents feel it would be an intrusion: on holidays, Sundays, or during major sports events.

Mailed questionnaires

Advantages

Mailing questionnaires to respondents is by far the cheapest method of the three; in Siemiatycki's study (1979), the average cost was $6.08, as opposed to $7.10 for telephone interviewing and $16.10 for home interviewing. In the past, the major drawback has been a relatively low response rate, jeopardizing the generalizability of the results. Over the years, various techniques have been developed, which have resulted in higher rates of return. Dillman (1978), one of the most ardent spokesmen for this interviewing method, has combined many of them into what he calls the *Total Design Method*. He believes that response rates of over 75 per cent are possible with a general mailing to a heterogeneous population, and of 90 per cent to a targeted group, such as family practitioners.

As with telephone interviews, mailed questionnaires can be coordinated from one central office, even for national or international studies. In contrast, personal interviews usually require an office in each major city, greatly increasing the expense. Further, since there is no interviewer present, either in person or at the other end of a telephone line, social desirability bias tends to be minimized.

Disadvantages

However, there are a number of drawbacks with this method of administration. First, if a subject does not return the questionnaire, it is almost impossible to get any demographic information, obviating the possibility of comparing responders with non-responders. Second, subjects may omit some of the items; it is quite common to find statements in articles to the effect that 5–10 per cent of the returned questionnaires were unusable due to omitted, illegible, or invalid responses (e.g. Nelson *et al.* 1986). Third, while great care may have been taken by the investigator with regard to the sequence of the items, there is no assurance that the subjects read them in order. Some people may skip to the end first, or delay answering some questions because they have difficulty interpreting them.

A fourth difficulty is that, to ensure a high response rate (over 80 per cent), it is often necessary to send out two or three mailings to some subjects. If the identity of the respondent is known, then this necessitates some form of book-keeping system, to record who has returned the questionnaire and who should be sent a reminder. If anonymity is desired, then reminders and additional copies must be sent to all subjects, increasing the cost of the study. Fifth, there may be a delay of up to three months until all the questionnaires that will be returned have been received. Last, there is always the possibility that some or all of the questionnaires may be delayed by a postal strike.

Increasing the return rate

Many techniques have been proposed to increase the rate of return of mailed questionnaires, although not all have proven to be effective. These have included:

1. *A covering letter.* Perhaps the most important part of a mailed questionnaire is the letter accompanying it. It will determine if the form will be looked at or thrown away, and the attitude with which the respondent will complete it. A detailed description of letters and their contents is given by Dillman (1978), who stresses their importance. The letter should begin with a statement which emphasizes two points: why the study is important; and why that person's responses are necessary to make the results interpretable, in that order. Common mistakes are to indicate in the opening paragraph that a questionnaire (a word he says is to be avoided) is enclosed; that it is part of a survey (another 'forbidden' word); identifying who the researcher is before stating why the research is being done; or under whose auspices (again, best left for later in the letter). Other points that should be included in the letter are a promise of confidentiality, a description of how the results will be used, and a mention of any incentive. The letter should be signed by hand, with the name block under the signature indicating the person's title and affiliation. Since subjects are more likely to respond if the research is being carried out by a university or some other respected organization, its letterhead should be used whenever it is appropriate. Bear in mind, though, that the letterhead itself may affect the answers, as it influences respondent's inferences regarding what the questionnaire developer is interested in. Norenzayan and Schwarz (1999), for example, asked respondents about the motivations of mass murderers. When the letterhead said 'Institute of

Personality Research', the answers focused on personality factors; when it said 'Institute of Social Research', they stressed social-contextual ones. The letter itself should fit onto one page; coloured paper may look more impressive, but does not appear to influence the response rate.

Based on a meta-analysis of 292 randomized trials, Edwards *et al.* (2002) state that mentioning a university affiliation has an odds ratio (OR) for increasing the response rate of 1.31; and the meta-analysis by Fox *et al.* (1988) found it to be the most powerful factor affecting response rate. Using coloured ink had an OR of 1.39 (Edwards *et al.* 2002). However, there were no effects of stressing the benefit to the respondent, to the sponsor, or to society. Other factors that did not influence the response rate were giving a deadline (Edwards *et al.* 2002; Fox *et al.* 1988; Henley 1976) and having instructions. Giving the respondent an option to opt out of the study significantly decreased the response rate (OR = 0.76).

2. *Advance warning that the questionnaire will be coming.* A letter is seen as less of an intrusion than a form that has to be completed, especially one that arrives unannounced. The introductory letter thus prepares the respondent for the questionnaire, and helps differentiate it from junk mail. Edwards *et al.* (2002) report an OR of 1.54 for increased return rate with precontact, and that it does not matter if the contact is by letter or telephone; and Fox *et al.* (1988) found it to be one of the strongest factors in increasing response rate. Unfortunately for the researcher, many 'give away' offers now use the same technique; an official-looking letter announcing the imminent arrival of a packet of chances to win millions of dollars. This makes the wording of the covering letter even more critical, in order to overcome the scepticism that often greets such unsolicited arrivals.

3. *Giving a token of appreciation.* Most often, this is a sum of money, which significantly increases the return rate (Edwards *et al.* 2002; Fox *et al.* 1988; Yammarino *et al.* 1991). However, the relationship between the amount of the incentive and the return rate flattens out quite quickly; amounts as low as $0.50 or $1.00 doubles it, but $15.00 increases the return rate only 2.5 times (Edwards *et al.* 2002). For those who are mathematically inclined, they give the formula for the return rate as:

$$Log_e(\text{OR}) = 0.69 + 0.084\ Log_e(\text{Amount in US\$}).$$

A cost-effective method is to send cheques rather than cash, as James and Bolstein (1992) found that only 69 per cent of cheques for $5 were actually cashed. The promise of an incentive when the questionnaire is returned, as expected, has a much smaller effect, and some have said that it does not improve the response rate at all (Church 1993). For example, James and Bolstein (1992) found that the promise of $50 did not result in any increase in response rate. Other incentives that have been used with varying degrees of success have included lottery tickets, a chance to win a savings bond or a prize, pens or pencils (a favourite among census bureaus), tie clips, unused stamps, diaries, donations to charity, key rings, golf balls, and letter openers, but these seem to be much less powerful than cold, hard cash (Blomberg and Sandell 1996; Edwards *et al.* 2002; Warriner *et al.* 1996; Yammarino *et al.* 1991).

4. *Anonymity.* The literature on the effect of anonymity on response rate is contradictory. If the person is identifiable on questionnaires that ask for confidential information, such as income, sexual practices, or illegal acts, then the response rate is definitely jeopardized. In a meta-analysis by Singer *et al.* (1995) of 113 studies, assurances of confidentiality improved response rates to sensitive information. However, promises of confidentiality for non-sensitive material does not increase compliance. In fact, when the data are not sensitive, such assurances may make people more suspicious and result in an increased refusal rate (Singer *et al.* 1992), although they may be required by the research ethics board. If it is necessary to identify the respondent, in order to link the responses to other information or to determine who should receive follow-up reminders, then the purpose of the identification should be stated, along with guarantees that the person's name will be thrown away when it is no longer needed, and kept under lock and key in the meantime; and that in the final report, no subject will be identifiable.

5. *Personalization.* Envelopes addressed to 'Occupant' are often regarded as junk mail, and are either discarded unopened, or read in a cursory manner; the same may be true of the salutation on the letter itself. However, some people see a personalized greeting using their name as an invasion of privacy and a threat to anonymity. This problem can be handled in a number of ways. First, the letter can be addressed to a group, such as 'Dear Colleague', 'Resident of . . . Neighbourhood', or 'Member of . . .'; the personalization is given with a handwritten signature. Maheux *et al.* (1989) found that adding a handwritten 'thank you' note at the bottom of the covering letter increased the response rate by 41 per cent. (Again, with the wide use by politicians and advertisers of machines that produce signatures, which resemble handwriting, this may become less effective with time.) Another method to balance anonymity and personalization is to have the covering letter personalized, and to stress the fact that the questionnaire itself has no identifying information on it.

Other aspects of personalization include typed addresses rather than labels, stamps rather than metered envelopes, and regular envelopes rather than business reply ones. The former alternatives are usually associated with junk mail, and the latter with important letters. Based on their meta-analysis of 34 published and unpublished studies, Armstrong and Lusk (1987) found that stamped, first-class mail had a return rate on average of 9.2 per cent higher than when business replies were used. Interestingly, using a number of small-denomination stamps on the envelope yielded slightly better results (by 3.5 per cent) than using one stamp with the correct postage. Overall, though, the difference between using stamps as opposed to metered postage is small and may not be worth the effort (Fox *et al.* 1988).

6. *Enclosing a stamped, self-addressed envelope.* Asking the respondents to complete the questionnaire is an imposition on their time; asking them to also find and address a return envelope and pay for the postage is a further imposition, guaranteed to lead to a high rate of non-compliance. In what appears to be the only empirical study of this, Ferriss (1951) obtained a response rate of 90.1 per cent with an enclosed stamped return envelope; this dropped to 25.8 per cent when the envelope was omitted. Surprisingly, the 'active ingredient' seems to be the envelope itself, rather

than the stamp. Armstrong and Lusk (1987), after reviewing six articles comparing stamped versus unstamped return envelopes, found a difference of only 3 per cent in favour of using stamps; and the meta-analyses by Edwards *et al.* (2002) and Yammarino *et al.* (1991) similarly found non-significant increases in the return rate by putting a stamp on the return envelope.

7. *Length of the questionnaire.* It seems logical that shorter questionnaires should lead to higher rates of return than longer ones. However, the research is mixed and contradictory in this regard. Yu and Cooper (1983) showed that length is a relatively weak factor affecting return rate in comparison to others, but Edwards *et al.* (2002) found an OR of 1.86—that is, the odds of a response to a single page questionnaire is about twice that for a three page questionnaire—and Yammarino *et al.'s* meta-analysis (1991) concluded that response rates were significantly lower with questionnaires over four pages as compared to those with fewer pages. When the questionnaire is long (over roughly 100 items or 10 pages), each additional page reduces the response rate by about 0.4 per cent. Up to that point, the content of the questionnaire is a far more potent factor affecting whether or not the person will complete it (Goyder 1982; Heberlein and Baumgartner 1978). In fact, there is some evidence that lengthening the questionnaire by adding interesting questions may actually increase compliance and lead to more valid answers (Burchell and Marsh 1992; Dillman 1978). Thus, it seems that once a person has been persuaded to fill out the form, its length is of secondary importance.

8. *Pre-coding the questions.* Although this does not appear to appreciably increase compliance, pre-coding does serve a number of useful purposes. First, open-ended questions must at some point be coded for analysis; in other words, coding must take place at one time or another. Second, subjects are more likely to check a box rather than write out a long explanation. Last, handwritten responses may be illegible or ambiguous. On the other hand, subjects may feel that they want to explain their answers, or indicate why none of the alternatives apply (a sign of a poorly designed question). The questionnaire can make provisions for this, having optional sections after each section or at the end for the respondent to add comments.

9. *Follow-ups.* As important as the letter introducing the study is the follow-up to maximize returns. Dillman (1978) outlines a four-step process:

♦ Seven to ten days after the first mailing, a postcard should be sent, thanking those who have returned the questionnaire, and reminding the others of the study's importance. The card should also indicate to those who have mislaid the original where they can get another copy of the questionnaire.

♦ Two to three weeks later, a second letter is sent, again emphasizing why that person's responses are necessary for this important study. Also included are another questionnaire and return envelope. This can lead to a problem, though, if it is sent to all subjects, irrespective of whether or not they sent in the first form; very compliant or forgetful subjects may complete two of them.

- The third step, which is not possible in all countries, is to send yet another letter, questionnaire, and envelope via registered or special delivery mail. The former alternative is less expensive, but some people may resent having to make a special trip to the post office for something of no direct importance to them.

- The last step, often omitted because of the expense, is to call those who have not responded to the previous three reminders. This may be impractical for studies that span the entire country, but may be feasible for more local ones.

Some researchers have maintained that while the individual effect of each of these procedures may be slight (with the exception of the initial letter, return envelope, and follow-up, where major effects are seen), their cumulative effect is powerful.

The necessity of persistence

Even when all the techniques are used to maximize the return rate of a mailed questionnaire or to talk to the designated respondent on the telephone, the initial response rate is usually too low to permit accurate conclusions to be drawn. Consequently, most surveys call for follow-up mailings or calls in order to contact most of the subjects. The experience of one typical telephone survey is presented in Fig. 13.1, based on data from Traugott (1987). After three follow-up calls, about two-thirds of the respondents were contacted; one particularly elusive person required a total of 30 calls before he was reached.

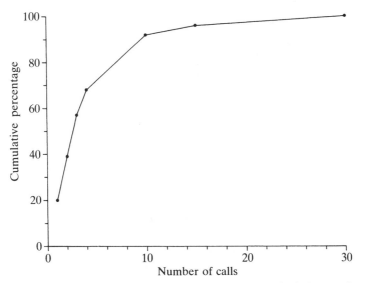

Fig. 13.1 Cumulative contact rate as a function of the number of telephone calls.

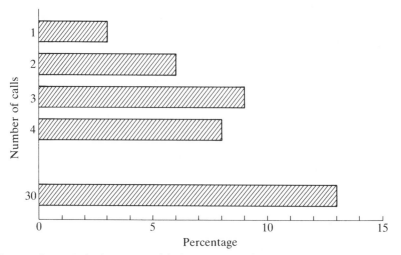

Fig. 13.2 Reagan's lead over Mondale in 1984, as a function of the number of calls required to reach the respondent.

The necessity of persistence in follow-up has been demonstrated in a number of studies, which have shown that people who are easier to contact are different in some important ways from those who are more difficult to find or who require more reminders before they return a questionnaire. Traugott (1987) found that during the 1984 Presidential campaign, Democrats were more accessible than Republicans. As Fig. 13.2 shows, people who were found after one telephone call favored Reagan by 3 per cent; the lead increased to nine points when the sample included people who were reached after three calls; and the total sample gave Reagan a 13-point advantage. He concluded that 'through persistence, the sample became younger and more male' (p. 53). Similar results were found in the health field by Fowler *et al.* (2002). An initial mailed survey to people enrolled in a health plan yielded a 46 per cent return rate. Phoning the non-responders raised this to 66 per cent. Of the 24 comparisons between those who responded by mail and those who were later contacted by telephone, 21 were significantly different. The former group was older, had a greater proportion of women, consistently reported more health problems, were more likely to have been hospitalized and to have seen a physician two or more times, took more prescription medication, and used more medical services than those who did not return the survey. In the same vein, Stallard (1995) found that non-respondents to a psychotherapy follow-up survey were more likely to have dropped out of therapy, and were more dissatisfied with the process than survey responders. Rao (1983) and Converse and Traugott (1986) summarize a number of characteristics which are different between early and late responders.

However, Keeter *et al.* (2000) found that while the demographic characteristics of the sample changed with more 'rigorous' attempts to contact people, the results of a survey focusing on engagement in politics, social and political attitudes, and social trust and connectedness were roughly the same for those easier and harder to find. Similarly, Siemiatycki and Campbell (1984) found relatively few differences between those who responded to initial mail and telephone surveys and those who needed further follow-up before they responded, and little evidence of nonresponse bias. Despite these negative findings, though, the weight of the evidence supports the conclusion that any survey is suspect that bases its results solely on responders to initial mailings or first telephone contacts.

Computer-assisted administration

Microcomputers are now ubiquitous, found in most offices and many homes. There are now computers small enough to be placed on one's lap, which far exceed the power of the original mainframes. Within the past few years, it has become feasible to present even the longest questionnaires on these portable machines. Whereas just a few years ago, computer-administered questionnaires had to be given in the researcher's office, the situation has since changed, and computer-assisted interviewing (CAI) is now fairly commonplace.

Advantages

There are at least four major advantages to computerized administration. First, it can free the interviewer to do other things, or to administer the scale to a number of people simultaneously. Second, every time data are transferred from one medium to another, there is the potential for transcription and entry errors. When the subject is interviewed in person, there are many steps where these errors can creep in: the subject means to say one answer but gives another; the interviewer mishears the response; means to write one thing but puts down something else; errs in transcribing a check mark in one box to a number; or finally keys the wrong number into the computer. Having the person enter his or her responses directly into the machine eliminates all sources of error but one—unknowingly hitting the wrong key. With so many steps eliminated, there is also a commensurate saving of time and money to the researcher.

A third advantage is that neither the subject nor the interviewer can inadvertently omit items or questions. As we have already discussed, a related advantage is that the skip patterns can be automated, eliminating another source of error.

Last, people may be more honest in reporting unacceptable or undesirable behaviours to an impersonal machine than to a human. A number of studies have shown that people admit to more drinking when seated in front of a computer console than an interviewer (e.g. Lucas *et al.* 1977; Skinner and Allen 1983).

Disadvantages

One potential disadvantage of computerizing scales stems from the direct transfer of existing instruments to a computerized format. In most cases, it has not been established whether or not the translation has adversely affected their reliability and validity. Paper-and-pencil questionnaires allow subjects to see how many items there are and to pace themselves accordingly; to skip around, rather than answering the questions in sequence; and to go back easily to earlier questions, in order to change them or to check for their own consistency. While scale-developers may deplore these deviations from the way the instrument was intended to be taken, the results of the original reliability and validity studies were conducted with these factors possibly playing a role. Modifying these factors *may* affect the psychometric properties of the scale. However, the evidence to date suggests that if there are any differences between the paper-and-pencil and the computerized versions, they are very small (e.g. Merten and Ruch 1996; Pinsoneault 1996; Watson *et al.* 1990).

A second, again potential, disadvantage is the belief, especially among health care workers, that some subjects or patients may be apprehensive about computers. These machines still retain the mystique of 'giant brains', which can, nevertheless, be brought to their knees by the press of a wrong key. However, their apprehension about subjects' reactions to these machines are probably not well founded. Most studies have found that far more people are comfortable in front of a terminal or microcomputer than are uncomfortable. Indeed, in many studies, a majority of responders preferred the machine to a human (for a review of this see Stein 1987). A related problem is that attitudes toward computerized interviewing may be sex-related: men tend to be more comfortable 'talking' to machines about sensitive material than to a human interviewer, while the reverse is true for women (e.g. Skinner and Allen 1983). At present, there is insufficient information to indicate whether this is due to the greater use of computers by men, or whether this attitude transcends familiarity with the machines. In either case, though, the sex difference tends to be small.

Implementation

In implementing a computerized scale or questionnaire, some considerations should be kept in mind. First, there should be an ability for the subject to interrupt the testing, and return later to the place where he or she stopped, without either losing the original data or having to go through questions already answered. This is particularly true for long scales, when it is one of many scales, or when the person may become tired or distracted easily. Second, there must be a provision for the subjects to modify their answers, both to the item they are completing at the time, and to previous ones. Respondents should be able to review their earlier answers, modify them if desired, and return to the same place in the instrument. Last, there must be a way for the subject to indicate that he or she cannot or does not want to answer a question. This option is often missing on paper-and-pencil questionnaires, since the person can simply leave the offending item out. If the subject cannot proceed to the next question without entering some response into the machine, the option must be explicit. When he was in the university town of Madison, Wisconsin, one of the pioneers in computerized interviewing, Warner Slack (cited in Fishman 1981), used the phrase 'None of your damn business' as the option the person could use to avoid a question. This was changed to 'Skip that one' when Slack moved to Boston, emphasizing the importance of cultural factors.

Using e-mail and the Web

Despite all its advantages, CAI has a number of shortcomings. If the computer is used to prompt the interviewer, who then enters the responses into the machine, then only one person can be assessed at a time. If the respondent sits at the computer, reading the items and using the keyboard to enter his or her answers, then the person must travel to where the computer is located, and again only a limited number of people can be accommodated at any one time. The explosive growth of the internet and the World Wide Web has eliminated both of these problems. Questionnaires can now be sent to literally thousands of people simultaneously.

Many of the advantages, disadvantages, and implementation issues discussed under CAI apply to Web-based scales. However, other issues must also be considered. The primary one is locating the sample. On the positive side, there are thousands of list servers and 'chat rooms' composed of people with similar interests, concerns, or disorders; and there is even a Web site that indexes them (www.tile. net/tile/listserv/index.html). Cinà and Clase (1999), for example, used the Web to administer the Illness Intrusiveness Rating Scale (Devins *et al.* 1983–84) to 68 patients with a relatively rare disorder, hyperhidrosis. Before the advent of the Web, it would have been almost impossible to locate such a group of people who are scattered all over the world. (Various ways to find samples on the Internet, and to administer scales and surveys, are discussed by Bradley 1999.)

The opposite side of the coin, though, is that it is often difficult to determine how many people received the questionnaire, meaning that it is equally hard to establish the response rate. By the same token, care must be taken to ensure that people do not respond a number of times, especially if the questionnaire taps an area about which the respondents feel very strongly. A Web-based survey about events in the Middle East, for example, had to be cancelled when it was found that some groups were flooding the Web site with thousands of copies of their answers. Both of these problems can be obviated if the researcher has the names of all eligible respondents. For example, Dhalla *et al.* (2002) and Kwong *et al.* (2002) were able to obtain the e-mail addresses for over 95 per cent of Canadian medical students, and assigned each one a unique code number, which was needed to open up the questionnaire. This meant that each person could respond only once.

There are two ways to administer questionnaires using the internet: either sending it directly by e-mail, or posting it on a Web site. There are a number of advantages to using the Web. The questionnaire can be designed to have 'drop-down windows' for each question, giving it a less cluttered look, and reducing the possibility of erroneous responses. The responses themselves are entered into a data base automatically, eliminating another source of error. However, this requires that there is someone with computer knowledge who can design the questionnaire and the database. There are other problems with this approach. First, various Web browsers have different capabilities; a scale that looks well-formatted on one may have items wrapped around onto a second line, or elements that are no longer aligned, with a different browser (Weinman 1996). Then, people have to know that the questionnaire exists. This could involve sending e-mails to people, with links to the Web page with the questionnaire; posting links on existing sites that are likely to be read by the intended audience; or simply hoping that people will stumble on the site. Third, because the site is available for anyone to see, more control must be exercised if it is to be completed only by specific people. Finally, the rule of thumb is that if more than three mouse clicks are needed to get to the questionnaire, people will become frustrated and leave.

A questionnaire sent directly by e-mail is a 'low tech' method that avoids some of these problems, but may introduce others. Web browsers are not required, eliminating the issue of incompatibility. However, without careful design, entering the responses into the questionnaire may in itself alter the format of the page and result in lines being split. Because drop-down menus cannot be used, the questionnaire may appear more cluttered, and there is more chance for entering erroneous answers. Finally, the answers have to be entered manually into the database.

Another consideration for both ways of using the internet is that many people pay for the time they are connected. This imposes yet another burden on them, which must be overcome in order to ensure compliance. Also, with the exponential increase in the number of 'junk' and 'spammed' messages, there is growing resentment over unsolicited and unannounced e-mail. One study, cited by Kaye and Johnson (1999), drew so many hostile messages from their mailing that it had to be aborted. Some suggestions for improving the quality of internet-based questionnaires are given by Kaye and Johnson (1999).

To date, there are limited data comparing questionnaires completed by e-mail or on the Web to more traditional methods of administration. It does not seem as if completing scales electronically introduces any additional biases (Pettit 2002), but response rates appear to be lower to e-mail than to postal mail (Eley 1999; Jones and Pitt 1999; Raziano et al. 2001).

In summary, there is no one method of administration that is ideal in all circumstances. Factors such as cost, completion rate, and the type of question asked must all be taken into account. The final decision will, to some degree, be a compromise, in that the disadvantages of the technique that is chosen are outweighed by the positive elements.

References

Aneshensel, C. S., Frerichs, R. R., Clark, V. A., and Yokopenic, P. A. (1982). Measuring depression in the community: A comparison of telephone and personal interviews. *Public Opinion Quarterly*, **46**, 110–21.

Armstrong, J. S. and Lusk, E. J. (1987). Return postage in mail surveys: A meta-analysis. *Public Opinion Quarterly*, **51**, 233–48.

Backstrom, C. H. and Hursh-Cesar, G. (1981). *Survey research* (2nd edn). Wiley, New York.

Beerten, R. and Martin, J. (1999). Household ownership of telephones and other communication links: Implications for telephone surveys. *Survey Methodological Bulletin*, **44**, 1–7.

Blomberg, J. and Sandell, R. (1996). Does a material incentive affect response on a psychotherapy follow-up questionnaire? *Psychotherapy Research*, **6**, 155–63.

Bradley, N. (1999). Sampling for Internet surveys: An examination of respondent selection for Internet research. *Journal of the Market Research Society*, **41**, 387–95.

Burchell, B. and Marsh, C. (1992). The effect of questionnaire length on survey response. *Quality and Quantity*, **26**, 233–44.

Church, A. H. (1993). Estimating the effect of incentives on mail survey response rates: A meta-analysis. *Public Opinion Quarterly*, **57**, 62–79.

Cinà, C. and Clase, C. M. (1999). The Illness Intrusiveness Rating Scale: A measure of severity in individuals with hyperhidrosis. *Quality of Life Research*, **8**, 693–8.

Colombotos, J., Elinson, J., and Loewenstein, R. (1968). Effect of interviewers' sex on interview responses. *Public Health Reports*, **83**, 685–90.

Converse, P. E. and Traugott, M. W. (1986). Assessing the accuracy of polls and surveys. *Science*, **234**, 1094–98.

Devins, G. M., Binik, Y. M., Hutchinson, T. A., Hollomby, D. J., Barre, P. E., and Guttmann, R. D. (1983–84). The emotional impact of end-stage renal disease: Importance of patients' perception of intrusiveness and control. *International Journal of Psychiatry and Medicine*, **13**, 327–43.

Dhalla, I. A., Kwong, J. C., Streiner, D. L., Baddour, R. E., Waddell, A. E., and Johnson, I. L. (2002). Characteristics of first-year students in Canadian medical schools. *Canadian Medical Association Journal*, **166**, 1029–35.

Dillman, D. A. (1978). *Mail and telephone surveys: The total design method.* Wiley, New York.

Edwards, P., Roberts, I., Clarke, M., DiGuiseppi, C., Pratap, S., Wentz, R., and Kwan, I. (2002). Increasing response rate to postal questionnaires: Systematic review. *BMJ*, **324**, 1183–5.

Eley, S. (1999). Nutritional research using electronic mail. *British Journal of Nutrition*, **81**, 413–6.

Ferriss, A. L. (1951). A note on stimulating response to questionnaires. *American Sociological Review*, **16**, 247–9.

Finkel, S. E., Guterbock, T. M., and Borg, M. J. (1991). Race-of-interviewer effects in a pre-election poll: Virginia 1989. *Public Opinion Quarterly*, **55**, 313–30.

Fishman, K. D. (1981). *The computer establishment.* Harper and Row, New York.

Fowler, F. J., Gallagher, P. M., Stringfellow, V. L., Zaslavsky, A. M., Thompson, J. W., and Cleary, P. D. (2002). Using telephone interviews to reduce nonresponse bias to mail surveys of health plan members. *Medical Care*, **40**, 190–200.

Fox, R. J., Crask, M. R., and Kim, J. (1988). Mail survey response rate: A meta-analysis of selected techniques for inducing response. *Public Opinion Quarterly*, **52**, 467–91.

Glasser, G. J. and Metzger, G. D. (1972). Random digit dialling as a method of telephone sampling. *Journal of Marketing Research*, **9**, 59–64.

Glasser, G. J. and Metzger, G. D. (1975). National estimates of nonlisted telephone households and their characteristics. *Journal of Marketing Research*, **12**, 359–61.

Goyder, J. C. (1982). Further evidence on factors affecting response rate to mailed questionnaires. *American Sociological Review*, **47**, 550–3.

Groves, R. M. and Fultz, N. H. (1985). Gender effects among telephone interviewers in a survey of economic attitudes. *Sociological Methods and Research*, **14**, 31–52.

Heberlein, T. A. and Baumgartner, R. (1978). Factors affecting response rate to mailed questionnaires: A quantitative analysis of the published literature. *American Sociological Review*, **43**, 447–62.

Henley, J. (1976). Response rate to mail questionnaires with a return deadline. *Public Opinion Quarterly*, **40**, 374–375.

Hornik, J. (1982). Impact of pre-call request form and gender interaction on response to a mail survey. *Journal of Marketing Research*, **19**, 144–51.

Hutchinson, K. L. and Wegge, D. G. (1991). The effects of interviewer gender upon response in telephone survey research. *Journal of Social Behavior and Personality*, **6**, 573–84.

Hyman, H. H., Cobb, W. J., Feldman, J. J., Hart, C. W., and Stember, C. H. (1954). *Interviewing in social research*. University of Chicago Press, Chicago.

James, J. M. and Bolstein, R. (1992). Large monetary incentives and their effects on mail survey response rates. *Public Opinion Quarterly*, **56**, 442–53.

Jones, R. and Pitt, N. (1999). Health surveys in the workplace: Comparison of postal, email and World Wide Web methods. *Occupational Medicine (Oxford)*, **49**, 556–8.

Kaye, B. K. and Johnson, T. J. (1999). Research methodology: Taming the cyber frontier. *Social Science Computer Review*, **17**, 323–37.

Keeter, S. (1995). Estimating telephone noncoverage bias in a telephone survey. *Public Opinion Quarterly*, **59**, 196–217.

Keeter, S., Miller, C., Kohut, A., Groves, R. M., and Presser, S. (2000). Consequences of reducing nonresponse in a national telephone survey. *Public Opinion Quarterly*, **64**, 125–48.

Kwong, J. C., Dhalla, I. A., Streiner, D. L., Baddour, R. E., Waddell, A. E., and Johnson, I. L. (2002). Effects of rising tuition fees on medical school class composition and financial outlook. *Canadian Medical Association Journal*, **166**, 1023–8.

Locander, W. B. and Burton, J. P. (1976). The effect of question form on gathering income data by telephone. *Journal of Marketing Research*, **13**, 189–92.

Lucas, R. W., Mullin, P. J., Luna, C. B. X., and McInroy, D. C. (1977). Psychiatrists and a computer as interrogators of patients with alcohol-related illness: A comparison. *British Journal of Psychiatry*, **131**, 160–7.

Maheux, B., Legault, C., and Lambert, J. (1989). Increasing response rates in physicians' mail surveys: An experimental study. *American Journal of Public Health*, **79**, 638–9.

Meislin, R. (1987). Racial divisions seen in poll on Howard Beach attack. *New York Times*, January 8.

Merten, T. and Ruch, W. (1996). A comparison of computerized and conventional administration of the German versions of the Eysenck Personality Questionnaire and the Carroll Rating Scale for Depression. *Personality and Individual Differences*, **20**, 281–91.

Monsees, M. L. and Massey, J. T. (1979). Adapting a procedure for collecting demographic data in a personal interview to a telephone interview. *Proceedings of the American Statistical Association, Social Statistics Section*, 130–5.

Moreland, K. L. (1987). Computerized psychological assessment: What's available. In *Computerized psychological assessment* (ed. J. N. Butcher), pp. 26–49. Basic Books, New York.

Nelson, N., Rosenthal, R., and Rosnow, R. L. (1986). Interpretation of significance levels and effect sizes by psychological researchers. *American Psychologist*, **41**, 1299–301.

Norenzayan, A. and Schwarz, N. (1999). Telling what they want to know: Participants tailor causal attributions to researchers' interests. *European Journal of Social Psychology*, **29**, 1011–20.

Nicolaas, G. and Lynn, P. (2002). Random-digit dialling in the UK: Viability revisited. *Journal of the Royal Statistical Society, A*, **165**, Part 2, 297–316.

Oldendick, R. W. and Link, M. W. (1994). The answering machine generation: Who are they and what problem do they pose for survey research? *Public Opinion Quarterly*, **58**, 264–73.

Pettigrew, T. F. (1964). *A profile of the Negro American*. Van Nostrand, Princeton, NJ.

Pettit, F. A. (2002). A comparison of World-Wide Web and paper-and-pencil personality questionnaires. *Behavior Research Methods, Instruments, & Computers*, **34**, 50–4.

Pinsoneault, T. B. (1996). Equivalency of computer-assisted and paper-and-pencil administered versions of the Minnesota Multiphasic Personality Inventory-2. *Computers in Human Behavior*, **12**, 291–300.

Pollner, M. (1998). The effects of interviewer gender in mental health interviews. *Journal of Nervous and Mental Disease*, **186**, 369–73.

Quine, S. (1985). 'Does the mode matter?': A comparison of three modes of questionnaire completion. *Community Health Studies*, 9, 151–6.

Rao, P. S. R. S. (1983). Callbacks, follow-ups, and repeated telephone calls. In *Incomplete data in sample surveys. Vol. 2: Theory and bibliographies* (ed. W. G. Madow, I. Olkin, and D. B. Rubin), pp. 33–44. Academic Press, New York.

Raziano, D. B., Jayadevappa, R., Valenzula, D., Weiner, M., and Lavizzo-Mourey, R. (2001). E-mail versus conventional postal mail survey of geriatric chiefs. *The Gerontologist*, 41, 799–804.

Rice, S. A. (1929). Contagious bias in the interview. *American Journal of Sociology*, 35, 420–3.

Rogers, E. M. and Bhowmik, D. K. (1970). Homophily-heterophily: Relational concepts for communication research. *Public Opinion Quarterly*, 34, 523–38.

Saltier, J. (1970). Racial 'experimenter effects' in experimentation, interviewing and psychotherapy. *Psychological Bulletin*, 73, 137–60.

Siemiatycki, J. (1979). A comparison of mail, telephone, and home interview strategies for household health surveys. *American Journal of Public Health*, 69, 238–45.

Siemiatycki, J. and Campbell, S. (1984). Nonresponse bias and early versus all responders in mail and telephone surveys. *American Journal of Epidemiology*, 120, 291–301.

Singer, E., Hippler, H. J., and Schwarz, N. (1992). Confidentiality assurances in surveys: Reassurance or threat? *International Journal of Public Opinion Research*, 4, 256–68.

Singer, E., von Thurn, D. R., and Miller, E. R. (1995). Confidentiality assurances and response: A quantitative review of the experimental literature. *Public Opinion Quarterly*, 59, 66–75.

Skinner, H. A. and Allen, B. A. (1983). Does the computer make a difference? Computerized versus face-to-face versus self-report assessment of alcohol, drug, and tobacco use. *Journal of Consulting and Clinical Psychology*, 51, 267–75.

Smith, T. W. (1990). Phone home? An analysis of household telephone ownership. *International Journal of Public Opinion Research*, 2, 369–90.

Stallard, P. (1995). Parental satisfaction with intervention: Differences between respondents and non-respondents to a postal questionnaire. *British Journal of Clinical Psychology*, 34, 397–405.

Stein, S. J. (1987) Computer-assisted diagnosis for children and adolescents. In *Computerized psychological assessment* (ed. J. N. Butcher), pp. 145–58. Basic Books, New York.

Thornberry, O. T. (1987). An experimental comparison of telephone and personal health interview surveys. *Vital and Health Statistics*. Series 2, No. 106. DHHS Pub. No. (PHS) 87–1380.

Traugott, M. W. (1987). The importance of persistence in respondent selection for preelection surveys. *Public Opinion Quarterly*, 51, 48–57.

Waksberg, J. (1978). Sampling methods for random digit dialling. *Journal of the American Statistical Association*, 73, 40–6.

Warriner, K., Goyder, J., Gjertsen, H., Hohner, P., and McSpurren, K. (1996). Charities, no; lotteries, no; cash, yes. *Public Opinion Quarterly*, 60, 542–62.

Watson, C. G., Manifold, V., Klett, W. G., Brown, J., Thomas, D., and Anderson, D. (1990). Comparability of computer- and booklet-administered Minnesota Multiphasic Personality Inventories among primarily chemically dependent patients. *Psychological Assessment*, 2, 276–80.

Weinman, L. (1996). *Designing Web graphics*. New Riders, Indianapolis, IN.

Weiss, C. H. (1975). Interviewing in evaluation research. In *Handbook of evaluation research*, Vol. 1 (ed. E. L. Struening and M. Guttentag), pp. 355–95. Sage Publications, Beverly Hills.

Yammarino, F. J., Skinner, S. J., and Childers, T. L. (1991). Understanding mail survey response behavior. *Public Opinion Quarterly*, 55, 613–39.

Yu, J. and Cooper, H. (1983). A quantitative review of research design effects on response rates to questionnaires. *Journal of Marketing Research*, 20, 36–44.

Chapter 14

Ethical considerations

For the most part, ethical discussions concerning the development and administration of tests have centred around assessments conducted within clinical, educational, or employment settings, and where the results would directly affect the person being evaluated. These situations would include, for example, intelligence, achievement, and aptitude testing in schools; personality and neurocognitive evaluations of patients; and ability testing of job applicants.

Initially, the major focus of the professional organizations was on establishing standards for the tests themselves. In 1895, the American Psychological Association (APA) began looking at the feasibility of standardizing 'mental' and physical tests (Novick 1981). The first formal set of guidelines appeared in 1954—the *Technical Recommendations for Psychological Tests and Diagnostic Techniques*, published by the APA—and these were followed a year later by the *Technical Recommendations for Achievement Tests*, prepared by the American Educational Research Association (AERA) and the National Council on Measurement in Education (NCME). These two sets of recommendations set standards for the assessment and reporting of the psychometric properties of tests, and for the first time set forth the requirements for reliability and validity testing. Later revisions modernized the definitions of reliability and validity, and put greater emphasis on the qualifications of the test user.

Tests that are used only for research purposes, however, are usually considered to be exempt from these standards. This does not mean that there are no ethical problems in devising and using instruments for primarily research questions. Consider the following situations:

Example A. While filling out a questionnaire enquiring about various mood states, one respondent writes in the margin of the answer sheet that she is feeling very despondent, and has recently been thinking of taking her own life. Another subject, while not as explicit about his suicidal thoughts, scores in a range indicative of severe emotional turmoil.

Example B. You are developing a test of marital relationships, and have assured the respondents that their answers will remain confidential, especially since some of the items tap issues of infidelity. One year later, the spouse of one of the respondents files for a divorce, and subpoenas the questionnaire to be used as evidence in court.

Example C. In order to validate a self-report measure of medical utilization, you need to examine the charts of subjects to see how much use they make of various hospital services. In order to ensure that the results are not biased by those who refused to participate in the study, you want to pull their charts to obtain some basic demographic information about them, and to determine their use of medical services.

Example D. Your aim is to develop a measure of self-esteem. One validity study would involve testing two groups of students before and after they make an oral presentation. Subjects in one group are told that they did very well, and those in the other group that they had done very badly and had made fools of themselves, irrespective of how they actually had performed. The students were enrolled in an Introductory Psychology class, and had to participate in three studies as part of the course requirements.

Example E. In order to develop a test of abstract reasoning ability, it is necessary to administer it to people ranging in age from 5 to 75 years, and to psychiatric patients who may exhibit problems in this area, such as schizophrenics and those with brain injuries.

These situations illustrate a number of ethical considerations which may be encountered, such as the use of deception, confidentiality, free and informed consent, and the proper balance between the researcher's need for data and the individual's right to privacy. In this section, we will discuss these and other issues, and see how they affect scale development. As with many aspects of ethics, there are few right or wrong answers. Rather, there are general considerations which must be weighed and balanced against each other, and the 'correct' approach may vary from one situation and institution to another.

The primary consideration in all discussions of ethics is *respect for the individual's autonomy.* This means that we treat people in such a way that they can decide for themselves whether or not to participate in a study. At first glance, this principle may seem so self-evident that one wonders why it is even mentioned; it appears as if it should be understood and accepted by everyone, both researchers and subjects. However, the implementation of the principle of autonomy can lead to some thorny issues.

To begin with, people cannot exercise autonomy unless they know what it is that they are agreeing to. This means that there must be *informed consent;* that is, the subjects must be told:

(a) that they are participating in a research study;

(b) what the study is about; and

(c) what they are being called upon to do.

In studies done for the purpose of scale development, these requirements are most often easy to meet and present no difficulties.

Example D, though, involves deception, in that the subjects are not told that the feedback about their performance is fallacious. Indeed, it could be argued that the study would be impossible if the students were told its true nature. Wilson and Donnerstein (1976) give examples of at least eight types of studies in which they feel deception was a necessary and integral part. Some professional organizations—mainly medical ones, which have little experience with psychosocial research methods—have a blanket prohibition against all studies that involve deception; and some people have argued that it is always possible to substitute observational procedures, which do not involve deception, for experiments which do (e.g. Shipley 1977). Others, such as the APA and the Medical Research Council of Canada (MRC), discourage its use, but recognize that there are some situations where it is required. If no alternative research strategy is possible, then the APA and MRC state that:

(a) the subjects must be told of the deception after their participation; and

(b) the researcher must be able to cope with any possible psychological sequelae that may result from the deception (American Psychological Association 1992; Medical Research Council of Canada 1987).

A different problem with free and informed consent is raised in Example E. How 'informed' can the consent be from minors or those whose cognitive processes are compromised because of some innate or acquired disorder? Some ethicists have argued that those who are unable to fully comprehend the nature of the study and to refuse to participate should never be used in research studies unless they benefit directly from their participation; even parents should not be able to give surrogate consent for their children. Adoption of this extreme view, though, would result in 'research orphans'; groups on whom no research can be done, even if it may result in potential benefit to other members of that group.

Although few people adhere to such an extreme position, it is widely recognized that special precautions must be taken with these vulnerable groups. For those who are legally minors (the age of majority varies between 16 and 18, depending on the jurisdiction), the consent of at least one parent is mandatory. Increasingly over the years, there has been legal recognition of a grey zone between the age of majority and some vaguely defined point where the child is capable of understanding that he or she is part of a study. Within this age frame, the child's *assent* is required in addition to the parent's consent. This means that the child must not object to being in the study, although actively saying 'I agree' is not necessary. If he or she does object, this overrides the consent of the parent. Unfortunately for the investigator, the lower age of this zone is rarely explicitly stated, in recognition of the fact that children mature at different rates; it is left to the judgement of the researcher to determine if the child is cognitively capable of understanding.

A rational guideline for what can be done with children is provided by the *Guidelines* of the MRC (1987). It states that (p. 29):

> ...society and parents should not expose children to greater risks, for the sake of pure medical research, than the children take in their everyday lives.... Parents may consent to inspection of their children's medical records for research....

Psychiatric patients pose a different set of problems. Having a diagnosed disorder, such as schizophrenia, does not necessarily mean that the person is incompetent and unable to give consent (or to deny it). Some institutions have taken the position that some mental health worker who does not have a vested interest in the research sign a portion of the consent form indicating that, in his or her opinion, the patient was able to understand what was being asked. In cases where the patient has been judged to be incompetent (e.g. suffering from some severe psychiatric disorders, Alzheimer's disease, mental retardation, and the like), consent is gained from the legal guardian or next-of-kin, such as a spouse, child, or parent.

The other aspect of autonomy, in addition to the informed part, *is freedom to not participate in* or to *withdraw from* the study (hence, it is often referred to as 'free and informed consent'). This component of consent can be violated in ways which range from the blatantly obvious to the sublimely subtle. Since flagrant violations are easy to detect and are usually patently unethical, we will devote most of the discussion to the less obvious situations, where researchers may not even be aware of the fact that they are trespassing on dangerous territory.

Having Introductory Psychology students participate in studies as a requirement of the course or for extra marks has been a long, if not hallowed, tradition. (Indeed, as far back as 1946, McNemar referred to psychology as 'the science of the behavior of sophomores'.) However, this clearly obviates the freedom to withdraw, since to do so would result in a lower mark or perhaps even a failing grade. Many universities have banned this practice entirely, or allow the student to perform some other activity, such as writing a paper, as an alternative to serving as a research subject (American Psychological Association 1992).

A more subtle form of coercion may exist when a clinician recruits his or her patients to be research subjects. Some subjects may agree to participate because they are concerned that, if they do not, they will not receive the same level of care, despite assurances to the contrary. At one level, they are probably correct. Even if the clinician does not intend to withdraw services or to perform them in a more perfunctory manner, it is natural to assume that his or her attitude toward the patient may be affected by the latter's cooperation or refusal. Other patients may agree to participate out of a sense of gratitude; as a way of saying 'Thank you' for the treatment received. There is considerable debate whether this is a mild form of coercion, capitalizing on the patient's sense of obligation, or a very legitimate form of *quid pro quo*, allowing the patient to repay a perceived debt. Perhaps the safest course to take is for consent to be sought by a person not directly involved in the patient's care: a research assistant, teaching fellow, or by another, disinterested clinician.

The use of hospital or agency charts without the express permission of the patient is another area in which there is no consensus of opinion. The most stringent interpretation of the principle of consent is that in the absence of it, the researcher is prohibited from opening them. This would ban access to patient charts in such circumstances as:

(a) gathering information to determine if those who refused to participate in a study differed in terms of demographic information from those who took part;

(b) wanting to correlate test data with clinical information, such as the number of times a patient presented at the emergency room or at an outpatient clinic; or

(c) even finding a group of patients who should later be approached to participate in a study (e.g. those with specific disorders, those who make frequent use of clinical services, or who have certain demographic characteristics).

It is obvious that this strict interpretation of consent would make some forms of research impossible, or at least extremely costly. A more liberal view is held by people such as Berg (1954), who states that (p. 109):

> If the persons concerned are not harmed by the use of their records and their identities are not publicly revealed, there is no problem and their consent for the professional use of their records is not necessary.

Most research ethics committees take an intermediate position, exemplified by the Ethical Principles of Research of the British Psychological Society (1977). It states that when there is any 'encroachment upon privacy', that the 'investigator should seek the opinion of experienced and disinterested colleagues', a role that is usually played now by the ethics committees of various institutions themselves. The Council for International Organizations of Medical Sciences (CIOMS 1993) adopts a similar position, explicitly stating that the review must be done by an ethical review committee, and further adds the stipulation that 'access ... must be supervised by a person who is fully aware of the confidentiality requirements' (p. 35).

This confidentiality of records continues after the data have been collected. The research guidelines of all psychological organizations have emphasized this point for both clinical and research findings (cf. Schuler 1982). Whenever possible, forms should be completed anonymously. However, this is not always feasible; it is sometimes necessary for the purposes of validity testing to link the results of the scale under development to other data or, when test–retest reliability is being determined, to scores on the same measure completed at some later date. When this is the case, then:

(a) the data should be kept in a locked storage cabinet, to which only the researcher has access; and

(b) the names should be removed and replaced by identification numbers as soon as possible.

Even when these precautions are taken, there may be circumstances (albeit admittedly rare) in which confidentiality cannot be maintained. In Example B, the data have been subpoenaed by a court. If the names have already been removed, and no key linking the names with the ID numbers exists, then there is no problem; the data are unretrievable in a form which can be linked to a specific individual. However, if the individual people are still identifiable for some of the reasons given above, then the test developer is legally obligated to provide the information, and can be cited for contempt of court if he or she does not. The rule of privileged communication does not apply in this case for a number of reasons. First, the researcher is most often not in a fiduciary or therapeutic relationship with the subject. Indeed, he or she may never have met the subject previously, and the contact was usually made at the researcher's initiative and for his or her purposes. Second, the rule is not universal, and rarely extends beyond lawyers and priests; psychologists, physicians, and other health providers are usually not protected.

Finally, there are situations where confidentiality must be violated by the researcher. These involve cases where the investigator believes that the subject is in imminent danger of harming him- or herself or other people. The person should be offered help and encouraged to seek professional advice. If the researcher feels that the danger is acute, and that the person is unwilling to be helped, then the 'duty to warn' supersedes the rules of confidentiality; this is called the Tarasoff rule, following the case of *Tarasoff v Regents of University of California* in 1974. Even if the test is not yet validated, so that the researcher is not sure that a high score truly reflects emotional disturbance, it is often better to err on the side of intervening than simply dismissing the test as 'under development'.

In conclusion, the major issue confronting the scale developer is that of the autonomy of the subject. If the person is seen as an autonomous individual, who has the right to privacy and to not participate in the study irrespective of the difficulties this may pose for the researcher, then most problems should be avoidable.

References

American Educational Research Association, National Council on Measurement in Education (1955). *Technical recommendations for achievement tests.* American Psychological Association, Washington DC.

American Psychological Association (1954). *Technical recommendations for psychological tests and diagnostic techniques.* American Psychological Association, Washington DC.

American Psychological Association (1992). Ethical principles of psychologists and code of conduct. *American Psychologist*, **47**, 1597–611.

Berg, I. A. (1954). The use of human subjects in psychological research. *American Psychologist*, **9**, 108–11.

British Psychological Society, Scientific Affairs Board (1977). Ethics of investigations with human subjects: A set of principles proposed by the Scientific Affairs Board. *Bulletin of the British Psychological Society*, **30**, 25–6.

Council for International Organizations of Medical Sciences (1993). *International ethical guidelines for biomedical research involving human subjects.* CIOMS, Geneva.

McNemar, Q. (1946). Opinion-attitude methodology. *Psychological Bulletin*, **43**, 289–374.

Medical Research Council of Canada. (1987). *Guidelines on research involving human subjects: 1987.* Medical Research Council of Canada, Ottawa, ON.

Novick, M. R. (1981). Federal guidelines and professional standards. *American Psychologist*, **36**, 1035–46.

Schuler, H. (1982). *Ethical problems in psychological research* (Trans. M. S. Woodruff and R. A. Wicklund). Academic Press, New York.

Shipley, T. (1977). Misinformed consent: An enigma in modern social science research. *Ethics in Science and Medicine*, **4**, 93–106.

Tarasoff *v* Regents of the University of California, 131 Cal. Rptr. 14, 551 P 2d 334 (1976).

Wilson, D. W. and Donnerstein, E. (1976). Legal and ethical aspects of nonreactive social psychological research. *American Psychologist*, **31**, 765–73.

Appendix A: Further reading

Chapter 1: Introduction

Colton, T. D. (1974). *Statistics in medicine*. Little Brown, Boston.
Freund, J. E. (1967). *Modern elementary statistics*. Prentice-Hall, Englewood Cliffs, NJ.
Huff, D. (1954). *How to lie with statistics*. W. W. Norton, New York.
Norman, G. R. and Streiner, D. L. (2000). *Biostatistics: The bare essentials* (2nd edn). B. C. Decker, Toronto.
Norman, G. R. and Streiner, D. L. (2003). *PDQ Statistics* (3rd edn). B. C. Decker, Toronto.

Chapter 2: Basic concepts

American Psychological Association (1985). *Standards for educational and psychological testing*. American Psychological Association, Washington.

Chapter 3: Devising the items

Brislin, R. W. (1970). Back-translation for cross-cultural research. *Journal of Cross-Cultural Psychology*, **1**, 185–216.
Del Greco, L., Walop, W., and Eastridge, L. (1987). Questionnaire development: 3. Translation. *Canadian Medical Association Journal*, **136**, 817–18.
Oppenheim, A. N. (1966). *Questionnaire design and attitude measurement*. Heinemann, London.
Payne, S. L. (1951). *The art of asking questions*. Princeton University Press, Princeton, NJ.
Roid, G. H. and Haladyna, T. M. (1982). *A technology for test-item writing*. Academic Press, New York.
Sudman, S. and Bradburn, N. M. (1982). *Asking questions*. Jossey-Bass, San Francisco.

Chapter 4: Scaling approaches

Dunn-Rankin, P. (1983). *Scaling methods*. Erlbaum, Hillsdale, NJ.
Guilford, J. P. (1954). *Psychometric methods*. McGraw-Hill, New York.
TenBrick, T. D. (1974). *Evaluation: A practical guide for teachers*. McGraw-Hill, New York.

Chapter 5: Selecting the items

Anastasi, A. (1982). *Psychological testing* (5th edn), Chapter 8. Macmillan, New York.
Jackson, D. N. (1970). A sequential system for personality scale development. In *Current topics in clinical and community psychology* (ed. C. D. Spielberger), Vol. 2, pp. 61–96. Academic Press, New York.

Kornhauser, A. and Sheatsley, P. B. (1959). Questionnaire construction and interview procedure. In *Research methods in social relations* (Revised edn), (ed. C. Selltiz, M. Jahoda, M. Deutsch, and S. W. Cook) pp. 546–87. Holt, Rinehart and Winston, New York.

Woodward, C. A. and Chambers, L. W. (1980). *Guide to questionnaire construction and question writing.* Canadian Public Health Association, Ottawa.

Chapter 6: Biases in responding

Berg, I. A. (ed.) (1967). *Response set in personality assessment.* Aldine, Chicago.

Couch, A. and Keniston, K. (1960). Yeasayers and naysayers: Agreeing response set as a personality variable. *Journal of Abnormal and Social Psychology*, **60**, 151–74.

Edwards, A. L. (1957). *The social desirability variable in personality assessments and research.* Dryden, New York.

Thorndike, E. L. (1920). A constant error in psychological ratings. *Journal of Applied Psychology*, **4**, 25–9.

Warner, S. L. (1965). Randomized response: Survey technique for eliminating evasive answer bias. *Journal of the American Statistical Association*, **60**, 63–9.

Chapter 7: From items to scales

Nunnally, J. C., Jr. (1970). *Introduction to psychological measurement*, Chapter 8 McGraw-Hill, New York.

Chapter 8: Reliability

Anastasi, A. (1982). *Psychological testing* (5th edn), Chapter 5. Macmillan, New York.

Cronbach, L. J. (1984). *Essentials of psychological testing* (4th edn), Chapter 6. Harper and Row, New York.

Nunnally, J. C., Jr. (1970). *Introduction to psychological measurement*, Chapter 5. McGraw-Hill, New York.

Chapter 9: Generalizability theory

Brennan, R. L. (1983). *Elements of generalizability theory.* American College Testing Program, Iowa City.

Chapter 10: Validity

Anastasi, A. (1982). *Psychological testing* (5th edn). Chapters 6 and 7. Macmillan, New York.

Nunnally, J. C., Jr. (1970). *Introduction to psychological measurement*, Chapter 6. McGraw-Hill, New York.

Chapter 11: Measuring change

Collins, L. M. and Horn, J. L. (ed.) (1991). *Best methods for the analysis of change.* American Psychological Association, Washington.

Collins, L. M. and Horn, J. L. (ed.) (2001). *New methods for the analysis of change.* American Psychological Association, Washington.

Nunnally, J. C., Jr. (1975). The study of change in evaluation research: Principles concerning measurement, experimental design, and analysis. In *Handbook of evaluation research* (ed. E. L. Struening and M. Guttentag) pp. 101–37. Sage, Beverly Hills.

Chapter 12: Item response theories

Allen, M. J. and Yen, W. M. (1979). *Introduction to measurement theory.* Wadsworth, Belmont, CA.

Bejar, I. I. (1983). *Achievement testing.* Sage, Beverly Hills.

Bond, T. G. and Fox, C. M. (2001). *Applying the Rasch model: Fundamental measurement in the human sciences.* Lawrence Erlbaum Associates, Mahwah, NJ.

Crocker, L. and Algina, J. (1986). *Introduction to classical and modern test theory.* Holt, Rinehart, and Winston, New York.

Embretson, S. E. and Reise, S. P. (2000). *Item response theory for psychologists.* Lawrence Erlbaum Associates, Mahwah, NJ.

Hambleton, R. K. (ed.) (1983). *Applications of item response theory.* Educational Research Institute of British Columbia, Vancouver.

Lord, F. M. (1980). *Application of item response theory to practical testing problems.* Erlbaum, Hillsdale, NJ.

Traub, R. E. and Wolfe, R. G. (1981). Latent trait theories and assessment of educational achievement. In *Review of research in education 9,* (ed. D. C. Berliner). American Educational Research Association, Washington DC.

Chapter 13: Methods of administration

Dillman, D. A. (1978). *Mail and telephone surveys: The total design method.* Wiley, New York.

Hyman, H. H., Cobb, W. J., Feldman, J. J., Hart, C. W., and Stember, C. H. (1954). *Interviewing in social research.* University of Chicago Press, Chicago.

Appendix B: Where to find tests

As mentioned in Chapter 3, a very useful place to find questions is to look at what others have done. Below is a partial listing of books and articles which are compendia of information about published and unpublished scales. We give a brief description of the books and articles we have been able to look at; others are just listed. We have not listed references for educational, intellectual, or achievement tests.

A. General

Piotrowski, C. and Perdue, B. (1999). Reference sources on psychological tests: A contemporary review. *Behavioral & Social Sciences Librarian*, 17, 47–58.

This article is a guide to print, online, and electronic reference sources, and gives examples of searches to find specific tests.

Behavioral Measurement Database Services. *Health and psychosocial instruments database* (HAPI). BRS Retrieval Service.

This is an on-line, computerized database, similar to MEDLINE or PsychInfo, containing over 120,000 documents (as of August 2003) which provides information on various instruments. It covers health, social sciences, organizational behaviour, and human resources. Coverage is comprehensive from 1985 to the present, with many earlier measures included on a more haphazard basis. At the current time, the cost to use it is $55 US, or $88 Canadian per hour.

The mental measurements yearbooks. Buros Institute of Mental Measurements, Lincoln.

The first eight editions of the *MMY* were edited by Oscar Buros, and the set is often referred to as 'Buros'. After his death, there have been various editors of this excellent series. The latest volume, the 12th in the series, is edited by Conoley and Impara. Only published tests are listed, and most are reviewed by two or more experts in the field. The articles also include a fairly comprehensive list of published articles and dissertations about the instruments. The yearbooks, which are not published annually, are cumulative: tests reviewed in one edition are not necessarily reviewed in subsequent ones.

The same group has also brought out more focused indices: *Reading tests and reviews, Tests in print*, and *Personality tests*. The latter two volumes do not have reviews, but the reader is directed back to the *MMY*.

Cattell, R. G. and Warburton, F. (1967). *Objective personality and motivation tests.* University of Illinois Press, Urbana, IL.

Although dated now, this book lists over 600 personality tests for adults and children. The psychometric properties of each are given, along with some sample test items.

Keyser, D. J. and Sweetland, R. C. *Test critiques.* Test Corporation of America, Kansas City, MO.

As of 1994, there were 10 volumes in this series of critical evaluations of published tests; there do not appear to have been any additions since then. Unlike the *MMY*, there is only one review per test, and the reference list is representative rather than exhaustive. However, the reviews tend to be considerably longer and more detailed, and follow a common format: introduction, practical applications and uses, technical aspects, and critique.

Sweetland. R. C. and Keyser, D. J. (1986). *Tests: A comprehensive reference for assessments in psychology, education, and business* (2nd edn). Test Corporation of America, Kansas City, MO.

The main volume and the *Supplement* are similar to *Tests in print*. A description is given of over 3000 published tests: purpose, format, description, appropriate population, approximate time to complete them, and where to order.

Directory of unpublished experimental measures. American Psychological Association, Washington.

One of the few comprehensive sources of scales that have appeared in journals but have not been published. The set consists of seven volumes; Volumes 1–3 (1996), edited by B. A. Goldman, J. L. Saunders, and J. C. Busch, are bound together; as are Volumes 4–5 (1996), edited by B. A. Goldman, W. L. Osborne, and D. F. Mitchell. Volume 6 (1995) is edited by B. A. Goldman and D. F. Mitchell; and Volume 7 (1997) by B. A. Goldman, D. F. Mitchell, and P. A. Egelson. Over 7,400 tests are described with one or two key articles cited for each; there are no reviews.

B. Social and attitudinal scales

Antonak, R. F. and Livneh, H. (1998). *The measurement of attitudes toward people with disabilities: Methods, psychometrics and scales*. C. C. Thomas, Springfield, IL.

Bearden, W. O., Netemeyer, R. G., and Mobley, M. F. (1993). *Handbook of marketing scales*. Sage, Newbury Park.

The focus of the book is on consumer behaviour and marketing research. However, it also covers tests of individual traits which may have a role in such behaviours, such as values, susceptibility to peer pressure, materialism, and the like. Over 100 scales are covered; for each, there is a brief review of the psychometric properties, as well as a copy of the tool itself.

Bonjean, C. M., Hill, R. J., and McLemore, S. D. (1967). *Sociological measurement*. Chandler, San Francisco.

Lists every scale used in four sociology journals between 1954 and 1965. Over 2000 measures are listed, with comprehensive references.

Heitzman, C. A. and Kaplan, R. M. (1988). Assessment of methods for measuring social support. *Health Psychology*, 7, 75–109.

This is a critical review of 24 of the more widely used social support scales. The scales themselves are not given, but the assessments of them are excellent.

Lester, P. E. and Bishop, L. K. (1997). *Handbook of tests and measurement in education and the social sciences*. Technomic Publishing Co., Lancaster, PA.

Miller, D. C. (1970). *Handbook of research design and social measurement* (2nd edn). McKay, New York.

Provides lists and examples of 36 sociometric scales in the areas of social status, group structure and dynamics, morale, job satisfaction, and the like.

Price, J. M. and Mueller, C. W. (1986). *Handbook of organizational measures.* Pitman, Marshfield, MA.

Although oriented toward people in businesses, this book also covers such topics as autonomy, communication, and satisfaction. There are a total of 30 areas, with usually one test per area reviewed. Representative items are given for some of the scales.

Robinson, J. P. and Shaver, P. R. (1973). *Measures of social political attitudes.* Institute for Social Research, Ann Arbor, MI.

Robinson, J. P., Shaver, P. R., and Wrightsman, L. S. (ed.) (1991). *Measures of personality and social psychological attitudes.* Academic Press, San Diego, CA.

Robinson, J. P., Shaver, P. R., and Wrightsman, L. S. (ed.) (1999). *Measures of political attitudes.* Academic Press, San Diego, CA.

These three volumes from the ISR provide the actual items comprising the various scales. Each volume lists between 30 and 90 scales, with a short critique of each.

Shaw, M. E. and Wright, J. M. (1967). *Scales for the measurement of attitudes.* Institute of Social Research, Ann Arbor.

Altogether176 scales are described and listed, covering such areas as international and social issues, social practices and problems, political and religious attitudes, and so forth.

C. **Personality and behaviour**

Burn, B. and Payment, M. (2000). *Assessments A to Z: A collection of 50 questionnaires, instruments, and inventories.* Jossey-Bass/Pfeiffer, San Francisco, CA.

Chéné, H. (1986). *Index des variables mesurées par les tests de personalité* (2nd edn). Les Presses de l'Université Laval, Laval Quebec.

Brief, non-evaluative descriptions of primarily published tests. In French.

Chun, K-T., Cobb, S., and French, J. R. P., Jr. (1975). *Measures for psychological assessment: A guide to 3, 000 original sources and their applications.* Institute of Social Research, Ann Arbor.

A listing of 3000 articles which have used various psychological tests, keyed back to the original scales.

Guion, R. M. (1998). *Assessment, measurement, and prediction for personnel decisions.* Lawrence Erlbaum Associates, Mahwah, NJ.

Lake, D. G., Miles, M., and Earle, R. (1973). *Measuring human behavior.* Teachers College Press, New York.

This book gives psychometric data on 84 tests in the areas of personal attributes, interpersonal and organizational relationships, and the like. The tests themselves are not given.

Newmark, C. S. (1996). *Major psychological assessment instruments* (2nd edn). Allyn & Bacon, Boston, MA.

D. **Child and family**

L'Abate, L. and Bagarozzi, D. A. (1993). *Sourcebook of marriage and family evaluation.* Brunner/Mazel, New York.

Center for the Study of Evaluation. (1970). *Elementary school test evaluations.* Author, Los Angeles.

Center for the Study of Evaluation. (1971). *Preschool/kindergarten test evaluations.* Author, Los Angeles.

The above two volumes are designed for both professionals and school administrators. Critical evaluations are provided for tests focussed on educational objectives.

Filsinger, E. E. (ed.) (1983). *Marriage and family assessment: A sourcebook for family therapy.* Sage, Beverley Hills, CA.

Fredman, N. and Sherman, R. (1987). *Handbook of measurements for marriage and family therapy.* Brunner/Mazel, New York.

This book gives the psychometric properties and has the scales themselves in the areas of satisfaction and adjustment (nine scales), communication and intimacy (seven scales), special family assessment scales (eight scales), and the seven scales that comprise the Minnesota Family Inventories.

Grotevant, H. D. and Carlson, C. I. (1989). *Family assessment: A guide to methods and measures.* Guilford, New York.

Johnson, O. G. (1976). *Tests and measurements in child development: Handbooks I and II.* Jossey-Bass, San Francisco.

This is an update of Johnson and Bommarito's earlier book, which was subtitled simply, *A handbook*. The two volumes now cover 1200 non-commercial tests which are appropriate for those under 19 years of age. A wide variety of areas are covered, and the psychometric properties of each test are described.

Levy, P. and Goldstein, H. (eds). (1984). *Tests in education: A book of critical reviews.* Academic Press, London.

Similar in design and intent to the *MMY* and *Test critiques*, this volume is oriented toward published tests available in England, which do not need to be administered by a psychologist, and which cover children from nursery school through secondary school.

McCubbin, H. I. and Thompson, A. I. (ed.) (1991). *Family assessment inventories for research and practice* (2nd edn.). University of Wisconsin, Madison, WI.

Orvaschel, H., Sholomskas, D., and Weissman, M. M. (1980). *The assessment of psychopathology and behavioral problems in children: A review of scales suitable for epidemiological and clinical research (1967–1979).* NIMH, Rockville, MD.

Orvaschel, H. and Walsh, G. (1984). *The assessment of adaptive functioning in children: A review of existing measures suitable for epidemiological and clinical services research.* NIMH, Rockville, MD.

The above two monographs list and critique unpublished scales which can be used with children under the age of 18.

Straus, M. A. and Brown, B. W. (1978). *Family measurement techniques: Abstracts of published instruments, 1935–1974* (Revised edn). University of Minnesota Press, Minneapolis.

This book consists of descriptions of 813 family behaviour measures, culled from journals in psychology, education, and sociology, and covering husband-wife interactions, parent-child and sibling interactions, and sex and premarital relations. Each scale is described, with a few representative items given.

Touliatos, J., Perlmutter, B. F., Straus, M. A., and Holden, G. W. (ed.) (2001). *Handbook of family measurement techniques*, Vols 1–3. Sage, Thousand Oaks, CA.

Walker, D. K. (1973). *Socioemotional measures for preschool and kindergarten children.* Jossey-Bass, San Francisco.

This covers published and unpublished, copyrighted and freely available tests for children between the ages of 3 and 6. There are psychometric data given for 143 instruments.

E. **Health**

American Psychiatric Association. (2000). *Handbook of psychiatric measures.* American Psychiatric Association, Washington.

Bowling, A. (1997). *Measuring health: A review of quality of life measurement scales* (2nd edn). Open University Press, Philadelphia.

The book reviews scales in five areas: functional ability, health status, psychological well-being, social networks and support, and life satisfaction and morale. Each test is described and evaluated, and representative items given for each.

Bowling, A. (2001). *Measuring health: A review of disease specific quality of life measurement scales* (2nd edn). Open University Press, Philadelphia.

There is a description of the scales, their psychometric properties, and examples of items from each.

Cohen, S., Kessler, R. C., and Gordon, L. U. (1995). *Measuring stress: A guide for health and social scientists.* Oxford University Press, Oxford.

This book discusses and assesses stress questionnaires in such areas as life events, chronic stressors, and stress appraisal. The scales themselves are not printed.

Comrey, A. L., Backer, T. E., and Glaser, E. M. (1973). *A sourcebook for mental health measures.* Human Interaction Research Institute, Los Angeles.

Consists of over 1000 abstracts of mental health measures. Some reliability and validity data are given for each scale; the scales themselves are not reproduced.

Corcoran, K. J. and Fischer, J. (2000). *Measures for clinical practice: A sourcebook* (3rd ed.). Free Press, New York.

The first volume of this excellent set has scales that can be used with children, couples, and families; the second volume has scales for adults. For each scale, there is one page describing its norms, scoring system, reliability, validity, and availability; the scales themselves are also given, although the scoring keys are not. An excellent scourcebook for scales and items.

Frank-Stromborg, M. and Olsen, S. J. (ed.) (1997). *Instruments for clinical health-care research* (2nd edn). Jones and Bartlett, Sudbury, MA.

Hersen, M. and Bellack, A. S. (ed.) (1988). *Dictionary of behavioral assessment techniques.* Pergamon, New York.

The book covers many different techniques to measure attributes such as anxiety, assertiveness, beliefs, and skills. Some of the techniques are scales, while others are structured tasks or even pieces of electronic equipment. The psychometric characteristics of each procedure are given, but the scales themselves are not reproduced.

McDowell, I. and Newell, C. (1996). *Measuring health* (2nd edn). Oxford University Press, Oxford.

This book reviews 88 scales in the areas of physical disability, psychological well-being, social health, depression, pain, general health and quality of life, and mental status. Each scale is described in detail, often with example questions, and its reliability and validity are reviewed. An excellent guide.

Reader, L. G., Ramacher, L., and Gorelnik, S. (1976). *Handbook of scales and indices of health behavior.* Goodyear Publishing, Pacific Palisades, CA.

For each test within the areas of health behaviour, health status, and utilization, psychometric data are presented, as well as copies of the scales themselves.

Redman, B. K. (ed.) (1998). *Measurement tools in patient education.* Springer, New York.

Redman, B. K. (2002). *Measurement instruments in clinical ethics.* Sage, Thousand Oaks, CA.

Salek, S. (1998). *Compendium of quality of life instruments,* Vols 1–5. Wiley, Chichester, England.

Spilker, B. (ed.) (1990). *Quality of life assessments in clinical trials.* Raven Press, New York.

Stewart, A. L. and Ware, J. E. (ed.) (1992). *Measuring functioning and well-being.* Duke University Press, Durham, NC.

This book focuses on the tests used in a very large study, the Medical Outcome Study. Within this limited scope, it provides useful information on some indices for social and role functioning, psychological distress, pain, sleep, and the like.

Wilkin, D., Hallam, L., and Doggett, M. A. (1992). *Measures of need and outcome for primary health care.* Oxford University Press, Oxford.

This book covers tests in seven areas: functioning, mental health and illness, social support, patient satisfaction, disease-specific questionnaires, multi-dimensional tests, and miscellaneous. A number of tests in each area are reviewed. For copyrighted ones, a representative item is presented; for others, the whole test is shown.

Zalaquett, C. P. and Wood, R. J. (ed.) (1997). *Evaluating stress: A book of resources.* Scarecrow, Lanham, MD.

F. Gerontology

Burns, A., Lawlor, B., and Craig, S. (1999). *Assessment scales in old age psychiatry.* Martin Dunitz, London.

Kane, R. A. and Kane, R. L. (1981). *Assess the elderly: A practical guide to measurement.* Lexington Books, Lexington, MA.

Mangen, D. and Peterson, W. (ed.) (1982). *Research instruments in social gerontology: Vol 2. Social roles and social participation.* University of Minnesota Press, Minneapolis, MN.

McKeith, I., Cummings, J., Lovestone, S., Harvey, R., and Wilkinson, D. (ed.) (1999). *Outcome measures in Alzheimer's disease.* Martin Dunitz, London.

G. Nursing

Beaton, S. R. and Voge, S. A. (1998). *Measurements for long-term care: A guidebook for nurses.* Sage, Thousand Oaks, CA.

This book lists over 100 instruments that can be used by nurses in long-term care facilities. There is a brief description of each, with a short summary of its psychometric properties. For most scales, one or two sample items are given.

Frank-Stromborg, M. (ed.) (1988). *Instruments for clinical nursing research.* Appleton & Lange, Norwalk, CN.

Each of the book's 24 chapters covers a different functional area or clinical problem, such as quality of life, sleep, dyspnoea, pain, or spirituality. Numerous scales are briefly mentioned within each chapter, and most get only one or two paragraphs. A good source of tests, but weak on evaluation.

Waltz, C. F. and Strickland, O. L. (ed.) (1988). *Measurement of nursing outcomes: Vol. I. Measuring client outcomes.* Springer, New York.

Strickland, O. L., and Waltz, C. F. (ed.) (1988). *Measurement of nursing outcomes: Vol. II. Measuring nursing performance: practice, education, and research.* Springer, New York.

The first volume consists of 25 chapters, covering such topics as illness-oriented measures, measuring wellness, quality of care, and factors in community based care. Each chapter focuses on and reproduces usually one or two measures, with some psychometric data. The second volume looks at measuring professionalism, clinical performance, and educational outcomes, using a similar format.

Waltz, C. F. and Jenkins, L. S. (2001). *Measurement of nursing outcomes* (2nd edn). Springer, New York.

Ward, M. J. and Fetler, M. E. (1979). *Instruments for use in nursing education research.* Western Interstate Commission for Higher Education, Boulder, CO.

A wide variety of instruments is presented, ranging from achievement tests of nursing knowledge to attitudes toward nursing and toward various patient groups, learning styles, and so on. Each test is shown in full, with some discussion of its psychometric properties.

Ward, M. J. and Lindeman, C. A. (ed.) (1979). *Instruments for measuring nursing practice and other health care variables*, Vols 1–2. Bureau of Health Manpower; Division of Nursing, Hyattsville, MD.

H. **Sex and gender**

Beere, C. A. (1990). *Gender roles: A handbook of tests and measures*. Greenwood, Westport, CT.

Beere, C. A. (1990). *Sex and gender issues: A handbook of tests and measures*. Greenwood, Westport, CT.

Beere, C. A. (1979). *Women and women's issues: A handbook of tests and measures*. Josey-Bass, San Francisco.

Davis, C. M., Yarber, W. L., Bauserman, R., Scheer, G., and Davis, S. L. (1997). *Handbook of sexually-related measures*. Sage, Thousand Oaks, CA.

I. **Miscellaneous**

Jones, R. L. (1996). *Handbook of tests and measurements for black populations*, Vols 1–2. Cobb & Henry, Hampton, VA.

Ostrow, A. C. (1996). *Directory of psychological tests in the sport and exercise sciences* (2nd edn). Fitness Information Technology, Morgantown, WV.

Redman, B. K. (2002). *Measurement instruments in clinical ethics*. Sage, Thousand Oaks, CA.

Appendix C: A (very) brief introduction to factor analysis

Exploratory factor analysis

Assume you are developing a test to measure a person's level of anxiety. After following the steps in Chapter 3 (Devising the items), you come up with the following ten items:

1. I often avoid high places.
2. I worry a lot.
3. My hands often get sweaty.
4. I cross the street in order to avoid having to meet someone.
5. I have difficulty concentrating.
6. I can often feel my heart racing.
7. I find myself pacing when I'm under stress.
8. I frequently feel tense.
9. When I'm under stress, I tend to get headaches.
10. People tell me I have trouble letting go of an idea.

There are three hypotheses regarding the way these 10 items are related. At the one extreme, the first hypothesis is that they are totally unrelated, and tap 10 different, uncorrelated aspects of anxiety. The second, at the other extreme, is that they are all highly correlated with each other. The third hypothesis is somewhere in the middle: that there are groups of items that cluster together, with each cluster tapping a different aspect of anxiety. A natural place to begin is to look at the correlation matrix. If all of the correlations are high, it would favour the first hypothesis; while all low correlations would lead you to adopt the second; and groups of items that seem related to each other but uncorrelated with the other groups would support the last hypothesis. There are two problems, though, in simply examining a correlation matrix. First, it is unusual for correlations to be very close to 1.0 or to 0.0; most often, they fall in a more restricted range, making it more difficult to separate high correlations from low ones. Second, even with as few as 10 items, there are 45 unique correlations to examine; if there are 30 items, which is more common when we are developing a test, there will be 435 correlations to look at (the number of unique correlations is $n \cdot (n-1)/2$); far more than we can comfortably make sense of. However, we can turn to factor analysis to help us.

What factor analysis does with the correlation matrix is, as the name implies, to derive *factors*, which are weighted combinations of all of the variables. The first two factors will look like:

$$F_1 = w_{1,1}X_1 + w_{1,2}X_2 + \cdots w_{1,10}X_{10}$$
$$F_2 = w_{2,1}X_1 + w_{2,2}X_2 + \cdots w_{2,10}X_{10}$$

where the Fs are the factors, the Xs are the variables (in this case, the items), and the ws are weights. The first subscript for w indicates the factor number, and the second the variable, so that $w_{1,2}$ means the weight for Factor 1 and variable 2.

There are as many factors 'extracted' as there are variables, so that there would be 10 in this case. It may seem as if we have only complicated matters at this point, because we now have 10 factors, each of which is a weighted combination of the variables, rather than simply 10 variables. However, the factors are extracted following definite rules. The weights for first factor are chosen so that it *explains*, or *accounts for*, the maximum amount of the variability (referred to as the *variance*) among the scores across all of the subjects. The second factor is derived so that it:

(a) explains the maximum amount of the variance that remains (i.e. that is left unaccounted for after Factor 1 has been extracted); and

(b) is uncorrelated with (the technical term is *orthogonal to*) the first factor.

Each remaining factor is derived using the same two rules; account for the maximum amount of remaining variance, and be orthogonal to the previous factors. In order to completely capture all of the variance, we would need all 10 factors. But, we hope that the first few factors will adequately explain most (ideally, somewhere above 70% or so) of the variance, and we can safely ignore the remaining ones with little loss of information. There are a number of criteria that can be used to determine how many factors to retain; these are described in more detail in Norman and Streiner (2000, 2003).

At this point, the computer will print a table called the *factor loading matrix*, where there will be one row for each variable, one column for each retained factor, and where the cells will contain the ws. These weights are called the *factor loadings*, and are the correlations between the variables and the factors. After we have done this initial factor extraction, we usually find that:

(a) the majority of the items 'load' on the first factor;

(b) a number of the items load on two or more factors;

(c) most of the factor loadings are between 0.3 and 0.7; and

(d) each factor after the first has some items that have positive weights and other items with negative weights.

Mathematically, there is nothing wrong with any of these, but they make the interpretation of the factors quite difficult.

To try to overcome these four problems, the factors are *rotated*. In the best of cases, this results in:

(a) a more uniform distribution of the items among the factors that have been retained;

(b) items loading on one and only one factor;

Table C.1 An example of a rotated factor loading matrix for three factors and 10 variables

Item	Factor 1	Factor 2	Factor 3
1	0.12	0.75	0.33
2	0.81	0.11	−0.02
3	0.03	0.22	0.71
4	0.40	0.45	0.27
5	0.74	0.29	0.15
6	0.23	0.31	0.55
7	0.22	0.71	0.32
8	0.86	−0.18	0.17
9	0.33	0.19	0.66
10	0.72	0.21	0.05
Eigenvalue	2.847	1.622	1.581

(c) loadings that are closer to either 1.0 or 0.0; and

(d) all of the significant loadings on a factor having the same sign.

A hypothetical example of a rotated factor matrix with three factors is seen in Table C.1.

At the bottom of each column is a number called the *eigenvalue*, which is an index of the amount of variance accounted for by each factor. Its value is equal to the sum of the squares of all of the *w*s in the column, so for Factor 1, it is $(0.12^2 + 0.81^2 + \cdots + 0.72^2)$. Because all of the variables have been standardized to have a mean of zero and a standard deviation (and hence, a variance) of 1.0, the total amount of variance in the data set is equal to the number of variables; in this case, 10. Consequently, Factor 1 accounts for $2.847/10 = 28.47$ per cent of the variance, and the three factors together account for $(2.847 + 1.622 + 1.581)/10 = 6.050/10 = 60.5$ per cent of the variance; a bit low, but still acceptable.

The items that load highest on Factor 1 are 2, 5, 8, and 10, which appear to tap the *cognitive* aspect of anxiety. Similarly, Factor 2, composed of items 1, 4, and 7, reflects the *behavioural* component; and Factor 3, with items 3, 6, and 9, measures the *physiological* part of anxiety. Note also that, although item 4 loads most heavily on Factor 2, its loading on Factor 1 is nearly as high. This *factorially complex* item may warrant rewording in a revised version.

This is the older, more traditional form of factor analysis, and is generally what is meant when people use the term. Because a new form of factor analysis was later introduced (described in the next section), a way had to be found to distinguish the two. Consequently, this is now referred to as *exploratory* factor analysis (EFA). This reflects the fact that we start with no *a priori* hypotheses about the correlations among the variables, and rely on the procedure to explore what relationships do exist. This example was also somewhat contrived, in that the rotated solution was easily interpreted, corresponded to existing theory about the nature of anxiety (Lang 1971), did not have too many factorially complex items, nor any items that did not load on any of the extracted factors. Reality is rarely so generous to us. More often, the results indicate that more items should be rewritten, others discarded, and there may be factors which defy explanation.

Confirmatory factor analysis

Confirmatory factor analysis (CFA) is a subset of a fairly advanced statistical technique called *structural equation modeling* (see Norman and Streiner 2003 for a basic introduction, and Norman and Streiner 2000 for a more complete one). Although it has been around for many years, the earlier statistical programs required a high degree of statistical sophistication. Within the past decade or so, though, a number of programs have appeared that have made the process considerably easier and available to more researchers.

We said in the previous section that EFA is a *hypothesis generating* technique, used when we do not know beforehand what relationships exist among the variables. Thus, while it can be used to evaluate construct validity, the support is relatively weak because no hypotheses are stated *a priori*. As the name implies, though, CFA is a *hypothesis testing* approach, used when we have some idea regarding which items belong on each factor. So, if we began with Lang's conceptualization of the structure of anxiety, and specifically wrote items to measure each of the three components, it would be better if we were to use CFA rather than EFA, and identified which items should belong to which factor. At the simplest level, we can specify which items comprise each factor. If our hypotheses were better developed, or we had additional information (as explained in the next paragraph), we can 'constrain' the loadings to be of a given magnitude; for example, that certain items will have a high loading, and others a moderate one.

The technique is extremely useful when we are trying to compare two different versions of a scale (e.g. an original and a translated version), or to see if two different groups (e.g. men and women) react similarly to the items. We would begin by running an EFA on the target version in order to determine the characteristics of the items. Testing for equivalence could then be done in a stepwise fashion.

First, we would simply specify that the items on the second version (or with the second group of people) load on the same factors as the original. If this proves to be the case, we can make the test for equivalence more stringent, by using the factor loadings from the original as trial loadings in the second. If this more tightly specified model continues to fit the data we have from the second sample, we can proceed to the final step, where we see if the variances of each item are equivalent across versions. If all three steps are passed successfully, we can be confident that both versions of the test or both groups are equivalent. Various 'diagnostic tests' can tell us which items were specified correctly and which do not fit the hypothesised model. However, unlike EFA, CFA will not reassign an ill-fitting item to a different factor.

References

Lang, P. J. (1971). The application of psychophysiological methods. In *Handbook of psychotherapy and behavior change* (eds. S. Garfield and A. Bergin) pp. 75–125. Wiley, New York.

Norman, G. R. and Streiner, D. L. (2000). *Biostatistics: The bare essentials* (2nd ed.). B. C. Decker, Toronto.

Norman, G. R. and Streiner, D. L. (2003). *PDQ Statistics* (3rd ed.). B. C. Decker, Toronto.

Author Index

Subject Index